Scar-Less Surgery

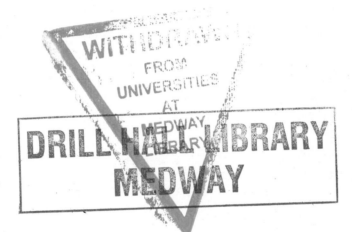

Abhay Rane • Jeffrey A. Cadeddu • Mihir M. Desai
Inderbir S. Gill
Editors

Scar-Less Surgery

NOTES, Transumbilical, and Others

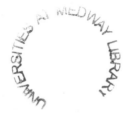

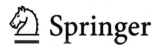

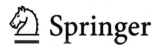 Springer

Editors

Abhay Rane, M.D.
Department of Urology
East Surrey Hospital
Redhill
United Kingdom

Mihir M. Desai, M.D.
Department of Urology
USC Institute of Urology
Los Angeles, California
USA

Jeffrey A. Cadeddu, M.D.
Department of Urology
University of Texas Southwestern
Medical Center
Dallas, TX
USA

Inderbir S. Gill, M.D.
Catherine and Joseph Aresty
Department of Urology
Keck School of Medicine of USC
University of Southern California
Los Angeles, California
USA

ISBN 978-1-84800-359-0   ISBN 978-1-84800-360-6   (eBook)
DOI 10.1007/978-1-84800-360-6
Springer London Heidelberg New York Dordrecht

Library of Congress Control Number: 2012947864
© Springer-Verlag London 2013

Printed on acid-free paper

Springer is part of Springer Science+Business Media (www.springer.com)

This book is dedicated to those minimally invasive surgeons who have always strived to push the proverbial envelope to its limit in order to get the best for our patients. These dedicated kindred souls have often had to brave withering criticism from peer skeptics, but have nevertheless managed to prove their point by maximizing minimally invasive surgery.

Such an effort would not be complete without acknowledging our better halves: those who have always "stood and waited": Ruta, Marlo, Rimple, and Neeti.

Finally, we formally wish to acknowledge the support from Melissa Morton at Springer, and the dedication and hard work put in by our developmental editor, Liz Corra.

Abhay Rane, M.D.
Jeffrey A. Cadeddu, M.D.
Mihir M. Desai, M.D.
Inderbir S. Gill, M.D.

Preface

Natural orifice translumenal endoscopic surgery (NOTES) and laparoendoscopic single-site (LESS) surgery are based on the premise that patients would significantly benefit in terms of recovery time, physical discomfort, pain, and cosmesis by a surgery performed without visible scarring. Over the last five to seven years, there has been a rapid expansion of LESS and NOTES procedures across surgical specialites, with hundreds of procedures reported in the literature ranging from cholecystectomy to radical prostatectomy. To date, there has not been a comprehensive text providing detailed information on the techniques, their limitations, instrumentation requirements, and results. Such a source is necessary to catalog progress to date, provide concise state-of-the-art technical information, and serve as a resource text as clinicians embark on this exciting new frontier.

The initial chapters in this text provide state-of-the-art reviews of the advances in surgical instrumentation that have increased the feasibility of these procedures. Nevertheless, the challenge for LESS and NOTES techniques is whether they can be utilized to improve patient outcomes without significantly increasing surgical cost, operative time, or complications. The balance of the text expertly addresses this issue. One must keep in mind that the benefits of LESS and NOTES procedures are incremental compared to the transition from open surgery to laparoscopy, where it was fairly easy to demonstrate an advantage in morbidity. Convalescence, hospital stay, and pain were consistently better with minimally invasive surgery. Even though it is conceptually obvious, those in practice at the time laparoscopy was introduced will recall that the acceptance of laparoscopy's benefits was neither immediate nor universal. The transition from conventional laparoscopy to LESS is more subtle. Pure NOTES where the access is commonly transoral (transgastric) or transvaginal may have greater advantages in this regard. There is no doubt that LESS and NOTES provide clear advantages in cosmesis. LESS, with its single scar often undetectable in the umbilicus, and NOTES, with its absence of transabdominal incisions, are clearly most appealing to our increasingly sophisticated patients.

LESS and NOTES techniques are gaining momentum as the next frontier in minimally invasive surgery. It is critically important that surgeons maintain their pioneering spirit and evaluate these new approaches. This text serves as the first comprehensive reference for general and urologic surgeons while also highlighting future developments and research needs.

Abhay Rane, M.D.
Jeffrey A. Cadeddu, M.D.
Mihir M. Desai, M.D.
Inderbir S. Gill, M.D.

Contents

Part IV Future Perspectives

Contributors

André Luis de Castro Abreu, M.D. Center for Advanced Robotic and Laparoscopy Surgery, USC Institute of Urology, Keck Medical Center of USC, University of Southern California, Los Angeles, CA, USA

Monish Aron, M.D., MCh, FRCS Center for Advanced Robotic and Laparoscopy Surgery, USC Institute of Urology, Keck Medical Center of USC, University of Southern California, Los Angeles, CA, USA

Antonio Alcaraz Asensio, M.D., Ph.D. Department of Urology, Hospital Clinic, University of Barcelona, Barcelona, Spain

Alexander R. Aurora, M.D., M.Sc. Department of General Surgery and Bariatrics, Harford Memorial Hospital, Upper Chesapeake Medical System, Havre de Grace, MD, USA

Riccardo Autorino, M.D., Ph.D., FEBU Urology Clinic, Second University of Naples, Piazza Miraglia, Naples, Italy

Center for Laparoscopic and Robotic Surgery, Glickman Urological and Kidney Institute, Cleveland Clinic, Cleveland, OH, USA

Maria Bergström, M.D., Ph.D. Department of Surgery and Urology, South Älvsborg Hospital, Boras, Sweden

Sara L. Best, M.D. Department of Urology, University of Texas Southwestern Medical Center, Dallas, TX, USA

Michael L. BluteJr M.D. The Smith Institute for Urology, The Hofstra-North Shore LIJ School of Medicine, New Hyde Park, NY, USA

Jeffrey A. Cadeddu, M.D. Department of Urology, University of Texas Southwestern Medical Center, Dallas, TX, USA

David Canes, M.D. Institute of Urology, Lahey Clinic Medical Center, Tufts University School of Medicine, Burlington, MA, USA

Jorge Correia-Pinto, M.D., Ph.D. Department of Pediatric Surgery, Hospital Braga, Braga, Portugal

Surgical Sciences Research Doman, Life and Health Sciences Research Institute, School of Health Sciences, University of Minho, Braga, Portugal

ICVS/3Bs – PT Government Associate Laboratory, Braga/Guimarães, Braga, Portugal

Bernard Dallemagne, M.D. Department of Digestive and Endocrine Surgery and IRCAD (Institut de Recherche contre les Cancers de l'Appareil Digestif), University Hospital of Strasbourg, Strasbourg, France

Oussama M. Darwish, M.D. Urology Institute, University Hospitals Case Medical Center, Cleveland, OH, USA

Mihir M. Desai, M.D. Department of Urology, Keck Medical Center, University of Southern California Institute of Urology, Los Angeles, CA, USA

Michele Diana, M.D. Department of Digestive and Endocrine Surgery and IRCAD (Institut de Recherche contre les Cancers de l'Appareil Digestif), University Hospital of Strasbourg, Strasbourg, France

Matthew T. Gettman, M.D. Department of Urology, Mayo Clinic, Rochester, MN, USA

Tania Gill, BS Department of Urology, Keck Medical Center, University of Southern California Institute of Urology, Los Angeles, CA, USA

Candace F. Granberg, M.D. Department of Urology, Mayo Clinic, Rochester, MN, USA

Melanie L. Hafford, M.D. Department of Surgery, University of Texas Southwestern, Dallas, TX, USA

Santiago Horgan, M.D., FACS Department of Minimally Invasive Surgery, University of California at San Diego, San Diego, CA, USA

John E. Humphrey, M.D. Institute of Urology, Lahey Clinic Medical Center, Tufts University School of Medicine, Burlington, MA, USA

Brian H. Irwin, M.D. Division of Urology, Department of Surgery, University of Vermont College of Medicine, Burlington, VT, USA

Jihad H. Kaouk, M.D. Department of Urology, Cleveland Clinic, Cleveland, OH, USA

The Laparoscopic and Robotic Surgery Institute, Cleveland, OH, USA

Rakesh Vijay Khanna, M.D. Department of Urology, SUNY Upstate Medical University, Syracuse, NY, USA

Nitin Kumar, M.D. Department of Gastroenterology, Harvard Medical School, Brigham and Women's Hospital, Boston, MA, USA

Humberto Kern Laydner, M.D. Department of Urology, Glickman Urological and Kidney Institute, Cleveland Clinic, Cleveland, OH, USA

Dennis J. Lee, M.D. Department of Urology, University of Southern California Institute of Urology, Los Angeles, CA, USA

Scott Leslie, B.Sc. (Med), MB BS (Hons), FRACS (Urol) Department of Urology, Keck Medical Center, University of Southern California Institute of Urology, Los Angeles, CA, USA

Estevao Lima, M.D., Ph.D. Department of Urology, Hospital Braga, University of Minho, Braga, Portugal

Life and Health Sciences Research Institute, School of Health Sciences, University of Minho, Braga, Portugal

ICVS/3Bs – PT Government Associate Laboratory, Braga/Guimarães, Braga, Portugal

Saniea F. Majid, M.D. Center for the Future of Surgery/Minimally Invasive Surgery, University of California at San Diego, San Diego, CA, USA

Magnus Jayaraj Mansard, M.S., DNB Department of Surgical Gastroenterology, Asian Institute of Gastroenterology, Hyderabad, Andhra Pradesh, India

Jacques Marescaux, M.D. (Hon), FRCS, FACS (Hon), JSES Department of Digestive and Endocrine Surgery, University Hospital of Strasbourg, Strasbourg, France

Matthew J. Maurice, M.D. Urology Institute, University Hospitals Case Medical Center, Cleveland, OH, USA

Shashikant Mishra, M.S., DNB (Urol) Department of Urology, Muljibhai Patel Urological Hospital, Nadiad, Gujarat, India

Per-Ola Park, M.D., Ph.D. Department of Surgery and Urology, South Älvsborg Hospital, Borås, Sweden

Silvana Perretta, M.D. Department of Digestive and Endocrine Surgery and IRCAD (Institut de Recherche contre les Cancers de l'Appareil Digestif), University Hospital of Strasbourg, Strasbourg, France

Melissa S. Phillips, M.D. Department of Surgery, University of Tennessee Health Science Center, Knoxville, TN, USA

Jeffrey L. Ponsky, M.D. Department of Surgery, University Hospitals Case Medical Center, Cleveland, OH, USA

Lee E. Ponsky, M.D., FACS Urology Institute, University Hospitals Case Medical Center, Cleveland, OH, USA

Urologic Oncology and Minimally Invasive Therapies Center, Case Western Reserve University School of Medicine, Cleveland, OH, USA

Soroush Rais-Bahrami, M.D. The Smith Institute for Urology, The Hofstra-North Shore LIJ School of Medicine, New Hyde Park, NY, USA

Jay D. Raman, M.D. Department of Surgery, Penn State Milton S. Hershey Medical Center, Hershey, PA, USA

Abhay Rane, M.D. Department of Urology, East Surrey Hospital, Redhill, Surrey, UK

G. Venkat Rao, M.S., FRCS, MAMS Department of Surgical Gastroenterology, Asian Institute of Gastroenterology, Hyderabad, Andhra Pradesh, India

Pradeep P. Rao, M.B., MNAMS, DNB (Urol), FRCSED Department of Urology, Mamata Hospital, Mumbai, Maharashtra, India

Prashanth P. Rao, M.S. (Bom), FRCS (Ed), FCPS, DNB, MNAMS, FICS, DLS (Fr), FIAGES, FMAS Department of Surgery, Mamata Hospital, Mumbai, Maharashtra, India

Department of GI and Minimal Access Surgery, Mamata Hospital, Mumbai, Maharashtra, India

D. Nageshwar Reddy, M.D., DM, DSc, FAMS, FRCP Department of Surgical Gastroenterology, Asian Institute of Gastroenterology, Hyderabad, Andhra Pradesh, India

Maria J. Ribal Caparros, M.D., Ph.D. Department of Urology, Hospital Clinic, University of Barcelona, Barcelona, Spain

Lee Richstone, M.D. The Smith Institute for Urology, The Hofstra-North Shore LIJ School of Medicine, New Hyde Park, NY, USA

Bryan J. Sandler, M.D., FACS Department of Surgery, University of California at San Diego Medical Center, La Jolla, CA, USA

Hagop Sarkissian, M.D. Division of Urology, Department of Surgery, University of Vermont College of Medicine, Burlington, VT, USA

Daniel J. Scott, M.D., FACS Southwestern Center for Minimally Invasive Surgery, Department of Surgery, University of Texas Southwestern, Dallas, TX, USA

Robert J. Stein, M.D. Center for Robotic and Image-Guided Surgery, Glickman Urological and Kidney Institute, Cleveland Clinic, Cleveland, OH, USA

Christopher C. Thompson, M.D., M.Sc., FACG, FASGE Division of Gastroenterology, Brigham and Women's Hospital, Boston, MA, USA

Michael A. White, DO, FACOS Department of Urology, Cleveland Clinic, . Cleveland, OH, USA

Part I
Overview

Chapter 1
Historical Perspectives of LESS and NOTES

Michael L. Blute Jr., Soroush Rais-Bahrami, and Lee Richstone

Keywords Laparoendoscopic single-site surgery • Natural orifice transluminal endoscopic surgery • Laparoscopy • Endoscopy

Introduction

The craft of surgery has undergone a remarkable transformation in a few short decades, evolving from traditional large incisions to smaller "keyhole" incisions characteristic of a minimally invasive approach. The drive toward minimally invasive techniques seeks to benefit patients by reducing pain and the physiologic responses to the stresses of open surgery. Smaller incisions limit disfigurement and improve upon cosmetic outcomes without compromising the exposure provided by open surgery with the advent of improved optical scopes and display mechanisms. Today, it is commonplace for patients to undergo major extirpative surgery through small incisions and enjoy a rapid recovery, with a brief hospitalization and quickened convalescence.

The introduction and diffusion of multiple-port, or "conventional," laparoscopy account for a large part of this revolution in the practice of surgery. This progress has been carried on by the development of robotic-assisted laparoscopy, which has allowed for the widespread diffusion of minimally invasive surgery, particularly for the lower urinary tract. More recently, the evolution of minimally invasive surgery has been characterized by the desire to perform completely scarless surgery. Two approaches to further improve the cosmetic outcomes of minimally invasive sugery,

M.L. Blute, Jr., M.D. • S. Rais-Bahrami, M.D. (✉) • L. Richstone, M.D.
The Smith Institute for Urology, The Hofstra-North Shore LIJ School of Medicine,
450 Lakeville Road Suite M41, New Hyde Park, NY 11040, USA
e-mail: mlblute@gmail.com; soroushraisbahrami@gmail.com; lrichsto@nshs.edu

A. Rane et al. (eds.), *Scar-Less Surgery*,
DOI 10.1007/978-1-84800-360-6_1, © Springer-Verlag London 2013

namely, natural orifice translumenal endoscopic surgery (NOTES) and laparoendo-scopic single-site (LESS) surgery, have developed in tandem during recent years. Natural orifice surgery represents perhaps the Holy Grail of minimally invasive surgery: extirpative and/or reconstructive surgery with no violation of the externally visible body integument. Although proven feasible for some procedures, limitations in current technology and instrumentation have delayed and/or prevented the incorporation of NOTES into common, everyday surgical practice. In this context, interest was stirred in the concept of transumbilical "single-port" surgery, offering nearly scarless surgery.

As laparoscopic and now robotic LESS surgeries have been explored for a wide variety of procedures, it seems like something old has become new again, as single-port laparoscopy had, in fact, been first reported decades prior [1]. It is in this basic context that LESS and NOTES have emerged as the latest techniques in the continued evolution of modern surgery toward the least invasive approach to surgical intervention. The history of these techniques is brief but lends insight into the progression away from large, invasive surgery with open wounds and the morbidities experienced with these traditional approaches.

History of NOTES

Endoscopic procedures have been performed in the intralumenal gastrointestinal tract dating back to the early part of the twentieth century and perhaps represent the starting point for "natural orifice surgery." Rigid scopes were used to remove foreign bodies, dilate strictures, and excise accessible lesions. By 1960, flexible endoscopes were developed, allowing more extensive and invasive intubation of the gastrointestinal tract [2]. Endolumenal procedures performed today using flexible endoscopes range from biopsies to ablation to extirpative surgery replacing traditionally open or conventional laparoscopic surgery. The most commonly recognized application of flexible endoscopy is the use of a colonoscope for diagnostic and therapeutic management of the large bowel pathologies [3]. Additionally, the advances in fiber optic technology and flexible scopes now provide the maneuverability to perform complex endoscopy into the upper gastrointestinal tract and into the pancreaticobiliary duct system, which requires a very fine caliber endoscope with multiple levels of deflection and procedural dexterity.

Combining the emerging technologies of improved flexible optical scopes and the goals of providing more complex surgeries via endolumenal approaches, NOTES was developed. The successes of endoscopic procedures for intralumenal pathologies via biopsies, tumor excisions, and ablations have evolved into procedures initiated through the natural orifices to address pathologies outside the gastrointestinal lumen.

Also, the use of endoscopy in the genitourinary system via cystoscopy, vaginoscopy, and hysteroscopy has paralleled the advances of gastrointestinal endoscopy. Similarly, biopsies, mass excisions, and ablative procedures performed through a cystoscope or hysteroscope have now evolved into procedures whereby these instruments are used via the natural portal of entry to allow access to extralumenal pathologies or provide routes of specimen extraction previously not harnessed as a means of minimizing skin incisions [4–6].

Employing a puncture through the gastrointestinal tract with an endoscope to access extralumenal organs of interest was first used in animal models. NOTES surgery first began through a transgastric approach. A transgastric approach was proven safe for diagnostic imaging of the peritoneal cavity and the therapeutic purpose of removing tissue and organs [7, 8].

In early studies, cholecystectomy was performed via a transgastric and simultaneous transvesical approach in seven anesthetized pigs [9, 10]. Access was obtained through the stomach and urinary bladder, and the cholecystectomy was performed with a gastroscope transgastrically and a ureteroscope passed transvesically. The surgical dissection was performed gastroscopically. Five of the seven cases were performed successfully without complications, while two had evidence of bile leak and hemorrhage from the liver surface. These initial studies demonstrated the feasibility of performing a cholecystectomy exclusively through natural orifices.

This proof of concept quickly expanded from animal models to cases of successful transgastric NOTES in human patients. One of the earliest accounts of NOTES for gastrointestinal pathology in humans date back to 2004, when an appendectomy was first performed via a transgastric approach [11].

Now, increasing numbers of subsequent therapeutic procedures are being performed using these transgastric NOTES techniques, including cholecystectomy, gastrojejunostomy, splenectomy, hysterectomy, and oophorectomy [12–16]. In essence, this provides patients with an outwardly scarless approach, replacing traditional open surgical or conventional laparoscopic techniques that render patients with visible cutaneous scars at incision sites.

Considering all human natural orifices, any one could possibly be used for this form of surgery. More recently, other routes of entry into the body have been used to gain better access to various intraabdominal and retroperitoneal organs. These additional portals of access include the transvesical, transcolonic, and transvaginal approaches [17–19].

Another natural orifice that has recently been utilized not only as an access portal but also as an extraction site for NOTES is the vagina. Again, this is a "rediscovery" of sorts, as the vaginal canal has served as a well-established extraction site for over a century. Gynecologic surgeons have been performing vaginal hysterectomies since the late 1800s, using the vaginal canal as the extraction site for extirpative surgery for both benign and malignant uterine pathologies [20].

In 2002, urologists reported on their series of patients who underwent laparoscopic nephrectomies and extracted the specimen through the vagina, saving patients large abdominal wounds [21, 22]. More recently, in 2007 Lima and colleagues reported on a nephrectomy performed completely via natural orifices in a porcine model [23]. The authors were able to demonstrate the successful completion of a nephrectomy using transgastric and transvesical access in six porcine models. Interestingly, the authors realized that they were able to operate with a low CO_2

pressure of approximately 3 mmHg. This was accounted for by the entrance of the instruments into the abdomen being parallel to the abdominal wall, which was used as a fulcrum during mobilization. Secondly, they noted that the magnification properties of the endoscopic instruments required decreased levels of pneumoperitoneum pressure, potentially decreasing the stresses incurred by the use of routinely higher pneumoperitoneum pressures.

Kaouk and colleagues reported their experience with NOTES transvaginal nephrectomy with Veress needle access initially obtained via the umbilicus for establishing the pneumoperitoneum followed by a direct vision colpotomy through which a transvaginal access port was placed. The entire operation was then completed via the transvaginal route [24]. More recently, the same group reported a pure NOTES transvaginal nephrectomy with no cutaneous violations [25].

The ability to surgically excise an organ of greater mass than the gallbladder and harbored within the retroperitoneum can be done through natural orifices. The problem that arises, especially in male patients, is how to remove an organ of such a size while maintaining exclusively scarless surgery. This concept has yet to be addressed definitively with a uniformly consensual solution. However, ideas such as specimen morcellation, extension of the transgastric incision, or transcolonic extraction routes have been proposed and tested as alternatives to transabdominal removal, which would render the patient with a scar at the cutaneous extraction site.

The practice of NOTES to date is relatively novel, and experience with the technique is still rapidly evolving. Like conventional laparoscopy did decades earlier, the development of NOTES offered a revolutionarily new surgical approach with the intent of improving patient outcomes postoperatively, in terms of both cosmesis and convalescence.

Following the earliest reports of translumenal procedures, leaders in the fields of laparoscopy and endoscopy met to discuss the flourishing development of NOTES as a feasible surgical technique. In 2005, this meeting, or the Natural Orifice Surgery Consortium for Assessment and Research (NOSCAR), set goals to facilitate the advancement of research in this field. The group established basic foundations for NOTES research, encouraging a multidisciplinary team approach, the advancement of minimally invasive surgical skill sets, the sharing of data among NOSCAR members at annual meetings, and the use of institutional review board approval for all NOTES procedures performed on humans [26]. Since that initial meeting, many papers have been published on NOTES proving its feasibility and safety in both animal models and human patient series. General surgeons, urologists, gynecologists, and gastroenterologists have worked in concert to apply NOTES techniques to a wide variety of intraabdominal procedures.

As demonstrated, this surgical technique has been born within the past decade and taken a stronghold in an academic realm as an area of investigation to test its applicability and methods of improving it further. The future of NOTES in mainstream surgical practice is unclear to date. However, it has safely and successfully been applied for extirpative and minor reconstructive procedures in human subjects. It may establish a realm of surgery, a true paradigm shift masking any outward evidence of undergoing surgery [19].

History of LESS

Much like NOTES, laparoendoscopic single-site (LESS) surgery is often acclaimed as a novel technique in its infancy, while, in fact, it is a popularization and application of previously applied techniques. LESS is now taking a stronghold as an evolutionary step beyond conventional laparoscopy to minimize incisions as an effort to improve convalescence and postoperative cosmesis. Publications regarding the contemporary LESS experience demonstrate the breadth of experience for which LESS techniques have been employed successfully to accomplish a wealth of operative cases in general surgery, urology, gynecology, and other surgical specialties.

In 2008, innovative leaders in the field of minimally invasive surgery gathered to establish a universally applied terminology for single-site surgical techniques. The Laparoendoscopic Single-Site Surgery Consortium for Assessment and Research (LESSCAR) agreed upon LESS as the accepted nomenclature for this field of surgery. This consolidation brought together "keyhole" surgery, single-site access (SSA) surgery, single-port surgery (SPS), single-incision laparoscopic surgery (SILS), embryonic natural orifice translumenal endoscopic surgery (E-NOTES), natural orifice transumbilical surgery (NOTUS), one-port umbilical surgery (OPUS), transumbilical endoscopic surgery (TUES), transumbilical laparoscopic-assisted (TULA) surgery, and other terminology that was used previously [27]. This was done in efforts to unify rather than fragment this evolving field, consolidate research efforts, improve educational training programs, and universalize reporting in the literature. Now, LESS encompasses many forms of minimally invasive surgery, all with the concerted effort to minimize or eliminate the incisions needed for operative access [28].

The earliest cases of LESS date back several decades to the initial publications describing laparoscopy. Basic laparoscopic procedures marginally expanded upon the well-described diagnostic laparoscopy of the time. These operative maneuvers were performed via a single trocar accommodating a laparoscope and working instrument or incision immediately adjacent to the laparoscopic access trocar. The initial reports of operative laparoscopy centered on needle biopsies performed under laparoscopic visualization by general surgeons and female sterilization by gynecologists [29, 30]. These limited uses of single-site laparoscopy continued to the present day. However, over this time period, more complex operative cases were attempted and proven safe to be performed laparoscopically with the use of additional access trocars. Multiport laparoscopy was adopted as a minimally invasive approach allowing for more complex extirpative, reconstructive, or diagnostic operations for surgeons in many fields [31–33]. At many institutions, laparoscopy surmounted the classic open technique as the standard operative approach for certain procedures [34].

A second wave of interest in LESS arose in the past decade, recognizing LESS as the next natural iteration of minimally invasive laparoscopic surgery. Modifications were made to attempt cases via a single entry incision. Otherwise, LESS techniques largely mirrored those of conventional multiport laparoscopy for nearly all surgical operations that were proven feasible via laparoscopy.

Some of the earliest contemporary cases of LESS date back to 2005. Hirano and colleagues reported one of the first minimally invasive adrenalectomies performed in this manner [35]. In their study, 54 patients underwent a retroperitoneoscopic adrenalectomy via a 4.5-cm incision in the midaxillary line. They were able to perform the surgery through a 4-cm resectoscopic tube using endoscopes without carbon dioxide insufflation. Still, as LESS developed further, attempts at more complex surgery and extirpative surgery for larger organs were made. In 2007, Raman and colleagues performed nephrectomies on pigs using a single incision through which subcentimeter trocars were inserted; once the technique was perfected in the porcine model, nephrectomy was successfully performed in three human subjects [36]. The authors demonstrated the feasibility of using articulating laparoscopic instruments to improve triangulation for their approach to dissecting and removing the kidney. As demonstrated by these early studies and additional small series, great advances have been made in the field of LESS by urologic surgeons [37–39]. Much of the available literature describes urologic LESS, including LESS nephrectomy, partial nephrectomy, nephroureterectomy, pyeloplasty, prostatectomy, sacral colpopexy, and ureteral reimplant [40–42].

In parallel with urologists who have embraced LESS as an innovative advancement of minimally invasive surgery, general surgeons and other surgical specialists have adopted these techniques and principles for their respective fields of surgery.

Just as the laparoscopic cholecystectomy was initially embraced by general surgeons a few decades ago, so too has the application of LESS for gallbladder removal. One of the initial studies that began in 2007 involved 29 patients who were offered LESS and compared to those undergoing multiport laparoscopic removal. When the authors compared LESS to multiport laparoscopy, there were no significant differences in operative time, blood loss, length of hospital stay, conversion to open surgery, or postoperative pain [43]. A retrospective case-control study comparing keyhole nephrectomy to standard laparoscopy failed to demonstrate any difference in surgical parameters. They showed no difference in operative time, blood loss, narcotic use, complications, and hospital stay [44]. Similarly, Fader and colleagues assessed LESS with regards to its feasibility to treat gynecologic oncology disease processes [45]. The authors performed LESS with both standard laparoscopic instruments as well as robot assistance with the DaVinci robotic platform and reported the successful resection of various gynecologic malignancies, including uterine and ovarian. They commented in the discussion that their patients required little postoperative narcotics for adequate analgesia. Other areas where LESS has been successfully applied include gastric banding, appendectomy, and robotic radical prostatectomy, all revealing safety, feasibility, and perioperative outcomes comparable to the well-accepted conventional laparoscopic techniques for each operation [46–48].

As evidenced, the initial reports regarding the success and feasibility of LESS support its presence as the next generation of minimally invasive surgery. LESS holds all the benefits of standard laparoscopy and affords the patient the added advantage of being left with at most one abdominal scar, often hidden periumbilically or below the waistline as a mini-Pfannenstiel incision. Thus far, most investigations show an equivalence in perioperative and convalescence outcomes compared to conventional multiport laparoscopy. However, additional studies are required to prove whether LESS offers improved postoperative pain parameters and patient satisfaction outcomes in head-to-head comparisons by case type. LESS approaches are launching surgery—once a practice of large open incisions now reduced to multiple trocar incisions—to yet the next step of being minimally invasive.

Conclusions

The historical accounts of both contemporary NOTES and LESS applied toward complex surgeries are limited; they are less than a decade old in either case. Both have been conceived from the continuous drive to make surgery less invasive while achieving at least equivalent results produced by traditional open and conventional laparoscopic techniques. These surgical approaches have evolved, providing patients with complex surgical procedures with either a single superficial wound for LESS or no scars by utilizing the body's natural orifices for NOTES.

References

1. Pelland PC. Sterilization by laparoscopy. Clin Obstet Gynecol. 1983;26(2):321–33.
2. Hirschowitz BI. The development and application of fiberoptic endoscopy. Cancer. 1988;61(10):1935–41.
3. Shinya H, Wolff W. Flexible colonoscopy. Cancer. 1976;37(1 Suppl):462–70.
4. Gettman MT, Blute ML. Transvesical peritoneoscopy: initial clinical evaluation of the bladder as a portal for natural orifice translumenal endoscopic surgery. Mayo Clin Proc. 2007;82(7):843–5.
5. Siegler AM. Therapeutic hysteroscopy. Acta Eur Fertil. 1986;17(6):467–71.
6. Pansadoro V, Pansadoro A, Emiliozzi P. Laparoscopic transvesical diverticulectomy. BJU Int. 2009;103(3):412–24.
7. Wagh MS, Merrifield BF, Thompson CC. Endoscopic transgastric abdominal exploration and organ resection: initial experience in a porcine model. Clin Gastroenterol Hepatol. 2005;3(9):892–6.
8. Kantsevoy SV, Jagannath SB, Niiyama H, Isakovich NV, Chung SS, Cotton PB, Gostout CJ, Hawes RH, Pasricha PJ, Kalloo AN. A novel safe approach to the peritoneal cavity for per-oral transgastric endoscopic procedures. Gastrointest Endosc. 2007;65(3):497–500.
9. Rolanda C, Lima E, Pêgo JM, Henriques-Coelho T, Silva D, Moreira I, Macedo G, Carvalho JL, Correia-Pinto J. Third-generation cholecystectomy by natural orifices: transgastric and transvesical combined approach. Gastrointest Endosc. 2007;65(1):111–7.
10. Rolanda C, Lima E, Correia-Pinto J. Searching the best approach for third generation cholecystectomy. Gastrointest Endosc. 2007;65(2):354.
11. Reddy N, Rao P. Peroral transgastric endoscope appendectomy in human. Paper presented at: 45th annual conference of the society of gastrointestinal endoscopy of India. 28–29 Feb 2004. Jaipur, India.
12. Merrifield BF, Wagh MS, Thompson CC. Peroral transgastric organ resection: a feasibility study in pigs. Gastrointest Endosc. 2006;63(4):693–7.

13. Bergström M, Ikeda K, Swain P, Park PO. Transgastric anastomosis by using flexible endoscopy in a porcine model (with video). Gastrointest Endosc. 2006;63(2):307–12.

14. Kantsevoy SV, Hu B, Jagannath SB, Vaughn CA, Beitler DM, Chung SS, Cotton PB, Gostout CJ, Hawes RH, Pasricha PJ, Magee CA, Pipitone LJ, Talamini MA, Kalloo AN. Transgastric endoscopic splenectomy: is it possible? Surg Endosc. 2006;20(3):522–5.

15. Kantsevoy SV, Jagannath SB, Niiyama H, Chung SS, Cotton PB, Gostout CJ, Hawes RH, Pasricha PJ, Magee CA, Vaughn CA, Barlow D, Shimonaka H, Kalloo AN. Endoscopic gastrojejunostomy with survival in a porcine model. Gastrointest Endosc. 2005;62(2):287–92.

16. Park PO, Bergström M, Ikeda K, Fritscher-Ravens A, Swain P. Experimental studies of transgastric gallbladder surgery: cholecystectomy and cholecystogastric anastomosis (videos). Gastrointest Endosc. 2005;61(4):601–6.

17. Granberg CF, Frank I, Gettman MT. Transvesical NOTES: current experience and potential implications for urologic applications. J Endourol. 2009;23(5):747–52.

18. Shin EJ, Kalloo AN. Transcolonic NOTES: current experience and potential implications for urologic applications. J Endourol. 2009;23(5):743–6.

19. Marescaux J, Dallemagne B, Perretta S, Wattiez A, Mutter D, Coumaros D. Surgery without scars: report of transluminal cholecystectomy in a human being. Arch Surg. 2007;142(9):823–6; discussion 826–7.

20. De Forest II HP. Richelot on the operative technique of vaginal hysterectomy. Ann Surg. 1893;18(3):334–44.

21. Gill IS, Cherullo EE, Meraney AM, Borsuk F, Murphy DP, Falcone T. Vaginal extraction of the intact specimen following laparoscopic radical nephrectomy. J Urol. 2002;167(1):238–41.

22. Gettman MT, Lotan Y, Napper CA, Cadeddu JA. Transvaginal laparoscopic nephrectomy: development and feasibility in the porcine model. Urology. 2002;59(3):446–50.

23. Lima E, Rolanda C, Pêgo JM, Henriques-Coelho T, Silva D, Osório L, Moreira I, Carvalho JL, Correia-Pinto J. Third-generation nephrectomy by natural orifice transluminal endoscopic surgery. J Urol. 2007;178(6):2648–54.

24. Kaouk JH, White WM, Goel RK, Brethauer S, Crouzet S, Rackley RR, Moore C, Ingber MS, Haber GP. NOTES transvaginal nephrectomy: first human experience. Urology. 2009;74(1):5–8.

25. Kaouk JH, Haber GP, Goel RK, Crouzet S, Brethauer S, Firoozi F, Goldman HB, White WM. Pure natural orifice translumenal endoscopic surgery (NOTES) transvaginal nephrectomy. Eur Urol. 2010;57(4):723–6.

26. Rattner D, Kalloo A. ASGE/SAGES Working Group on natural orifice transluminal endoscopic surgery. Surg Endosc. 2006;20(2):329–33.

27. Tracy CR, Raman JD, Cadeddu JA, Rane A. Laparoendoscopic single-site surgery in urology: where have we been and where are we heading? Nat Clin Pract Urol. 2008;5(10):561–8.

28. Gill IS, Advincula AP, Aron M, Caddedu J, Canes D, Curcillo 2nd PG, Desai MM, Evanko JC, Falcone T, Fazio V, Gettman M, Gumbs AA, Haber GP, Kaouk JH, Kim F, King SA, Ponsky J, Remzi F, Rivas H, Rosemurgy A, Ross S, Schauer P, Sotelo R, Speranza J, Sweeney J, Teixeira J. Consensus statement of the consortium for laparoendoscopic single-site surgery. Surg Endosc. 2010;24(4):762–8.

29. Platteborse R. Laparoscopy, laparophotography, punch biopsy of the liver, gallbladder punch biopsy and collection of specimens of the peritoneal organs through a single trocar. Acta Gastroenterol Belg. 1961;24:696–700.

30. Rioux JE. Operative laparoscopy. J Reprod Med. 1973;10(5):249–55.

31. Valle RF, Reichert JA. Laparoscopic surgery: an evolving revolution. JSLS. 2001;5(1):95–6.

32. Nguyen NT, Zainabadi K, Mavandadi S, Paya M, Stevens CM, Root J, Wilson SE. Trends in utilization and outcomes of laparoscopic versus open appendectomy. Am J Surg. 2004;188(6):813–20.

33. Kaouk JH, Gill IS. Laparoscopic reconstructive urology. J Urol. 2003;170(4 Pt 1):1070–8.

34. Lichten JB, Reid JJ, Zahalsky MP, Friedman RL. Laparoscopic cholecystectomy in the new millennium. Surg Endosc. 2001;15(8):867–72.

35. Hirano D, Minei S, Yamaguchi K, Yoshikawa T, Hachiya T, Yoshida T, Ishida H, Takimoto Y, Saitoh T, Kiyotaki S, Okada K. Retroperitoneoscopic adrenalectomy for adrenal tumors for a single large port. J Endourol. 2005;19(7):788–92.

36. Raman JD, Bensalah K, Bagrodia A, Stern JM, Cadeddu JA. Laboratory and clinical development of single keyhole umbilical nephrectomy. Urology. 2007;70(6):1039–42.
37. Raman JD, Cadeddu JA. Single access laparoscopic nephrectomy. Indian J Urol. 2008;24(4): 457–60.
38. Desai MM, Rao PP, Aron M, Pascal-Haber G, Desai MR, Mishra S, Kaouk JH, Gill IS. Scarless single port transumbilical nephrectomy pyeloplasty: first clinical report. BJU Int. 2008;101(1):83–8.
39. Rané A, Rao P, Rao P. Single-port-access nephrectomy and other laparoscopic urologic procedures using a novel laparoscopic port (R-port). Urology. 2008;72(2):260–3.
40. White WM, Haber GP, Goel RK, Crouzet S, Stein RJ, Kaouk JH. Single-port urological surgery: single-center experience with the first 100 cases. Urology. 2009;74(4):801–4.
41. Rais-Bahrami S, Montag S, Atalla MA, et al. Laparoendoscopic single-site surgery of the kidney with no accessory trocars: an initial experience. J Endourol. 2009;23(8):1319–24.
42. Desai MM, Berger AK, Brandina R, Aron M, Irwin BH, Canes D, Desai MR, Rao PP, Sotelo R, Stein R, Gill IS. Laparoendoscopic single-site surgery: initial hundred patients. Urology. 2009;74(4):805–12.
43. Hodgett SE, Hernandez JM, Morton CA, Ross SB, Albrink M, Rosemurgy AS. Laparoendoscopic single site (LESS) cholecystectomy. J Gastrointest Surg. 2009;13(2):188–92.
44. Raman JD, Bagrodia A, Cadeddu JA. Single-incision, umbilical laparoscopic versus conventional laparoscopic nephrectomy: a comparison of perioperative outcomes and short-term measures of convalescence. Eur Urol. 2009;55(5):1198–204.
45. Fader AN, Escobar PF. Laparoendoscopic single-site surgery (LESS) in gynecologic oncology: technique and initial report. Gynecol Oncol. 2009;114(2):157–61.
46. Teixeira J, McGill K, Koshy N, McGinty J, Todd G. Laparoscopic single-site surgery for placement of adjustable gastric band – a series of 22 cases. Surg Obes Relat Dis. 2010;6(1):41–5.
47. Vidal O, Valentini M, Ginestà C, Martí J, Espert JJ, Benarroch G, García-Valdecasas JC. Laparoendoscopic single-site surgery appendectomy. Surg Endosc. 2010;24(3):686–91.
48. White MA, Haber GP, Autorino R, Khanna R, Forest S, Yang B, Altunrende F, Stein RJ, Kaouk JH. Robotic laparoendoscopic single-site radical prostatectomy: technique and early outcomes. Eur Urol. 2010;58(4):544–50.

Chapter 2
Overview: Rationale and Terminology

Hagop Sarkissian and Brian H. Irwin

Keywords LESS • Laparoendoscopic single-site surgery • Single site • Nomenclature
• NOTES • Natural orifice translumenal endoscopic surgery

Introduction

In the last several decades, with the advent of the Internet and globalization, the world has seen unprecedented information dissemination and exchange. Accompanying this explosion of information has been an unquestionable and previously unparalleled increase in the development and propagation of technology and techniques in medicine and, in particular, in minimally invasive surgery.

Urology has long remained at the forefront of the development and implementation of such technologies. Its involvement in the improvement and distribution of these techniques worldwide is not surprising. Urology has long been a discipline with a dependence on innovative technology to minimize the invasive nature of our procedures. The nature of the urinary tract within the human body seems to spur innovation and has allowed urologists to keep at the leading edge of minimally invasive technological revolutions. In their simplest forms, single-site surgery and even NOTES procedures have been used by urologists for decades with the use of percutaneous nephrolithotomy via a single small incision and a multitude of transurethral endoscopic procedures. The application of similar principles to surgeries traditionally performed via open, or more recently laparoscopic and robotic-assisted, approaches is simply a natural extension of the urologist's current armamentarium to continue on his or her quest to minimize access-related trauma and improve outcomes.

H. Sarkissian, M.D. • B.H. Irwin, M.D. (✉)
Division of Urology, Department of Surgery, University of Vermont College of Medicine,
111 Colchester Ave, ACC EP5 Urology, Burlington, VT 05401, USA
e-mail: hagop.sarkissian@vtmednet.org; brian.irwin@vtmednet.org

A. Rane et al. (eds.), *Scar-Less Surgery*,
DOI 10.1007/978-1-84800-360-6_2, © Springer-Verlag London 2013

In the early 1990s, when conventional laparoscopy (CL) was in its infancy and Clayman performed the first laparoscopic nephrectomy [1], a revolution of surgical approach and thought occurred very rapidly. As it became clear that even the most complex of urologic reconstructive and oncologic procedures could be performed in ways that would allow for earlier recovery and minimization of morbidity, the scope of minimally invasive urology exploded. Today, the technology and techniques utilized during conventional laparoscopy have matured. These surgical approaches have evolved and, as a direct result, have given the minimally invasive community two progeny that are very much interrelated: natural orifice translumenal endoscopic surgery (NOTES) and laparoendoscopic single-site (LESS) surgery.

Prior to delving further into the world of urologic minimally invasive techniques and procedures, it is important to understand the history and rationale behind the development of these techniques, and the evolution of the standardization of their nomenclature. Current advances and issues that these approaches face, based on currently published white papers, clinical trials, and patient attitudes toward the new breed of minimally invasive surgical techniques, will also be reviewed.

Nomenclature

While the clinical applications of LESS have largely outshined those of NOTES mainly due to technical challenges related to access and instrumentation, the nomenclature and original studies of NOTES actually predate those of LESS. For this reason, most discussions of NOTES and LESS prefer to address them chronologically rather than the order in which they have been adopted into the clinical surgical repertoire.

NOTES

NOTES is the acronym used to describe procedures performed via natural orifice translumenal endoscopic surgery.

In its purest intended form, NOTES entails using one or more naturally occurring openings of the human body (i.e., mouth, nares, vagina, urethra, and anus) with the intention of puncturing through the wall of the accessed hollow organ (stomach, vagina, urinary bladder, and/or colon) to gain access to another body cavity/space (peritoneum, retroperitoneum, thorax, etc.). Following access, the surgeon then proceeds with the specific task of the intended operation using instruments introduced through the opening.

Other criteria related to the definition of NOTES have also been generally accepted and are as follows [2]:

- If instruments or ports are used transabdominally along with the natural orifice opening, but greater than 75 % of the dissection and operation is performed via the natural orifice, then the procedure is deemed a hybrid NOTES procedure.

- If the natural orifice is used only for additional port placement, but the majority of the operation is conducted via transabdominal ports, then the procedure takes on the designation of NOTES-assisted.
- If the natural orifice is used as an extraction point only, it is not considered NOTES.
- The umbilicus is not considered a natural orifice for purposes of NOTES designation.

LESS

LESS is also an acronym describing an endoscopic procedure. It stands for laparoendoscopic single-site surgery.

LESS procedures rely on a single access site, usually involving the transabdominal or retroperitoneal placement of ports. Because of the breadth of potential applications, the definition has become slightly more involved. It has been generally accepted that LESS also adheres to the following [2, 3]:

- A single, a multiple, or a single multi-port platform used through the single incision.
- If the umbilicus is used for access, the letter "U" shall be placed in front of the procedure, e.g., "U-LESS."
- Enlarging an incision for specimen retrieval does not exclude the procedure from being considered a LESS procedure.
- The adjunctive use of small needlescopic instruments/ports is encouraged if they enhance the surgeon's confidence and the patient's safety.
- A single incision with multiple fascial openings is not excluded from the LESS definition.

As seen, these are highly specific terminology and definitions that have been attached to a myriad of surgical procedures. The acronyms NOTES and LESS are the currently agreed-upon versions of a minimally invasive primordial alphabet soup that existed prior to 2006.

Nomenclature History

Prior to the consensus statement by the NOTES Working Group in 2008, the nomenclature used above for the procedures was referred to by several different combination and acronyms, a few of which can be seen in Table 2.1.

The lack of standardization of terminology led to confusion in the academic examinations of these techniques. It became difficult to perform meaningful literature searches and define inclusion criteria, making it impossible to report consistent results. Many centers were duplicating work due to the inability to accurately

Table 2.1 Descriptive terms and corresponding acronyms used in the literature

Descriptives	Acronyms
Natural orifice surgery	NOS
Natural orifice transluminal endoscopic surgery	NOTES
Natural orifice transluminal endoscopic surgery nephrectomy	
Embryonic NOTES	E-NOTES
Hybrid natural orifice transluminal endoscopic surgery	H-NOTES
Robotic NOTES	R-NOTES
Robot assisted single port access	
Umbilical natural orifice transluminal endoscopic surgery	U-NOTES
Laparoendoscopic single-site surgery	LESS
One port umbilical surgery	OPUS
Single access-site laparoscopic surgery	SAS
Single incision laparoscopy	SIL
Single Incision laparoscopic surgery	SILS
Single port access	SPA
Single port access surgery	
Transumbilical laparoscopic assisted surgery	TULA
Visibly scarless urologic surgery	VSUS
Combined single port access	
Pure single port access	
Pure natural orifice transluminal endoscopic surgery	
Scarless single port transumbilical surgery	
Single keyhole surgery	

describe these new techniques. It became clear that standardization was necessary. As an example of the resulting confusion, Box et al. [2] described a Medline/PubMed and ARGH online acronym database searches in which 8,710 and 11,010 citations, respectively, were obtained, using 720 different definitions of the searched acronyms to describe what would, some time later, be termed NOTES and LESS procedures. Fortunately for the urologist, 362 of the PubMed articles and only 5 of the ARGH acronyms pertained to urology from a period spanning 1990–2008. There seemed to have been a significant overlap with other specialties and keywords associated with alternative nonsurgical meanings. In a similar manner, Sanchez-Salas et al. [4] reported on 412 manuscripts, with 64 pertaining to urology, while searching PubMed for descriptive words of single port, single site, NOTES, LESS, and single-incision surgery from 2002 to 2009.

In 2006, the Natural Orifice Surgery Consortium for Assessment and Research (NOSCAR) Working Group convened to address the problem of confusion of nomenclature in the literature. The working group was a joint initiative between the American Society for Gastrointestinal Endoscopy (ASGE) and the Society of American Gastrointestinal and Endoscopic Surgeons (SAGES) [2, 5]. As a result of this meeting, the term NOTES was coined and adopted as the accepted standard for the procedures falling into the previously described definitions. Subsequently, the term was trademarked by the same entity.

In urology, the Urologic NOTES Working Group was established in 2007 not only to address the nomenclature, but also to aid in the safe implementation of clinical research and to help standardize outcomes reporting and training for these new techniques [2, 4–6]. This working group was composed of members of the Endourological Society as an ad hoc gathering of individuals interested in NOTES. The group's vision was one of the safe and systematic implantation of NOTES along a defined pathway from conception of procedures to bench research to animal lab protocols, ultimately culminating in improvements in patient care through clinical trials. It was felt the new techniques in development should at the very least match, if not exceed, the efficacy, economy, and safety of the current standard of care for minimally invasive procedures. But, above all else, all agreed that patient safety was of the utmost importance.

The other working group that was influential in defining the role of LESS was LESSCAR, or Laparo-Endoscopic Single-Site Surgery Consortium for Assessment and Research. They have taken the helm in the standardization of nomenclature and implementation of LESS procedures. Most of the members of the Urologic NOTES Working Group are also the founding members of LESSCAR, formed in 2008 [3, 7]. Their consensus statement in 2010 further delineated and specified the nomenclature, research, and outcomes reporting procedures. For example, the 2010 consensus statement requires the inclusion of clear and full standards of reporting procedures, called "mandatory descriptive second line," for research publications. This brief statement should be included in all manuscripts and should state the following information in a concise manner [3]:

- Single incision length and location (abdominal, thoracic, etc.)
- Approach (percutaneous intralumenal, transperitoneal, etc.)
- Number and type of ports used
- Type of surgery (laparoscopic, endoscopic, robotic)
- Type of laparoscope used (flexible, straight)
- Type of instruments used (straight, curved, articulating, etc.)
- Whether or not a 2-mm needlescopic instrument was used

The LESSCAR group has also taken steps in trademarking the acronym LESS with a similar rationale of the NOSCAR Group's. It is to ensure that the acronym can have universal availability to the surgical and/or medical community and that industry does not have exclusive rights and benefits for profiting or marketing from its usage.

We owe a tremendous debt of gratitude to the thought leaders in the NOSCAR, Urologic NOTES Group, and LESSCAR working groups. Aside from the standardization of the nomenclature to the procedures, a daunting task in itself, they also set forth guidelines for research, publication, and ultimately patient safety regarding NOTES and LESS. Due to their efforts, a clear increase in interest and in the number of publications can be seen in the literature in both single-site and NOTES surgery, as shown in Figs. 2.1 and 2.2.

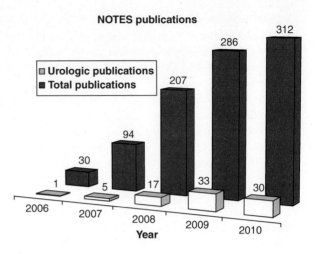

Fig. 2.1 Number of NOTES publications found as a result of PubMed search on the following terms: "natural orifice transluminal endoscopic surgery OR Robotic NOTES OR natural orifice surgery OR umbilical NOTES OR embryonic NOTES" (*red*) and with the addition of the search term "AND urology" (*white*)

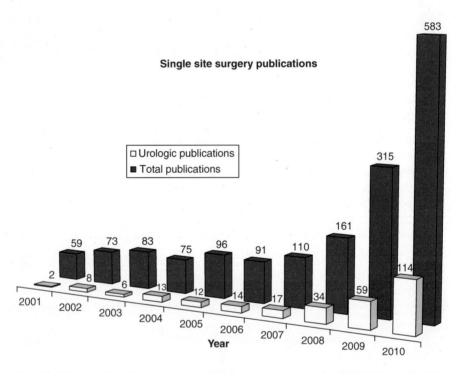

Fig. 2.2 Number of single-site surgery publications found as a result of PubMed search on the following terms: "laparoendoscopic single site surgery OR single port access surgery OR single port access OR single incision laparoscopic surgery OR single port laparoscopy OR single port laparoscopic surgery OR single incision laparoscopy OR one port umbilical surgery OR single trocar laparoscopic surgery OR keyhole surgery (*red*)" and with the addition of the search term "AND urology" (*white*)

Evolution of Procedures

Gettman et al. described the first application and feasibility of NOTES by success-fully completing transvaginal nephrectomy in a porcine model [6, 8]. Note that the procedure predates the acronym NOTES. The first NOTES series (transgastric liver biopsies in a porcine model) was published by Kalloo et al. in 2004 [9]; it was not until 2006 that the official name, NOTES, entered the surgical lexicon. Subsequently, there have been hybrid and pure NOTES procedures in both animal and human cases, including appendectomies, cholecystectomies, nephrectomies, and others.

Advanced LESS in urology, on the other hand, which describes a single transab-dominal incision as its mainstay, was pioneered early on by two groups, the University of Texas Southwestern Medical Center and the Cleveland Clinic [6]. Today, LESS has gained momentum in pyeloplasty, nephrectomy, and even pros-tatectomy and has been adopted at centers worldwide.

The first case reports of NOTES and LESS in porcine models showed the feasi-bility of the techniques and set the stage for the evolution of CL toward NOTES and LESS. It started a paradigm shift in thought leading to changes in technique and innovation in surgical specialties.

In 2006 at the SAGES conference, Rao et al. presented the first transgastric NOTES appendectomy in humans [5, 7]. In 2009, Marescaux et al. described the first transvagi-nal NOTES cholecystectomy [5, 10]. Urologically, as mentioned, in 2002 Gettman et al. reported their experimental case series of transvaginal NOTES nephrectomies in the porcine model. It was not until 2007 that there was a resurgence of NOTES in urologic procedures with publications by Clayman [11] and Lima [12], in animal mod-els. The experimental stages in the animal models and the success that followed helped move the procedures to the human cadaveric realm, where Aron et al. [13] explored the idea of transvaginal NOTES nephrectomies. Prior to this, hybrid NOTES procedures were successfully completed in humans by Gill et al. [14] and Branco et al. [15]. On the heels of Aron's transvaginal NOTES nephrectomies, Kaouk et al. reported the first successful human pure NOTES transvaginal nephrectomy procedure in 2009 [16].

Addressing LESS in urology, the first two cases of single-port surgery were reported by Rane et al. in 2007 at the 25th World Congress of Endourology and sub-sequently in *Urology,* of five human subjects using an R-port (two simple nephrecto-mies, one orchidopexy, one orchidectomy, and one ureterolithotomy) [17]. Raman et al. presented a case series of 7 nephrectomies, 4 in a porcine model and 3 in humans, using a single access site termed "single keyhole umbilical nephrectomy" [18]. In 2009, Barret et al. reported their experience with LESS extraperitoneal radi-cal prostatectomy in a cadaveric model [19]. Since the initial case series above, well over 300 upper and lower urinary tract procedures have been described in the world literature using a single access site in humans. The earliest ones include Desai et al.'s single-port transumbilical nephrectomy [20], Rane et al.'s LESS nephrectomies [21], Stolzenburg et al.'s 10 LESS radical nephrectomies [22], and Gill et al.'s four single-port transumbilical live-donor nephrectomies [23]. In fact, two large series involving as many as 100 cases each exist in the LESS literature [24, 25].

Table 2.2 The evolution of surgical techniques and the anticipated benefits to the patient, surgeon, and technology

	Open surgery	Conventional laparoscopy	Robot-assisted laparoscopy	LESS	Robotic LESS
Patient	+	+++		(+)	(+)
Surgeon	+	−	+	− −	(+)
Technology	+	++	+++	(++)	(+++)

It is clear that with each step forward, improvements are possible and necessary, but to date they have not all been realized (shown in parentheses)

Rationale

The move from open procedures to conventional laparoscopy was a huge paradigm shift that allowed a large positive leap forward in the reduction of patient morbidity. Patient safety; reduction in blood loss, pain, length of stay, and convalescence; and an increase in quality of life are consistently shown as advantages of conventional laparoscopy over open procedures. Has this same leap forward been seen with the advent of NOTES and/or LESS? To date, the answer is no. This is in part due to the concept of diminishing returns. Since the leap from open surgery to conventional laparoscopy was so radical, much of the benefit from the minimization of access has already been realized. Advances now are largely centered on providing ergonomic benefit to the surgeon and improving technology, while incremental benefits to the patient remain quite small, as shown in Table 2.2.

Currently, there is a lack of large prospective clinical trials or substantial case series to compare conventional laparoscopy to NOTES/LESS procedures with regard to patient safety and outcomes. The path for NOTES and LESS procedures does diverge here somewhat. NOTES procedures, by their very nature, have much higher technological constraints (i.e., inadequate instrumentation, visceral closure shortcomings, etc.). This has led to the inability of the vast majority to be able to perform these procedures clinically in humans. The only true comparative studies that exist in the current literature compare LESS to conventional laparoscopy. Irwin et al. presented a multicenter experience of complications and subsequent conversion from LESS to open in upper tract urinary procedures [26]. A total of 125 patients underwent LESS, comprising 13.3 % of urologic laparoscopic procedures at these institutions. Only 5.6 % of LESS were converted to CL due to a variety of reasons (facilitate dissection, reconstruction, or homeostasis). Complications were noted in 15.2 % of patients undergoing LESS (urine leak, DVT, hemorrhage). Subset analysis revealed a higher rate of complication in reconstructive cases compared to extirpative ones. Before we dismiss LESS as too difficult to be performed safely, historical data tell us that conversion rates for laparoscopic cholecystectomy during its infancy ranged from 4 % to 5 % as well [26–29]. In urology, conversion rates from CL to open procedures during laparoscopic nephrectomy ranged from 8 % to 10 % in early series [26, 30–32].

Two prospective randomized trial comparing LESS to CL have been very recently published, showing similar results and suggesting some improvement with regard to convalescence in patients undergoing LESS procedures [33, 34].

The above does not show the superiority of LESS over conventional laparoscopy, at least not during the early phases of the procedure's adoption. But does it need to? As the LESSCAR group mentions in their consensus statement, the goal is to have at least equal efficacy and patient safety in comparison to CL. Simply showing the noninferiority of the technique would be adequate to justify continued study into these techniques. In mentioning this, we should not neglect the needs and wants of our patients. While patient safety, efficacy, and cost are of paramount consideration, patient perception of surgical outcomes and body image are important as well.

Bucher et al. tried to evaluate the perception and/or preferences of women in Geneva regarding different operative modalities (CL, U-LESS, and transvaginal NOTES). Of the respondents, 87 % preferred umbilical LESS vs. 4 % transvaginal NOTES vs. 8 % CL. Eighty-two percent preferred NOTES/LESS due to cosmesis. Ninety-six percent responded with apprehension regarding the transvaginal approach/access for fear of dyspareunia, short-term sexual abstinence, decreased sensation during intercourse, and infertility [35]. The same author conducted another study wherein the expectations for surgical treatment and surgical approach preference were queried. The first concern of the respondents was that of safety or risk of complications (92 % of respondents). At 74 %, cure was the overwhelming concern for the respondents compared to cosmesis at 3 %. But, when asked for their preference if operative risk was similar, 90 % preferred scarless surgery (i.e., LESS and NOTES) [36]. These numbers represent a cross section of a European population. While cross-continental differences may exist, a regional stratification of preferences may be even more prevalent in certain parts of the United States, lending importance to cosmesis in cities where body image has higher perceived social cost to the patient. A similar North American study regarding patient preference of these surgical approaches might lend further credence to NOTES and LESS especially if noninferiority in comparison to conventional laparoscopy can be shown.

Shortcomings

The basic concepts of exposure, visualization retraction/countertraction, and triangulation learned from our collective experience with conventional laparoscopic surgery pose serious technical issues when applied to either NOTES or LESS procedures. By limiting the access point, the nature of the procedure becomes one of an in-line surgical procedure. NOTES and LESS suffer from the lack of triangulation and clashing of instruments or robotic arms with current technologies and platforms. As with many new procedures, they also suffer from a lack of instrument specificity. Recently, the development of better docking platforms, access ports, specialized instruments, and improved optics have allowed new procedures to evolve and move forward. New innovations such as low-profile robotic arms, miniature intraabdominal robotic devices, camera holding robots, magnetically anchored instruments and scopes, articulating instrumentation and improved tissue closure devices have and will need to continue to contribute to the successful transition of NOTES and LESS from the lab and animal models toward the generalizability of their use in hospitals and in human trials. Further prospective clinical trials are needed to address improvements made in technique, instrumentation, and patient outcomes in comparison to CL.

Current Trends and Future Directions

As conventional laparoscopy was in its infancy 25 years ago, NOTES and LESS are currently in theirs. Since LESS represents a more direct evolution from conventional laparoscopy, it has had a shallower learning curve and a much more extensive early clinical adoption than NOTES. Anatomical and access similarities suggest LESS will evolve slightly faster than NOTES.

Bench research, technological advancements set forward by industry, animal research, and prospective human studies conducted within the guidelines set forth by NOSCAR and SCARLESS are crucial in the growth of these novel minimally invasive techniques. Aside from the above, we still do not know how to teach these techniques due to their novelty. It is assumed that today's surgeon has a working knowledge of conventional laparoscopic techniques and instrumentation, but where do we go from there? Do trainees learn most effectively from animal models, virtual reality or mechanical trainers, under the direct supervision of another surgeon during live patient procedures, or a combination of these methods? What is the optimal way of learning these techniques and implementing them into the urologist's practice in a safe and efficacious manner? This point is crucial if the technological advancements in NOTES and LESS are to be incorporated into mainstream surgical practice.

Today, the working groups continue to meet, evolve, modify, and refine their goals and standards. They are actively moving the minimally invasive surgical procedures of NOTES and LESS toward their maturity. But ultimately, lest we forget, it is the patient who will benefit from these procedures.

References

1. Clayman RV, et al. Laparoscopic nephrectomy: initial case report. J Urol. 1991;146(2): 278–82.
2. Box G, et al. Nomenclature of natural orifice translumenal endoscopic surgery (NOTES) and laparoendoscopic single-site surgery (LESS) procedures in urology. J Endourol. 2008;22(11): 2575–781.
3. Gill IS, et al. Consensus statement of the consortium for laparoendoscopic single-site surgery. Surg Endosc. 2010;24(4):762–8.
4. Sanchez-Salas RE, et al. Current status of natural orifice trans-endoscopic surgery (NOTES) and laparoendoscopic single site surgery (LESS) in urologic surgery. Int Braz J Urol. 2010;36(4):385–400.

5. Autorino R, et al. Current status and future perspectives in laparoendoscopic single-site and natural orifice transluminal endoscopic urological surgery. Int J Urol. 2010;17(5):410–31.
6. Gettman MT, et al. Consensus statement on natural orifice transluminal endoscopic surgery and single-incision laparoscopic surgery: heralding a new era in urology? Eur Urol. 2008;53(6): 1117–20.
7. Rao GV, Reddy N. Transgastric appendectomy in humans. Oral presentation at: Society of American Gastrointestinal and Endoscopic Surgeons (SAGES) Conference; 2006; Dallas, TX, USA 26–29.
8. Gettman MT, et al. Transvaginal laparoscopic nephrectomy: development and feasibility in the porcine model. Urology. 2002;59(3):446–50.
9. Kalloo AN, et al. Flexible transgastric peritoneoscopy: a novel approach to diagnostic and therapeutic interventions in the peritoneal cavity. Gastrointest Endosc. 2004;60(1):114–7.
10. Marescaux J, et al. Surgery without scars: report of transluminal cholecystectomy in a human being. Arch Surg. 2007;142(9):823–6; discussion 826–7.
11. Clayman RV, et al. Rapid communication: transvaginal single-port NOTES nephrectomy: initial laboratory experience. J Endourol. 2007;21(6):640–4.
12. Lima E, et al. Third-generation nephrectomy by natural orifice transluminal endoscopic surgery. J Urol. 2007;178(6):2648–854.
13. Aron M, et al. Transvaginal nephrectomy with a multichannel laparoscopic port: a cadaver study. BJU Int. 2009;103(11):1537–41.
14. Gill IS, et al. Vaginal extraction of the intact specimen following laparoscopic radical nephrectomy. J Urol. 2002;167(1):238–41.
15. Branco AW, et al. Hybrid transvaginal nephrectomy. Eur Urol. 2008;53(6):1290–4.
16. Kaouk JH, et al. Pure natural orifice translumenal endoscopic surgery (NOTES) transvaginal nephrectomy. Eur Urol. 2010;57(4):723–6.
17. Rane AP, Rao P. Single-port-access nephrectomy and other laparoscopic urologic procedures using a novel laparoscopic port (R-port). Urology. 2008;72(2):260–3; discussion 263–4.
18. Raman JD, et al. Laboratory and clinical development of single keyhole umbilical nephrectomy. Urology. 2007;70(6):1039–42.
19. Barret E, et al. A transition to laparoendoscopic single-site surgery (LESS) radical prostatectomy: human cadaver experimental and initial clinical experience. J Endourol. 2009;23(1):135–40.
20. Desai MM, et al. Scarless single port transumbilical nephrectomy and pyeloplasty: first clinical report. BJU Int. 2008;101(1):83–8.
21. Rane A, et al. Single-port "scarless" laparoscopic nephrectomies: the United Kingdom experience. BJU Int. 2009;104(2):230–3.
22. Stolzenburg JU, et al. Technique of laparoscopic-endoscopic single-site surgery radical nephrectomy. Eur Urol. 2009;56(4):644–50.
23. Gill IS, et al. Single port transumbilical (E-NOTES) donor nephrectomy. J Urol. 2008;180(2):637–41; discussion 641.
24. Desai MM, et al. Laparoendoscopic single-site surgery: initial hundred patients. Urology. 2009;74(4):805–12.
25. White WM, et al. Single-port urological surgery: single-center experience with the first 100 cases. Urology. 2009;74(4):801–4.
26. Irwin BH, et al. Complications and conversions of upper tract urological laparoendoscopic single-site surgery (LESS): multicentre experience: results from the NOTES Working Group. BJU Int. 2011;107(8):1284–9.
27. Delaitre B, et al. Complications of cholecystectomy by laparoscopic approach. Apropos of 6512 cases. Chirurgie. 1992;118(1–2):92–9; discussion 100–2.
28. Peters JH, et al. Safety and efficacy of laparoscopic cholecystectomy. A prospective analysis of 100 initial patients. Ann Surg. 1991;213(1):3–12.
29. Scott TR, Zucker KA, Bailey RW. Laparoscopic cholecystectomy: a review of 12,397 patients. Surg Laparosc Endosc. 1992;2(3):191–8.
30. Eraky I, et al. Laparoscopic nephrectomy: an established routine procedure. J Endourol. 1994;8(4):275–8.

31. Eraky I, el-Kappany HA, Ghoneim MA. Laparoscopic nephrectomy: Mansoura experience with 106 cases. Br J Urol. 1995;75(3):271–5.
32. Wilson BG, et al. Laparoscopic nephrectomy: initial experience and cost implications. Br J Urol. 1995;75(3):276–80.
33. Kurien A, et al. First prize: standard laparoscopic donor nephrectomy versus laparoendoscopic single-site donor nephrectomy: a randomized comparative study. J Endourol. 2011;25(3): 365–70.
34. Tugcu V, et al. Laparoendoscopic single-site surgery versus standard laparoscopic simple nephrectomy: a prospective randomized study. J Endourol. 2010;24(8):1315–20.
35. Bucher P, et al. Female population perception of conventional laparoscopy, transumbilical LESS, and transvaginal NOTES for cholecystectomy. Surg Endosc. 2011;25(7):2308–15.
36. Bucher P, et al. Population perception of surgical safety and body image trauma: a plea for scarless surgery? Surg Endosc. 2011;25(2):408–15.

Chapter 3
Visualization Options

Prashanth P. Rao, Shashikant Mishra, and Pradeep P. Rao

Keywords LESS • Single-port laparoscopy • Optics • LESS optics • SILS • Chip-on-tip laparoscope • LESS ergonomics

Introduction

Minimal access surgery has come of age over the last 30 years. Urologists have been practicing minimal access surgery that has been genuinely scarless for more than 80 years [1]. However, those scarless surgeries (and genuinely natural orifice endoscopic surgeries) were performed using the portal of the urethra to access the genitourinary organs. Since the first laparoscopic cholecystectomy by Muhe in 1985, laparoscopic surgery has been used to operate on every organ within the abdominal cavity using multiple small incisions ranging from 3 to 15 mm [2]. These were all performed using rigid rod-lens endoscopes for visualizing the abdominal cavity. In open surgery the vision was binocular and the visual axis and the operating hands

P.P. Rao, M.S. (Bom), FRCS (Ed), FCPS, DNB, MNAMS, FICS, DLS (Fr), FIAGES, FMAS
Department of Surgery, Mamata Hospital,
P43, Phase 2, MIDC, Dombivli East, Mumbai 421203, Maharashtra, India

Department of GI and Minimal Access Surgery, Mamata Hospital,
P43, Phase 2, MIDC, Dombivli East, Mumbai 421203, Maharashtra, India
e-mail: pprao2@mac.com

S. Mishra, M.S., DNB (Urol)
Department of Urology, Muljibhai Patel Urological Hospital,
Dr. Virendra Desai Road, Nadiad 387001, Gujarat, India
e-mail: mishra@mpuh.org

P.P. Rao, M.B., MNAMS, DNB (Urol), FRCSED (⊠)
Department of Urology, Mamata Hospital,
Dombivli East, Mumbai, Maharashtra 421203, India
e-mail: pprao@mac.com

A. Rane et al. (eds.), *Scar-Less Surgery*,
DOI 10.1007/978-1-84800-360-6_3, © Springer-Verlag London 2013

were in line, causing an acute and equal azimuth angle (defined in laparoscopic surgery as the angle between the visual axis and the operating or working axis) and allowing movements to be automatic, ingrained, and intuitive. In laparoscopy, the magnification and reproduction of the image on a monitor via a closed-circuit system significantly alter the image, influencing visual perception and causing a peripheral convexity or barrel distortion, called the fish-eye effect. Coupled with a widening and at times obtuse azimuth angle, this made laparoscopic surgery difficult and necessitated a great deal of mental processing, including learning hand-eye coordination, interpretation of the dimensions, and tissue recognition and depth perception based on the visual clues provided by this enhanced apparent image [3]. However, this "Nintendo Surgical Revolution," which began in 1987, was something that the "Nintendo" generation or the twenty-first-century surgeon could relate to, and by the turn of the century, laparoscopy was the accepted gold standard for most routine abdominal surgery [4].

With the advent of the new century and technological advances in endoscopes as well as instruments, there have been significant developments toward increasingly minimally invasive surgery [5–7]. These include surgeries under the umbrella of the terms NOTES [8] and LESS [9]. While NOTES uses the natural orifice, LESS is done through a single site (usually the umbilicus, which is a preexisting cicatrix and has even been described as an embryonic natural orifice), to minimize any visible scars at the end of the surgical procedure [10].

Visualization Options in LESS

Laparoendoscopic single-site (LESS) surgery, by definition, uses only a single site, either to use a multiportal access device [7] or multiple trocars [11] through a single site, usually the umbilicus. These surgeries necessitate insertion of the endoscope through a point that may not otherwise be the preferred site for laparoscopy. This gives rise to an unnatural viewing angle from the surgeon's perspective. Also, due to the crowding of the instruments and telescope and without adequate triangulation, space is at a premium. The insertion of the optics and the operating instruments through the same incision causes a very acute and almost absent azimuth angle, which is a far cry from the 45–75° angle considered ideal for laparoscopic surgery [12].

To overcome these disadvantages, there was a need to use modifications of existing instruments as well as optics in a way that would maximize ease of surgery through a confined space. Pioneers of single-port surgery mixed, matched, and modified instruments to make this feasible [13]. The instruments needed to be bent, articulating, and of various lengths, and this has been discussed elsewhere. We will discuss the various optics available and their advantages during LESS.

Conventional modern-day rod-lens laparoscopes offer excellent vision and are more than adequate to visualize all the structures in the abdominal cavity. They have a perpendicular shaft for the connection of the light cable, which is positioned at

Fig. 3.1 The "chopsticks effect"

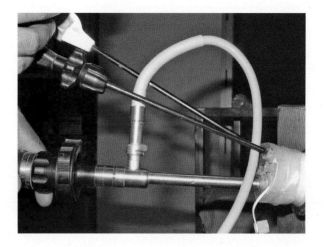

either 12 o'clock or 6 o'clock or can be altered during the course of surgery when using an angled scope, to optimize visualization. Within a confined space, this tends to get in the way and leads to clashing of the light cable with the instrument, the so-called chopsticks effect (Fig. 3.1). This tends to damage and break the light cable and hinders performance of the surgery by limiting movement of the instruments [13].

There are five ways of getting around this problem:

- Using a telescope with a coaxial light cable
- Using a telescope of a different length enabling the light guide to be away from the handles of the working instruments
- Modifying the telescope's light guide to keep the cable out of the way
- Using a regular or modified flexible endoscope as the optics
- Using a operative laparoscope with an instrument channel

There are solutions available incorporating one or more of these solutions, such as allowing these newer surgery techniques to be performed with a modicum of comfort.

Flexible Scopes and Chip-on-Tip Telescopes

Gastrointestinal endoscopists have long been using flexible endoscopes with the chip-on-tip technology, video endoscopes. Urologists and laparoscopic surgeons have been slower to adopt this technology primarily due to the availability of excellent rod-lens technology. With the advent of LESS and NOTES, it became convenient to use telescopes with an integrated light cable, placed coaxially to the shaft of the telescope (Fig. 3.2). This ensured that the instruments being used in a crowded space would not clash with the light cable, preventing damage to the cable as well

Fig. 3.2 The EndoEye™

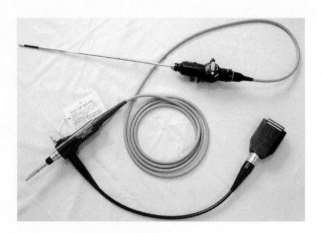

as improving the ergonomics of the operation. The chip-on-tip technology has other significant advantages. The optical device (CCD or CMOS chip), being at the tip of the telescope, is closer to the organ being operated upon and gives the most clarity, and the image is always in focus as the telescope integrates the camera within the tip. Having only a cable carrying the video signal allows the telescope to be smaller in diameter while offering an equivalent image to a larger-dimension rod-lens image. The EndoEye™ (Olympus Medical Systems, Tokyo, Japan) family of video endoscopes was originally developed for conventional laparoscopy but provides an elegant solution to the problems of overcrowding experienced in LESS [14]. The 5-mm rigid EndoEye™ videoscope is available in 30° or 0° depending on the surgery to be performed. The 30° lens allows the assistant to hold the telescope away from the operative field. The real advance in this technology, however, is seen with the EndoEye LTF-VP™ (Olympus Medical Systems, Tokyo, Japan). This is a 5-mm video laparoscope with a flexible tip, which allows the viewing of both 0° and 30° (or more) views without changing the telescope.

Palanivelu and others showed in 2009 that the same flexible endoscopes that gastroenterologists used could be inserted via an umbilical incision or a trocar, for visualization and dissection in a single-incision cholecystectomy [15]. However, they noted that flexible endoscopes had the problems of being floppy and easily movable in the capacious peritoneal cavity and thus provided an unstable surgical platform, one that required multiple operators manipulating the wheels and instruments. The other problem was that there was no effective means of sterilizing these. Current sterilizing devices above 50 °C could damage these scopes. Furthermore, the cable connecting the scopes to the processor was short, making it ergonomically difficult [16]. Cosmesis is one of the primary advantages of LESS procedures. To improve cosmesis, the portal of entry is not always that which would be used during conventional laparoscopy [17, 18]. Operating from a different perspective is always challenging for a surgeon and predicates a steep learning curve. The EndoEye LTF-VP™ is unique in that

Fig. 3.3 Flexible-tip
EndoEye™

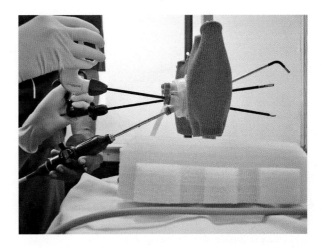

it allows the assistant to place the telescope in such a manner that allows the surgeon to get a more conventional view of the operative field, while at the same time placing the telescope away from the operating instruments (Fig. 3.3). The assistant holding the camera can also use the four-way deflection at the tip to offer the surgeon appropriate views of the structure being dissected. The regular use of a flexible-tip endoscope is one of the advances afforded by the development of LESS.

Modified Scopes and Light Guides

Standard laparoscopic scopes are 30 cm in length; this length has served surgical purposes in the past. Advances in the development of bariatric surgery have led to the development of longer scopes that are anywhere between 42 and 55/56 cm in length (Fig. 3.4). Newer technology and better lens systems ensure that even longer and thinner scopes end up giving better resolution and light than the thicker and shorter scopes available in the past. This has two advantages. Using a thinner, 5-mm scope that would give the same vision as a 10-mm scope in the past leaves extra space in the access device for more instruments. Using a longer scope ensures that the bulky camera head does not clash with the instrument handles at the port of entry. Having the assistant holding the camera while sitting down also alters the axis of the telescope and camera head from the point of maximum clashing at the point of entry of the access device or the single incision. Right-angled adapters applied at the insertion of the light guide can also mimic a coaxial light cable although they are not as ergonomic. They do, however, prevent damage to the light cable (Fig. 3.5).

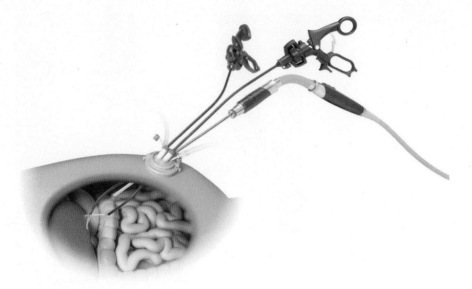

Fig. 3.4 The gooseneck telescope

Operative Laparoscope

Gynecologists have been doing single-port surgery for a long time. They have traditionally used the single-puncture operative laparoscope with a working channel for tubal ligations and ovarian cyst punctures (Fig. 3.6). Kawahara et al. successfully used the operating laparoscope to do one-trocar laparoscopy-aided gastrostomy in children in 2006 [19]. More recently, Khosla and Ponsky revisited this forgotten tool and used the prototype Frazee operative laparoscope (Karl Storz, Tuttlingen, Germany) for a series of successful single-incision surgeries in children [20]. The scope is a 6° 8-mm 30-cm scope with a 5-mm working channel that accommodates a standard laparoscopic 36-cm instrument. They noted that shorter laparoscopes with longer instruments going through the working channel would be ideal for such cases.

Newer Optics

Some newer scopes that were designed for other uses may also offer certain advantages to suit this technique. One such scope is the EndoCAMeleon™ (Karl Storz, Tuttlingen, Germany), which allows the user to change between a 0° and 120° viewing angle, allowing for an enhanced view from a single entry point. This also negates the necessity of scope changes or turning of the scope, which may be difficult in single-incision surgery. It also comes in a longer length of 42 cm, which could reduce clashing in LESS [21].

Fig. 3.5 Right-angled light guide adapter (Courtesy of Karl Storz, Tuttlingen, Germany)

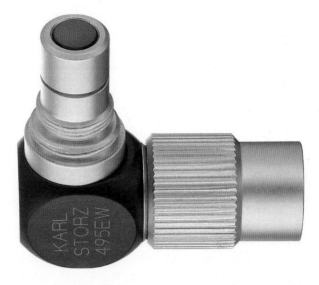

Fig. 3.6 Single-puncture operative laparoscope (Courtesy of Karl Storz, Tuttlingen, Germany)

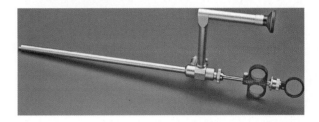

In vitro studies have shown in the past that 3D vision enhances the operative efficiency on Endotrainer models [22]. Robotic systems have used this to great advantage as in the Da Vinci® system (Intuitive Surgical, Sunnyvale, CA), and this 3D vision has been found to be advantageous in complex urological procedures [23]. With the development of new 3D optics as in the Einstein Vision System™ (Scholly Fiberoptic, Denzlingen, Germany), the advantage that the robotic systems had in terms of visualization may now be used in standard laparoscopic procedures. It remains to be seen whether this will make an impact on visualization in standard laparoscopy and by extension in LESS [24].

Visualization and NOTES

The quest for the Holy Grail of scarless surgery led to inroads into surgery through natural orifices of the vagina, mouth, and anus. Buess showed as early as 1988 that transanal surgery, a form of natural orifice surgery (NOS), was feasible using a special 40-cm stereoscopic telescope and standard operating techniques after gas dilatation of the rectum [25, 26]. This could then be extrapolated to transluminal access through the same entry point. Buess used a rigid transanal endoscopic microsurgery (TEM) device. Tremendous advances have been made in recent years addressing the key obstacles to safe performance and the introduction of human natural orifice translumenal endoscopic surgery (NOTES). These transvaginal, transgastric, and transrectal surgeries, though largely experimental, have been used successfully in human models [27–30].

Animal studies have focused on identifying optimal solutions to the obstacles, in particular, methods of creating translumenal access, safe closure of the point of access, and the development of a multitasking platform with dedicated instruments. The NOTES white paper released in 2005 stated that a number of key issues had to be overcome before NOTES could be fully implemented in human subjects [31].

NOTES has been traditionally done by endoscopists and surgeons working together, using a regular or modified flexible endoscope. The problem for surgeons has been getting used to an endoscopic image during surgery. The rigid rod-lens system used for laparoscopy gives an excellent depth of vision and a 10-mm scope gives about 380 lm. Conversely, a standard endoscope with 3-mm fiber bundles gives about 25 lm. Though the endoscopic magnification is better, it is excellent for near vision but lacks the distant visualization for abdominal explorations and complex surgeries. Surgeons are also used to a fixed horizon, while an endoscope provides a flexible, inverted, and rotating platform, which gastroenterologists have become accustomed to in the narrow bowel lumen [32]. Furthermore, in most cases, the odd angle of insertion through the natural orifice ensures that the endoscope is not necessarily in line with the organ of interest, and the endoscope has to be retroflexed for proper visualization. To avoid the limited maneuverability of a retroflexed endoscope, one will need to consider the access organ and the effect on the in-line position of the endoscope. Theoretically, the transgastric approach should facilitate in-line positioning of the endoscope to pelvic organs, while the transrectal, transvaginal, and transvesical routes provide good forward views of the upper abdominal structures. In an in vivo study by Voermans et al. involving 12 swine, transgastric peritoneoscopy was found to be inferior to laparoscopy in detecting simulated peritoneal metastasis, in particular for those located in the liver [33]. In another study, they also found that both transgastric and transcolonic routes provided similar degrees of visualization and access efficacy to the liver and the peritoneal cavity [34]. More studies are required to determine the best access route for performing a particular abdominal NOTES procedure, and it is likely that the preference is governed by the nature of the procedures.

Since in NOTES the optical and operating platform is built into a single flexible endoscope, it is generally agreed that a multitasking flexible endoscope-based platform designated for NOTES is essential for replication of complex laparoscopic surgical maneuvers, including dissection and suturing. This has spurred the development of a number of different platforms, including the EndoSAMURAI™ (Olympus Corp., Tokyo, Japan), the Anubis® (Karl Storz, Tuttlingen, Germany), the Direct Drive Endoscopic System (DDES) (Boston Scientific, Boston, MA), and the

TransPort™ Multi-lumen Operating Platform (USGI Medical, San Clemente, CA) [35–37]. The aim of these platforms is to provide a flexible, yet stable, system through which NOTES procedures can be performed universally through any of the transluminal approaches. Furthermore, these systems should provide a stable image of the operating field comparable to that in laparoscopic surgery and be independent of the movements of the working arms. More importantly, ergonomic user interfaces are available to control the movements of the arms (some of them are capable of up to five degrees of freedom). In a benchtop simulation setting, both the EndoSAMURAI and the DDES have been shown to significantly enhance performance times and accuracy in complex surgical tasks compared to using the double-channeled endoscope [35, 36]. Twelve participants, who included experienced surgeons, medical students, and research assistants, were able to complete a suture using the EndoSAMURAI. The DDES was also shown to allow the performance of complex tasks, such as cutting, grasping, suturing, and knot tying [37]. An added advantage of DDES is that it can be operated by a single operator. Performance data of the other multitasking platforms, however, are still lacking, and outcomes from human studies are still awaited.

It stands to reason that if one cannot see well, one cannot operate well. Endoscopic surgery is technology-intensive in that one relies on a lot of equipment, including cameras, telescopes, light sources, and fiber optics to convey in two dimensions what would have been seen in three dimensions by the naked eye in open surgery. Hence, optics is the most important aspect of laparoscopic and endoscopic surgery and is even more significant when the working hand clashes with the optics as in single-point entry procedures. This has the double jeopardy of compromising vision and the finesse of hand movements at the same time, threatening to destabilize the entire surgical platform. Pioneering work with access devices and innovative thinking led to the development and usage of modified instruments and optics to facilitate these procedures [13]. Luckily, industry has kept pace with the developments of LESS, and the surgeon now has a wide array of different options to facilitate visualization during these procedures. Future development of robotics and 3D optics and their application to LESS procedures may ease these even further [24]. NOTES still remains largely experimental or within the ambit of certain clinical trials due to its inherent problems, and industry has yet to come up with ideal optics and instrumentation [38, 39].

References

1. Walker KM. Transurethral resection of the prostate. Br Med J. 1937;1(3982):901–3.
2. Reynolds Jr W. The first laparoscopic cholecystectomy. JSLS. 2001;5(1):89–94.
3. Cuschieri A. Visual displays and visual perception in minimal access surgery. Semin Laparosc Surg. 1995;2(3):209–14.
4. Marohn MR, Hanly EJ. Twenty-first century surgery using twenty-first century technology: surgical robotics. Curr Surg. 2004;61(5):466–73.
5. Rao GV, Reddy DN, Banerjee R. NOTES: human experience. Gastrointest Endosc Clin N Am. 2008;18(2):361–70; x.

6. Kalloo AN, Singh VK, Jagannath SB, et al. Flexible transgastric peritoneoscopy: a novel approach to diagnostic and therapeutic interventions in the peritoneal cavity. Gastrointest Endosc. 2004;60(1):114–7.

7. Rane A, Rao P. Single-port-access nephrectomy and other laparoscopic urologic procedures using a novel laparoscopic port (R-Port). Urology. 2008;72(2):260–3; discussion 263–4.

8. Rattner D, Kalloo A. ASGE/SAGES Working Group on natural orifice translumenal endoscopic surgery. October 2005. Surg Endosc. 2006;20(2):329–33.

9. Gill IS, Advincula AP, Aron M, et al. Consensus statement of the consortium for laparoendoscopic single-site surgery. Surg Endosc. 2010;24(4):762–8.

10. Desai MM, Stein R, Rao P, et al. Embryonic natural orifice transumbilical endoscopic surgery (E-NOTES) for advanced reconstruction: initial experience. Urology. 2009;73(1):182–7.

11. Raman JD, Bensalah K, Bagrodia A, Stern JM, Cadeddu JA. Laboratory and clinical development of single keyhole umbilical nephrectomy. Urology. 2007;70(6):1039–42.

12. Hanna GB, Shimi S, Cuschieri A. Optimal port locations for endoscopic intracorporeal knotting. Surg Endosc. 1997;11(4):397–401.

13. Rao PP, Bhagwat SM, Rane A. The feasibility of single port laparoscopic cholecystectomy: a pilot study of 20 cases. HPB (Oxford). 2008;10(5):336–40.

14. Rane A, Kommu S, Eddy B, et al. Clinical evaluation of a novel laparoscopic port (R-Port) and evolution of the single laparoscopic port procedure (SLiPP). J Endourol. 2007;21 Suppl 1:A22–3.

15. Palanivelu C, Rajan PS, Rangarajan M, et al. Transumbilical endoscopic appendectomy in humans: on the road to NOTES: a prospective study. J Laparoendosc Adv Surg Tech A. 2008;18(4):579–82.

16. Binenbaum SJ, Teixeira JA, Forrester GJ, et al. Single-incision laparoscopic cholecystectomy using a flexible endoscope. Arch Surg. 2009;144(8):734–8.

17. Desai MM, Rao PP, Aron M, et al. Scarless single port transumbilical nephrectomy and pyeloplasty: first clinical report. BJU Int. 2008;101(1):83–8.

18. Andonian S, Herati AS, Atalla MA, et al. Laparoendoscopic single-site Pfannenstiel donor nephrectomy. Urology. 2010;75(1):9–12.

19. Kawahara H, Kubota A, Okuyama H, et al. One-trocar laparoscopy-aided gastrostomy in handicapped children. J Pediatr Surg. 2006;41(12):2076–80.

20. Khosla A, Ponsky TA. Use of operative laparoscopes in single-port surgery: the forgotten tool. J Minim Access Surg. 2011;7(1):116–20.

21. Eskef K, Oehmke F, Tchartchian G, et al. A new variable-view rigid endoscope evaluated in advanced gynecologic laparoscopy: a pilot study. Surg Endosc. 2011;25(10):3260–5.

22. Tevaearai HT, Mueller XM, von Segesser LK. 3-D vision improves performance in a pelvic trainer. Endoscopy. 2000;32(6):464–8.

23. Iselin C, Fateri F, Caviezel A, et al. Usefulness of the Da Vinci robot in urologic surgery. Rev Med Suisse. 2007;3(136):2766–8, 2770, 2772.

24. Spana G, Rane A, Kaouk JH. Is robotics the future of laparoendoscopic single-site surgery (LESS)? BJU Int. 2011;108(6 Pt 2):1018–23.

25. Buess G, Kipfmuller K, Hack D, et al. Technique of transanal endoscopic microsurgery. Surg Endosc. 1988;2(2):71–5.

26. Buess G, Mentges B, Manncke K, et al. Technique and results of transanal endoscopic microsurgery in early rectal cancer. Am J Surg. 1992;163(1):63–9; discussion 69–70.

27. Hagen ME, Wagner OJ, Swain P, et al. Hybrid natural orifice transluminal endoscopic surgery (NOTES) for Roux-en-Y gastric bypass: an experimental surgical study in human cadavers. Endoscopy. 2008;40(11):918–24.

28. Auyang ED, Hungness ES, Vaziri K, et al. Human NOTES cholecystectomy: transgastric hybrid technique. J Gastrointest Surg. 2009;13(6):1149–50.

29. Moreira-Pinto J, Lima E, Correia-Pinto J, Rolanda C. Natural orifice transluminal endoscopy surgery: a review. World J Gastroenterol. 2011;17(33):3795–801.

30. Palanivelu C, Rajan PS, Rangarajan M, et al. NOTES: transvaginal endoscopic cholecystec-
    tomy in humans—preliminary report of a case series. Am J Gastroenterol. 2009;104(4):
    843–7.
31. ASGE/SAGES Working Group on natural orifice translumenal endoscopic surgery white
    paper, October 2005. Gastrointest Endosc. 2006;63(2):199–203.
32. Shaikh SN, Thompson CC. Natural orifice translumenal surgery: flexible platform review.
    World J Gastrointest Surg. 2010;2(6):210–6.
33. Voermans RP, Faigel DO, van Berge Henegouwen MI, et al. Comparison of transcolonic
    NOTES and laparoscopic peritoneoscopy for the detection of peritoneal metastases. Endoscopy.
    2010;42(11):904–9.
34. Voermans RP, van Berge Henegouwen MI, Bemelman WA, Fockens P. Feasibility of transgas-
    tric and transcolonic natural orifice transluminal endoscopic surgery peritoneoscopy combined
    with intraperitoneal EUS. Gastrointest Endosc. 2009;69(7):e61–7.
35. Spaun GO, Zheng B, Swanstrom LL. A multitasking platform for natural orifice translumenal
    endoscopic surgery (NOTES): a benchtop comparison of a new device for flexible endoscopic
    surgery and a standard dual-channel endoscope. Surg Endosc. 2009;23(12):2720–7.
36. Spaun GO, Zheng B, Martinec DV, et al. Bimanual coordination in natural orifice transluminal
    endoscopic surgery: comparing the conventional dual-channel endoscope, the R-Scope, and a
    novel direct-drive system. Gastrointest Endosc. 2009;69(6):e39–45.
37. Thompson CC, Ryou M, Soper NJ, et al. Evaluation of a manually driven, multitasking plat-
    form for complex endoluminal and natural orifice transluminal endoscopic surgery applica-
    tions (with video). Gastrointest Endosc. 2009;70(1):121–5.
38. Rao PP, Bhagwat S. Single-incision laparoscopic surgery—current status and controversies.
    J Minim Access Surg. 2011;7(1):6–16.
39. Flora ED, Wilson TG, Martin IJ, et al. A review of natural orifice translumenal endoscopic
    surgery (NOTES) for intra-abdominal surgery: experimental models, techniques, and applica-
    bility to the clinical setting. Ann Surg. 2008;247(4):583–602.

Chapter 4
LESS: Ports and Instrumentation

Michael A. White and Robert J. Stein

Keywords Laparoendoscopic single-site • Single port • Port • Robotic • Natural orifice • NOTES • LESS • Laparoscopic

Introduction

A new era in medicine, minimally invasive surgery, has been initiated since the implementation of laparoscopy. As this field evolves, so does the push to further reduce the invasiveness of laparoscopic surgery. To achieve this goal, surgeons have begun limiting the number of abdominal incisions with laparoendoscopic single-site surgery (LESS) or eliminating them completely through natural orifice translu-menal endoscopic surgery (NOTES) [1]. The latter has been demonstrated primarily in preclinical animal models with limited clinical experience [2–6], while LESS has undergone laboratory and clinical work and has proven to be feasible and applicable for human intervention [7–12].

LESS has been documented in the literature since 1997 for various specialties, including general surgery and gynecology [13, 14]. Limitations in technology at the time of its introduction severely limited its permeation throughout clinical practice.

M.A. White, DO, FACOS
205 Corolwood Dr, San Antonio, TX 78213, USA

Center for Robotic and Image-Guided Surgery,
Glickman Urological and Kidney Institute, Cleveland Clinic,
Q10, 9500 Euclid Avenue, Cleveland, OH 44195, USA
e-mail: mikeawhite@sbcglobal.net

R.J. Stein, M.D. (✉)
Center for Robotic and Image-Guided Surgery,
Glickman Urological and Kidney Institute, Cleveland Clinic,
Q10, 9500 Euclid Avenue, Cleveland, OH 44195, USA
e-mail: steinr@ccf.org

A. Rane et al. (eds.), *Scar-Less Surgery*,
DOI 10.1007/978-1-84800-360-6_4, © Springer-Verlag London 2013

Current innovations such as articulating instrumentation and novel multilumen ports have fostered a renaissance for LESS, with several recent clinical series reporting successful completion of a range of procedures [8–12]. The proposed benefits of LESS include improved cosmesis and reduced postoperative pain.

Ports

LESS is essentially laparoscopic surgery performed through a small incision at a single site. These procedures are commonly performed via a commercially made single port or through a single incision with multiple trocars. Additionally, standard trocars can be added adjacent to the commercially available single ports (Table 4.1) through the same skin incision but into a separate fascial stab. This is particularly helpful during robotic laparoendoscopic single-site surgery (R-LESS). There are several single-port devices available, each with its own advantages and disadvantages.

Multiple-Trocar Configuration

Piskun et al. were the first to report utilizing multiple trocars through a single transumbilical incision to perform a cholecystectomy [13]. Two separate 5-mm trocars were placed through an intraumbilical incision via two separate fascial stab incisions. The procedure was performed and the specimen extracted after the fasciotomies were joined, leaving a virtually scar-free appearance. Utilizing a similar approach, Raman et al. was able to complete two of three nephrectomies without adding additional trocars and found "the single trocar to be more cumbersome with fewer degrees of freedom than 3 adjacent trocars" [7]. While the above examples were performed with traditional 5-mm trocars, purpose-built low-profile kits are now available; see the discussion that follows.

AnchorPort™

AnchorPort™ (Surgiquest, Orange, CT) consists of a small and low-profile housing that allows three 5-mm cannulae to be placed close together. The ports contain an internal anchor that prevents the port from dislodging, and optical entry can be used not just on the first entry, but on all entries.

Multichannel Laparoscopic Ports

In an attempt to reduce abdominal wall trauma, multichannel laparoscopic ports were designed. These ports are placed through a single skin and fascial incision via an open (Hasson) technique primarily through the umbilicus.

Table 4.1 Available single-port devices

Access device	Features	Advantages	Disadvantages
TriPort™ advanced surgical concepts	Flexible multichannel valve; up to three instruments (1 × 12 mm; 2 × 5 mm); covered with an elastomer	Adapts to incision and abdominal wall thickness	Fragile when using 12-mm instruments; lubrication required; constrictive outer ring; gas leaking
QuadPort™ advanced surgical concepts	Flexible multichannel valve; up to four usable instruments (1 × 15 mm, 1 × 10 mm, 2 × 5 mm); covered with an elastomer	Adapts to incision and abdominal wall thickness	Fragile when using 12-mm instruments; lubrication required; constrictive outer ring; gas leaking
SILS™ Port Covidien	Flexible platform; up to three individual ports and instruments	Easy exchange of different size ports	Difficult to use with large abdominal wall
GelPOINT™ applied medical	Three components: GelSeal™ providing PseudoAbdomen™ platform; Alexis™ wound retractor; self-retaining trocars	Larger outer working profile for enhanced triangulation; adapts to incision and abdominal wall thickness	Fragile; gas leakage during prolonged procedures
AirSeal™ Surgiquest	Oval valve-less cannula with invisible pressure seal	Stable CO_2 pressure; multiple instrument insertion	Rigid; less freedom of movement; noisy
AnchorPort™ Surgiquest	Low-profile ports of various lengths placed in close proximity	Anchoring system; optical entry	Rigid; less freedom of movement
Homemade	Alexis™ wound retractor, latex glove, variable ports	Inexpensive, larger outer working profile for enhanced triangulation; adapts to incision and abdominal wall thickness	Must be built for each case
OctoPort™ DalimSurg	Wound retractor, three flexible caps, three cannulas, two channels for insufflation and smoke evacuation	Adapts to incision and abdominal wall thickness; multiple caps allow tailoring of procedure	Fragile when using 12-mm instruments; lubrication required; constrictive outer ring; gas leaking
SSL access system	Wound retractor, 360° rotation of the seal cap, three entry points, insufflation channel	Quick reorientation of instruments during procedures, reduced need for instrument exchanges	Rigid; less freedom of movement
X-Cone™ Storz	Two-piece design, flexible cap, three cannulas	Reusable; easy to place	Gas leakage from cap; the two pieces disengage

R-Port®/TriPort™/QuadPort™

The TriPort and QuadPort (Advanced Surgical Concepts, Wicklow, Ireland) represent an evolution of the R-Port and have been reported in LESS [8, 10, 12, 15–24]. The device consists of a wound protector and a valve. The valve component incorporates three or four inlets for the introduction of instruments. The three-inlet valve (TriPort) has one portal for a 12-mm instrument and two for 5-mm instruments. The larger version (QuadPort) has two inlets for 12-mm and two inlets for 5-mm instruments. Advantages include ease of placement even through very small incisions and easy introduction of instruments through the port. Disadvantages include possible tearing and insufflant leakage through the gel material covering the individual channels.

SILS™ Port

The SILS™ Port (Covidien, Cupertino, CA) is a flexible laparoscopic multichannel port that is made of soft foam designed to conform to the contours of the incision. It contains a built-in insufflation valve and three port sites that can accommodate two 5-mm cannulae and a single 12-mm cannula. Advantages include easy placement of ancillary trocars next to the port through a separate fascial stab [25, 26]. Disadvantages include difficult placement of the port through a very small (2-cm or less) incision [25, 26].

GelPort™/GelPOINT™/Alexis™

The GelPort™ (Applied Medical, Rancho Santa Margarita, CA) laparoscopic system combines a GelSeal™ cap with the Alexis™ wound retractor. Designed for hand-assisted laparoscopic procedures, the GelPort™ has been used during LESS and R-LESS procedures [27–29]. The GelPOINT™ (Applied Medical) represents the evolution of the GelPort™ and is designed specifically for LESS. It has a smaller gel cap and four premade self-retaining 5-mm trocars, though various-sized trocars can be placed similarly to the GelPort. Additionally, there is an insufflation port built into the side of the device, and the Alexis wound retractor is fitted with a tether for easier removal. Advantages include flexibility of port size and positioning through the GelCap as well as full utilization of larger incisions. Disadvantages include difficulty introducing instruments and tearing of the wound protector, which has largely been temporized with the development of a new instrument shield on the advanced access platform.

AirSeal™

AirSeal™ (Surgiquest, Orange, CT) is a technology that recirculates and filters peritoneal gas. There are no valves or gaskets required, so multiple instruments and a camera can be inserted without a reduction in pneumoperitoneum. At the time of this writing, only prototypes specifically designed for LESS use have been developed.

OCTO-Port™

The OCTO-Port™ (dalimSurgNET Corp., Seoul, South Korea) consists of an abdominal wall retractor that varies in size from 1 to 5 cm. Two configurations are available for single-site surgery, including a cap with two 10/12-mm cannulas and a single 5-mm cannula and a cap with one 10/12-mm cannula and two 5-mm cannulas. The cannulas are different heights to prevent external clashing, and the cap is flexible to allow for an improved range of motion.

Ethicon Endo-Surgery SSL Access System

The SSL Access System (Ethicon Endosurgery, Inc., Johnson and Johnson, Cincinnati, OH) is a single-port access device that consists of a wound retractor and a cap that has two 5-mm seals and a larger 15-mm seal in a low-profile design. Insufflation is achieved through an additional channel on the cap. The internal profile of the device is minimal because trocars are not required. The device is able to rotate 360° at the seal cap, enabling quick reorientation of instruments during procedures and reducing the need for instrument exchange.

X-Cone™

The X-Cone (Karl Storz Endoscopy America, El Segundo, CA) is a reusable access device for transumbilical laparoscopy that consists of a plastic, but flexible, cap with three channels that attach to a two-piece metal device. The device contains three working channels that permit the introduction of instruments up to 12.5 mm in size. Introduction is via a Hasson technique in two pieces that then easily assemble.

Homemade Single-Port Device

Commercially produced multichannel laparoscopic ports are not available worldwide and have pushed surgeons to create their own access devices [30–33]. The most widely reported of these devices consist of the Alexis™ wound retractor, a sterile surgical glove, and standard laparoscopic ports. The size seven surgical glove is attached to the wound retractor and three or four of the fingertips are removed so the cannulas can be inserted and tied in place. Insufflation is performed through the previously placed ports.

Multichannel Hybrid Laparoscopic Ports

The multichannel hybrid laparoscopic port has been conceived as much from natural orifice translumenal endoscopic surgery (NOTES) as it has from LESS. It is a complete system that behaves more as a surgical platform than a port alone. The multichannel hybrid laparoscopic ports require specialized instruments (flexible gastroscope, etc.) and are placed through a single skin and fascial incision using the Hasson technique.

SPIDER™

The SPIDER™ (Trans Enterix, Inc., Durham, NC) is designed to allow multiple surgical instruments to be advanced and manipulated through a single port. It consists of an insertion trocar and retractable sheath that guides the distal end into the abdominal cavity. There are four working channels (two rigid and two flexible). The two flexible channels, known as IDTs (instrument delivery tubes), facilitate motion to allow for a multidirectional and triangulated approach within the surgical field. Crossing of instruments is not necessary, and therefore the left hand controls the left instrument and vice versa with the right hand. Two rigid channels positioned vertically to the operative field accommodate the use of a scope and any other rigid surgical instrument. Three pneumoperitoneum ports exist to maintain pneumoperitoneum and facilitate insufflation and/or smoke evacuation. The SPIDER flexible instruments include wavy or fenestrated graspers, Maryland dissector, Hem-o-lock clip applier, shears, monopolar hook, and suction irrigator. There is a docking ball that attaches the device to the stabilizer and subsequently to the operating table.

TransPort™

The TransPort™ (USGI Medical, San Clemente, CA) provides stable access to the operating site via one of the body's natural orifices or an incision in the umbilicus. The TransPort has four large working channels, one for an endoscope and three others for large-diameter instruments. This device creates a multitasking platform and utilizes a flexible endoscope along with multiple flexible endoscopic instruments.

Laparoscopic Instrumentation

During LESS the laparoscopic instruments and the camera lens are in close proximity, resulting in intracorporeal instrument collision, hindering the surgeon from operating ergonomically. To minimize clashing, specifically designed instruments have been created, including instruments that are prebent and ones that articulate.

Prebent Instruments

In an attempt to improve ergonomics and reduce external crowding of instrumentation around the access site, prebent instruments (Olympus, Hamburg, Germany; Karl Storz, Tuttlingen, Germany) have been designed and are available. These instruments allow for triangulation and reduce internal and external clashing. When compared to flexible instrumentation in the laboratory setting, prebent instruments were less time-consuming and were found to have better maneuverability [34, 35].

Flexible Instruments

Autonomy Laparo-Angle™

The Autonomy series (Cambridge Endo, Framingham, MA) allows for seven degrees of freedom, full articulation, and a handle that locks at any angle and rotates. Additionally, the instrument tip can rotate 360° around its axis, thereby allowing simultaneous actions such as articulating downward while rotating. There are various instruments available, including Metzenbaum scissors, a Maryland dissector, monopolar hook cautery, and needle holders.

Real Hand™

Real Hand (Novare Surgical Systems, Cupertino, CA) instruments were designed with an EndoLink® mechanism, which affords seven degrees of freedom of movement. The full line of instruments includes a bipolar coagulator, various graspers, dissectors, and needle drivers. All have a locking mechanism that allows for use as a straight or up to 90° angulated instrument.

Roticulator™ Articulating Instruments

The Roticulator line of instruments (Covidien, Cupertino, CA) includes a grasper, shears, and dissector. The Roticulator offers 0–80° of articulation, 360° rotation at all articulation angles, spin-lock rotation position lock, ability to perform as a fully rigid straight instrument, and a diameter of 5 mm.

Standard Laparoscopic Instruments

Conventional laparoscopic instruments can effectively be used with a LESS approach. After surpassing a learning curve largely involved with minimizing clashing, many surgeons have noted that the use of standard instrumentation is feasible and not prohibitive. Advantages include significant cost savings, as articulating instruments tend to be single-use.

NOTES Instrumentation

Despite the fact that the concept of NOTES predates LESS, clinical experience in NOTES has lagged significantly. Reasons for this deliberate progress include considerations of safety as well as greater reliance on more complex instrumentation and technology. A large body of literature as well as industry support is dedicated to the development and description of concept and prototype equipment. Herein we aim to describe instrumentation that has been used clinically.

Flexible Instrumentation

Several clinical reports of hybrid and pure NOTES procedures have appeared in the literature and will be detailed further in other chapters of this book. The majority of initial work centered around the use of flexible instrumentation introduced through endoscopes, primarily gastroscopes. As these scopes were primarily designed for basic intraluminal work, only a single working channel was included, largely for instrumentation necessary for performance of biopsies. Due to the simultaneous need for working instrumentation along with an instrument for retraction during NOTES procedures, a dual-channel endoscope (Olympus GIF-2T 160) has preferentially been used.

Access differs based on the natural orifice chosen. Transvaginal access can be gained with direct incision of the vaginal fornix after exposure using a weighted speculum. The majority of reports discuss the use of a transumbilical port and laparoscope to ensure that the peritoneum is suitable in addition to providing guidance for access. A 2–3-mm needlescope can be used for this purpose [36].

Transgastric access requires the use of endoscopic techniques for scope entry. Use of a needle-knife for a full-thickness incision of the gastric wall is followed by balloon dilation over wire guide and, finally, scope entry. An overtube can then be advanced to maintain access. At the time of access, a closure system such as g-Prox® sutures (USGI, San Clemente, CA) can be preplaced for use in closure at the completion of the procedure [37]. The g-Prox instrument has a dual function as a flexible grasper for retraction along with suturing capabilities for delivery of tissue anchors through the g-Cath mechanism.

In terms of closure of the access site, standard open instrumentation and sutures are used for closure under direct vision of transvaginal defects. Transgastric sites, as noted above, can be closed using tissue anchors introduced with the G-prox mechanism or may be sutured using a system such as the OverStitch™ (Apollo Endosurgery, Austin, TX). The OverStitch is a single-use mechanism that is mounted to a dual-channel endoscope and can deliver full-thickness running or interrupted sutures. Despite the availability of these commercial products, thus far sole reliance on these closure mechanisms has not been practiced clinically. The use of standard laparoscopic sutured or stapled closure of the gastric entry site instead has been described due to the need for a reliable gastric closure.

A significant challenge when performing flexible NOTES is the lack of a stable platform. The orientation can often be difficult, and fine control of the endoscope during delicate dissection is ideal. Use of the TransPort™ steerable platform (USGI, San Clemente, CA) allows for fine manipulation of the scope at its distal end while the remainder of the shaft is maintained in a stable position [37]. This platform also includes three additional working channels for introduction of ancillary flexible instrumentation.

Once access is established and the endoscope is introduced into the peritoneum, a variety of flexible equipment can be used through the endoscopic channels, including needle-knife, scissors, a variety of graspers, snares, electrocautery hook, etc. Furthermore, through a transvaginal access, standard laparoscopic instruments or articulating instruments with a rigid shaft can be introduced alongside the endoscope. This may be especially useful to create some additional triangulation as well as more robust retraction.

Horgan et al. described use of an extra-long 75-cm articulating grasper (Novare Surgical Systems, Cupertino, CA), which was introduced transvaginally alongside the operating endoscope [37]. Alternatively, Davila et al. used the simple concept of percutaneously introduced marionette sutures in order to successfully complete a pure NOTES transvaginal cholecystectomy. These sutures are strategically placed percutaneously and then through the organ of interest and finally suspended using a clamp extracorporeally for effective retraction [38].

Rigid Instrumentation

Due to significant challenges in performing NOTES procedures with a classical flexible endoscopic approach, Aron and colleagues introduced the concept of using standard laparoscopic as well as rigid articulating instruments through a single-access device placed transvaginally [39]. Using this approach, the authors were able to perform nephrectomy in three cadavers. Thereafter, using a similar approach, Sotelo and colleagues and Kaouk and colleagues both performed hybrid NOTES nephrectomy [40, 41]. Kaouk et al. then reported the first pure NOTES nephrectomy in humans [42]. The group used the TriPort (Advanced Surgical Concepts, Wicklow, Ireland) as well as the GelPort (Applied Medical, Rancho Santa Margarita, CA) transvaginally. Articulating instruments (Novare Surgical Systems, Cupertino, CA), surgical staplers, as well as an extra-long electrosurgical hook were used for renal dissection. Benefits of the approach with rigid instrumentation include more robust retraction and working instrumentation, which is vital for bulkier organs such as the kidney (see Fig. 4.1).

Fig. 4.1 Illustration of rigid
laparoscopic instrumentation
introduced through a
single-access device in order
to perform NOTES
nephrectomy (Reprinted
with permission, Cleveland
Clinic Center for Medical
Art & Photography © 2011.
All rights reserved)

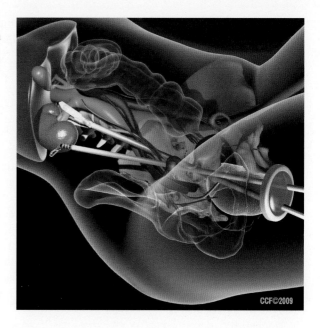

Conclusion

LESS is developing at a rapid pace, and as more surgeons adopt this laparoscopic approach, further refinement in technology will be identified. Significant improvements in the toolbox will likely allow LESS techniques to be disseminated more widely and include more complex procedures. NOTES is progressing at a more deliberate pace due to the considerable demands of access, closure, vantage point, and distance from target organ. Therefore, more substantial technological advancement is necessary in order to make these procedures more reproducible. Computer interface or robotic surgical instruments will likely greatly improve ergonomics and precision.

References

1. Raman JD, Cadeddu JA, Rao P, Rane A. Single-incision laparoscopic surgery: initial urological experience and comparison with natural-orifice transluminal endoscopic surgery. BJU Int. 2008;101:1493–6.
2. Swain P. Nephrectomy and natural orifice translumenal endoscopy (NOTES): transvaginal, transgastric, transrectal, and transvesical approaches. J Endourol. 2008;22:811–8.
3. Gettman MT, Cadeddu JA. Natural orifice translumenal endoscopic surgery (NOTES) in urology: initial experience. J Endourol. 2008;22:783–8.
4. Lima E, Rolanda C, Pêgo JM, et al. Third generation nephrectomy by natural orifice transluminal endoscopic surgery. J Urol. 2007;178:648–54.
5. Gettman MT, Lotan Y, Napper CA, Cadeddu JA. Transvaginal laparoscopic nephrectomy: development and feasibility in the porcine model. Urology. 2002;59:446–50.

6. Kaouk JH, Haber GP, Goel RK, et al. Pure natural orifice translumenal endoscopic surgery (NOTES) transvaginal nephrectomy. Eur Urol. 2009;57:723–6.
7. Raman JD, Bensalah K, Bagrodia A, et al. Laboratory and clinical development of single keyhole umbilical nephrectomy. Urology. 2007;70:1039–42.
8. Rane A, Rao P, Bonadio F, Rao P. Single port laparoscopic nephrectomy using a novel laparoscopic port (R-port) and evolution of single laparoscopic port procedure (SLIPP). J Endourol. 2007;21:A87.
9. White WM, Haber GP, Goel RK, et al. Single-port urological surgery: single-center experience with the first 100 cases. Urology. 2009;74:801–4.
10. Sotelo Noguera RJ, Astigueta JC, Carmona O, et al. Laparoscopic augmentation enterocystoplasty through a single trocar. Urology. 2009;73(6):1371–4.
11. Ponsky LE, Cherullo EE, Sawyer M, et al. Single access site radical nephrectomy: initial clinical experience. J Endourol. 2008;22:663–6.
12. Stolzenburg JU, Kallidonis P, Hellawell G, et al. Technique of laparo-endoscopic single-site surgery radical nephrectomy. Eur Urol. 2009;56:644–50.
13. Piskun G, Rajpal S. Transumbilical laparoscopic cholecystectomy utilizes no incisions outside the umbilicus. J Laparoendosc Adv Surg Tech A. 1999;9:361–4.
14. Ghezzi F, Cromi A, Fasola M, et al. One-trocar salpingectomy for the treatment of tubal pregnancy: a "marionette-like" technique. Br J Obstet Gynaecol. 2005;112:1417–9.
15. Aron M, Canes D, Desai MM, et al. Transumbilical single-port laparoscopic partial nephrectomy. BJU Int. 2008;103:516–21.
16. Gill IS, Canes D, Aron M, et al. Single port transumbilical (E-NOTES) donor nephrectomy. J Urol. 2008;180:637–41.
17. Rane A, Ahmed S, Kommu SS, et al. Single-port "scarless" laparoscopic nephrectomies: the United Kingdom experience. BJU Int. 2009;104:230–3.
18. Ganpule AP, Dhawan DR, Kurien A, et al. Laparoendoscopic single-site donor nephrectomy: a single-center experience. Urology. 2009;74:1238–40.
19. Desai MM, Rao PP, Aron M, et al. Scarless single port transumbilical nephrectomy and pyeloplasty: first clinical report. BJU Int. 2008;101:83–8.
20. Desai MM, Stein R, Rao P, et al. Embryonic natural orifice transumbilical endoscopic surgery (E-NOTES) for advanced reconstruction: initial experience. Urology. 2009;73:182–7.
21. Desai MM, Aron M, Canes D, et al. Single-port transvesical simple prostatectomy: initial clinical report. Urology. 2008;72:960–5.
22. Sotelo RJ, Astigueta JC, Desai MM, et al. Laparoendoscopic single-site surgery simple prostatectomy: initial report. Urology. 2009;74:626–30.
23. Noguera RJ, Astigueta JC, Carmona O, et al. Laparoscopic augmentation enterocystoplasty through a single trocar. Urology. 2009;73:1371–4.
24. White WM, Goel RK, Kaouk JH. Single-port laparoscopic retroperitoneal surgery: initial operative experience and comparative outcomes. Urology. 2009;73(9):1279–82.
25. Saber AA, El-Ghazaly TH, Minnick DB. Single port access transumbilical laparoscopic Roux-en-Y gastric bypass using the SILS Port: first reported case. Surg Innov. 2009;16(4):343–7.
26. Saber AA, El-Ghazaly TH. Early experience with single incision transumbilical laparoscopic adjustable gastric banding using the SILS Port. Int J Surg. 2009;7(5):456–9.
27. Fader AN, Escobar PF. Laparoendoscopic single-site surgery (LESS) in gynecologic oncology: technique and initial report. Gynecol Oncol. 2009;114(2):157–61.
28. Stein RJ, White WM, Goel RK, et al. Robotic laparoendoscopic single-site surgery using GelPort as the access platform. Eur Urol. 2010;57(1):132–6.
29. Ponsky LE, Steinway ML, Lengu IJ, et al. A Pfannenstiel single-site nephrectomy and nephroureterectomy: a practical application of laparoendoscopic single-site surgery. Urology. 2009;74(3):482–5.
30. Park YH, Kang MY, Jeong MS, et al. Laparoendoscopic single-site nephrectomy using a homemade single-port device for single-system ectopic ureter in a child: initial case report. J Endourol. 2009;23:833–5.
31. Ryu DS, Park WJ, Oh TH. Retroperitoneal laparoendoscopic single-site surgery in urology: initial experience. J Endourol. 2009;23:1857–62.

32. Jeong BC, Park YH, Han DH, Kim HH. Laparoendoscopic single-site and conventional lap-aroscopic adrenalectomy: a matched case–control study. J Endourol. 2009;23:1957–60.
33. Han WK, Park YH, Jeon HG, et al. The feasibility of laparoendoscopic single-site nephrec-tomy: initial experience using home-made single-port device. Urology. 2010;76(4):862–5.
34. Andonian S, Herati AS, Atalla MA, et al. Laparoendoscopic single-site Pfannenstiel donor nephrectomy. Urology. 2010;75(1):9–12.
35. Stolzenburg JU, Kallidonis P, Oh MA, et al. Comparative assessment of laparoscopic single-site surgery instruments to conventional laparoscopic in laboratory setting. J Endourol. 2010;24(2):239–45.
36. Palanivelu C, Rajan PS, Rangarajan M, et al. NOTES: transvaginal endoscopic cholecystec-tomy in humans—preliminary report of a case series. Am J Gastroenterol. 2009;104(4): 843–7.
37. Horgan S, Cullen JP, Talamini MA, et al. Natural orifice surgery: initial clinical experience. Surg Endosc. 2009;23(7):1512–8.
38. Davila F, Tsin DA, Dominguez G, et al. Transvaginal cholecystectomy without abdominal ports. JSLS. 2009;13(2):213–6.
39. Aron M, Berger AK, Stein RJ, et al. Transvaginal nephrectomy with a multichannel laparo-scopic port: a cadaver study. BJU Int. 2009;103(11):1537–41.
40. Sotelo R, de Andrade R, Fernández G, et al. NOTES hybrid transvaginal radical nephrectomy for tumor: stepwise progression toward a first successful clinical case. Eur Urol. 2010;57(1): 138–44.
41. Kaouk JH, White WM, Goel RK, et al. NOTES transvaginal nephrectomy: first human experi-ence. Urology. 2009;74(1):5–8.
42. Kaouk JH, Haber GP, Goel RK, et al. Pure natural orifice translumenal endoscopic surgery (NOTES) transvaginal nephrectomy. Eur Urol. 2010;57(4):723–6.

Chapter 5
Retraction Systems in Single-Incision Laparoscopic Surgery and NOTES

Melanie L. Hafford and Daniel J. Scott

Keywords Retraction systems • Single-incision laparoscopic surgery • Natural orifice transluminal endoscopic surgery • Magnetic anchoring guidance system Laparoscopic liver retraction • Endograb • Endolift • Suture retraction • Magnetic retraction systems

Introduction

As minimally invasive surgery techniques evolve to include methods such as single-incision laparoscopic surgery (SILS) and natural orifice translumenal endoscopic surgery (NOTES), a major challenge has been maintaining surgical exposure through limited incisions in which instruments are introduced within the same axis. One of the basic tenets of laparoscopic surgery is triangulation. This allows for maximal exposure of the surgical field and the optimal retraction required for tissue dissection. Difficulties adhering to these principles secondary to instruments entering the abdomen through a common port, and therefore a parallel alignment, have led to the development of several novel retraction systems. These systems provide the necessary exposure to safely perform the operation. The Natural Orifice Surgery Consortium for Assessment and Research (NOSCAR) was developed to address potential barriers to adoption of NOTES into clinical practice, one of which was

M.L. Hafford, M.D. (✉)
Department of Surgery, University of Texas Southwestern,
5323 Harry Hines Blvd, Dallas, TX 75390, USA
e-mail: mhaffordmd@gmail.com

D.J. Scott, M.D., FACS
Department of Surgery, University of Texas Southwestern,
5323 Harry Hines Blvd, Dallas, TX 75390, USA
e-mail: daniel.scott@utsouthwestern.edu

A. Rane et al. (eds.), *Scar-Less Surgery*,
DOI 10.1007/978-1-84800-360-6_5, © Springer-Verlag London 2013

49

Table 5.1 Comparison of retraction methods for SILS cholecystectomy

	Bile spillage	Supracostal retraction	Technical difficulty	Risk of adjacent organ injury	Expense
Percutaneous suture	+	−	+	+	−
Intracorporeal suture	+	+	++	−	−
Endoloop	−	−	−	−	+
Endograb™ (virtual ports)	−	+	−	−	++

found to be challenges with spatial orientation [1]. The subsequent NOSCAR white paper states that the incorporation of conventional laparoscopic principles, such as triangulation, may be necessary for safe NOTES operations [1]. The Laparoendoscopic Single Site Surgery Consortium for Assessment and Research (LESSCAR) released a consensus statement and identified similar challenges for retraction during SILS procedures [2]. Hence, much work has been done to develop retraction systems in this environment as well. The purpose of this chapter is to review established and developing innovations in retraction systems for SILS and NOTES procedures.

Retraction Systems in Cholecystectomy

Laparoscopic cholecystectomy is one of the most basic and commonly performed laparoscopic operations. Much of the work reported to date using novel retraction methods of the gallbladder during cholecystectomy have been during SILS procedures. In 1997 Navarra et al. first described a SILS cholecystectomy using transabdominal stay sutures to allow for gallbladder retraction [3]. A suture on a Keith or straight needle is introduced through the working trocar. The suture is passed through the gallbladder fundus and secured to the gallbladder by passing the needle through a loop tied on the end of the suture, cinching the loop down onto the tissue. The needle may then be passed through the abdominal wall subcostally, and the suture is secured externally using a clamp. Additional individual sutures are then placed in the same fashion through the gallbladder body and infundibulum to progressively gain suitable exposure. Whereas the upper fundic and body sutures serve to elevate the gallbladder, the infundibular suture(s) serve to lateralize the lower gallbladder and expand the triangle of Calot. The materials for this approach result in negligible costs, and numerous investigators have reported the use of this technique with good results [4–7].

However, there are several potential drawbacks (Table 5.1). With the lower sutures lateralizing the triangle of Calot, it may be difficult to dissect the attachments on the right side of the gallbladder; thus, it may be helpful to perform an initial dissection on this side prior to placement of the fundic suture. Bile spillage may occur due to penetration of the gallbladder by the needle, but in our experience the volume of bile spilled has been minimal and of no clinical significance. There is inherently some limitation in cephalad retraction of the gallbladder, as most surgeons are only comfortable externalizing the fundic retraction suture below the costal margin to avoid any risk of pneumothorax. Accordingly, this tissue is not retracted to the same cephalad extent as would be conventionally achieved using a rigid laparoscopic grasper. In some cases, complete exposure of Calot's triangle may be difficult to achieve, especially when very large, redundant gallbladders are encountered. Using several sutures to elevate the gallbladder progressively may overcome this problem. There is also the potential risk of bleeding from piercing abdominal wall blood vessels during passage of the needle externally, though this risk is minimal. While this technique is simple, reproducible, and can be taught relatively easily, advanced laparoscopic skills are required. Specifically, the Keith needle is 6 cm in length and may be particularly awkward to manipulate, especially given the parallel orientation of the instruments in the SILS environment and when instrument conflicts are encountered. Hence, care must be taken to avoid injuries to adjacent organs related to the use of this needle type.

It may also be cumbersome to pass the needle outside the abdominal cavity, so the needle transverses through a loop on the end of the suture, fixating the suture to the gallbladder. One alternative is to use the small rubber plunger from a 1-cc TB syringe [7] (Fig. 5.1). This plunger may be tied to the end of the suture prior to insertion of the needle into the abdominal cavity. The needle can then penetrate the gallbladder and be retrieved externally, and, when pulled tight, the plunger serves to anchor the suture against the gallbladder. While this technique is quite effective and obviates the time associated with needle passes through a trocar, the usage of the plunger may introduce concerns over a foreign body being retained inside the abdomen should the suture break or if the plunger somehow becomes dislodged. Hence, we might recommend the use of pledgets for this purpose, as they have been used for many years as adjuncts to suturing in the abdomen for surgical procedures.

One modification of the suture retraction technique involves the addition of endoclips on each side of the suture to allow for additional external control in a "puppeteering" fashion, as described by Rawlings et al. [8]. For this technique, a prolene suture on a Keith needle is passed through the gallbladder fundus and then through the abdominal wall in the midclavicular line, allowing for cephalad retraction. A second suture was placed in a similar fashion through the infundibulum and exteriorized in the right mid-axillary line. Endoclips were then placed on the infundibulum suture on each side of the gallbladder. This technique essentially allows the lower gallbladder to be retracted either laterally or medially, such that both sides of Calot's triangle may be exposed.

Intracorporeal suture retraction has also been described, which eliminates the need to pass a needle through the abdominal wall [7, 9] (Fig. 5.2). In this method, a long suture on a conventional curved (SH) needle is placed through the gallbladder fundus and then through the anterior-lateral peritoneum well above the costal margin. The two ends of the suture are externalized through a trocar and knots are tied extracorporeally using a knot pusher. This effectively elevates the gallbladder fundus cephalad, similar to using a standard rigid laparoscopic grasper. The infundibulum is sutured by encircling a bite of tissue within a pretied loop at the suture tail

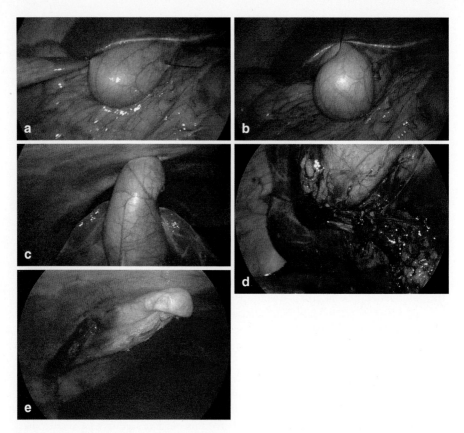

Fig. 5.1 Percutaneous suture retraction during SILS cholecystectomy. (**a**) The gallbladder is pierced at the fundus with a Keith needle. (**b**)The suture may be preattached to a rubber plunger that is then apposed against the gallbladder. (**c**) Percutaneous suture retraction of the fundus at the costal margin. (**d**) Exposure of Calot's triangle after placement of additional sutures at the infundibulum. (**e**) Completion of cholecystectomy with gallbladder suspended by percutaneous sutures

(the needle is passed through this loop). The needle is then passed through the lateral peritoneum and externalized though a trocar. The tail is left long and secured with a hemostat such that pulling on this tail retracts the infundibulum laterally, since the suture is created in a pulley configuration. Thus, dynamic retraction is facilitated, whereby tension may be progressively adjusted. While this method is advantageous for several reasons, it is relatively complex and difficult to teach.

Instead of suture, an endoloop may also be used as described by Mintz et al. [4, 10] (Fig. 5.3). This method involves placing an endoloop around the gallbladder fundus; a suture passer is then used to retract the endoloop transabdominally and provide anterior retraction. While simple and feasible, the endoloop is more costly than other suture materials. Additionally, the use of a suture passer usually requires a larger incision compared to the almost invisible scar associated with passage of a needle through the skin. And, as with percutaneous needle placement, there is a risk of bleeding with passage of the suture passer.

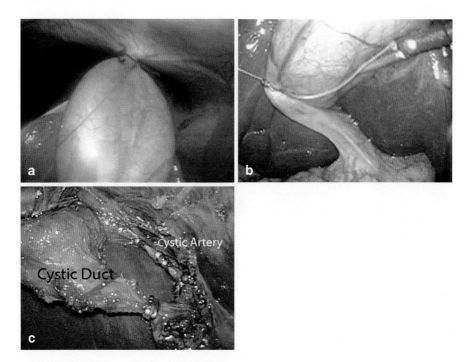

Fig. 5.2 Intracorporeal suture retraction during SILS cholecystectomy. (**a**) Fundus suture providing cephalad retraction. (**b**) Lateral suture retraction at infundibulum. (**c**) Resulting exposure of Calot's triangle using this technique (With kind permission from Springer Science+Business Media. Reproduced from Rivas et al. [7])

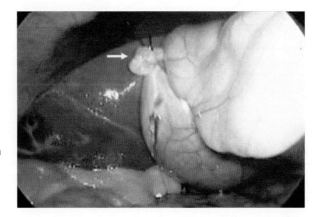

Fig. 5.3 Endoloop (*arrow*) retraction of fundus during SILS cholecystectomy (With kind permission from Springer Science+Business Media. Reproduced from Schlager et al. [4])

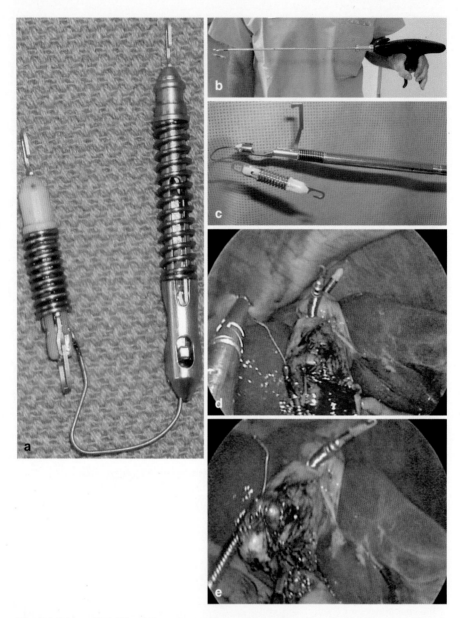

Fig. 5.4 Endograb™ (Virtual Ports, Inc., Misgav, Israel) retraction in SILS cholecystectomy. (**a**) Endograb device; (**b**) delivery device; (**c**) Endograb device and delivery tool demonstrating deployment; (**d**) placement of Endograb on fundus and infundibulum; (**e**) resulting exposure after placement of Endograb

Only one purpose-built FDA-approved device for gallbladder retraction is currently available in the United States. Namely, the Endograb™ (Virtual Ports, Inc., Misgav, Israel) device is a deployable retraction system that may be especially useful during SILS or even NOTES procedures [4, 9, 10] (Fig. 5.4). This system consists of a reusable hand instrument (insertion tool) and a disposable grasper unit. The hand instrument is introduced via a 5-mm port and the Endograb™ device is deployed into the abdominal cavity. The device consists of two spring-loaded graspers connected by a curved wire. For cholecystectomy, one of the graspers is attached to the gallbladder fundus and the other end is attached to the anterior-lateral peritoneum cephalad to the costal margin. A second Endograb™ is placed on the lower gallbladder and connected to the lateral peritoneum such that the infundibulum is retracted laterally, exposing Calot's triangle. The specific attachment points may be adjusted by simply opening the grasper and reattaching it to a different location. For instance, the infundibular grasper may be connected to a midline peritoneal location to expose the right side of the gallbladder. The connecting wire has sufficient memory such that a gentle continuous tension on the tissue may be afforded; thus, as the dissection progresses, the gallbladder is progressively lifted toward the anterior abdominal wall.

For SILS procedures, the Endograb™ is usually placed through a working trocar, and then this trocar may be used for other instrumentation. For NOTES procedures, the Endograb™ has been used during hybrid procedures in which a 5-mm umbilical trocar is available for introduction of the device. Because this device is deployable, it may be quite helpful in providing triangulation and relatively good exposure, including fundic retraction above the costal margin. Because of the spring-loaded design, occasionally part of the grasper device may obscure visualization of the operative field or simply prevent dissection of an area of interest. In this case, we have found that simply removing the grasper, rotating it 180°, and reattaching it tends to move the spring portion of the grasper out of the way and facilitate improved exposure.

Despite this device's utility, there is a potential risk of tissue shearing and hemorrhage at the grasper fixation locations (diaphragm or abdominal wall). However, in our experience and in the reported literature, this risk is minimal. There may also be potential for bile spillage should the gallbladder tear at the site of grasper fixation, but this has not been part of our experience. The primary disadvantage is cost; the reusable introducer device costs approximately $700 and each disposable Endograb™ device costs approximately $150, with two devices normally used per case.

The use of articulating instruments during NOTES cholecystectomy has been particularly helpful in facilitating tissue retraction. Horgan et al. reported on the use of an extra-long RealHand™ grasper (Novare, Inc., Cupertino, CA) to perform a hybrid transvaginal cholecystectomy [11, 12]. The RealHand™ instrument was advanced transvaginally through a trocar and used to retract and manipulate the gallbladder. The remainder of the dissection was performed via a 5-mm umbilical port and using the transvaginally placed flexible endoscope. Other groups in Europe have reported similar retraction strategies using extra-long laparoscopic graspers placed transvaginally during NOTES cholecystectomy [13]. Additionally, dedicated multifunctional single-access platforms are being developed by several manufactures, but are outside the purview of this chapter.

Fig. 5.5 Fundus retraction
using a magnet fixated with
endoclips to provide cephalad
retraction during NOTES
cholecystectomy (With kind
permission from Springer
Science+Business Media.
Reproduced from Scott et al.
[15])

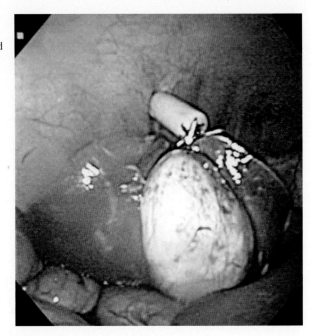

Magnetic Retraction Systems in Cholecystectomy

The use of magnets may be quite useful in retracting tissue during limited-access procedures. The Magnetic Anchoring and Guidance System (MAGS) was developed by Cadeddu and Scott. This group first developed the technology in 2001, well ahead of its time, in an effort to facilitate "trocarless" surgery. MAGS is an innovative method that aims to overcome limitations in spatial orientation and retraction inherent to NOTES and SILS. MAGS consists of a mobile magnet placed intraabdominally and then coupled to an extracorporeal handheld neodymium magnet across the abdominal wall. MAGS instruments, which include a camera, tissue retractors, and monopolar cautery, are then controlled transabdominally, allowing for unrestricted intraabdominal movement and improvement in spatial orientation and instrument spacing during SILS and NOTES. Alternatively, the internal magnet can be attached to an 18-gauge percutaneous needle lock, anchoring the platform to allow removal of the external magnet. This reduces unintended coupling between other magnetic instruments, permits hands-free control, and increases the force reaction capabilities of the intraabdominal instrument [14–16].

In one series, transvaginal NOTES cholecystectomy was performed in a porcine model using MAGS for gallbladder retraction [15] (Fig. 5.5). This was achieved by using either an attachable magnet or a flexible grasper cradle. In the former, an internal magnet was attached to a suture loop that was then secured to the gallbladder fundus with an endoclip deployed via a flexible endoscope. The internal magnet was then coupled with an external magnet, providing dynamic cephalad

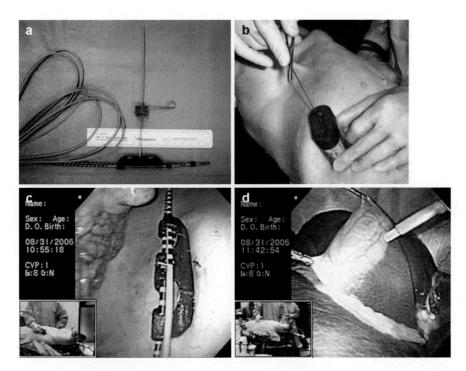

Fig. 5.6 MAGS retraction for NOTES cholecystectomy. (**a**) Flexible grasper cradle holding biopsy forceps that is secured in place by percutaneous needle anchor. (**b**) Placement of needle anchor after internal component is placed in desired position. (**c**) Intraabdominal view of grasper cradle that has been stabilized by needle anchor. (**d**) Biopsy forcep grasper retraction of gallbladder fundus and infundibulum (With kind permission from Springer Science+Business Media. Reproduced from Scott et al. [15])

retraction well above the costal margin. Positioning and deployment were performed without difficulty, as this configuration was quite simple; and cephalad retraction was excellent as the magnet could be positioned relatively high toward the diaphragm. However, infundibulum retraction was noted to be difficult due to problems associated with the use of flexible endoscopic equipment for this purpose. In addition, dislodgement of the endoclip during the case occurred relatively frequently, resulting in the need for laparoscopic suturing methods to provide more secure attachment.

The subsequent MAGS gallbladder grasper described was a flexible grasper cradle configured to allow two endoscopic biopsy forceps or rat-tooth graspers to transverse through it [15] (Fig. 5.6). This internal component contained a magnet such that the grasper could be positioned magnetically, and then stabilized with a percutaneous 18-gauge needle anchor. Retraction of the gallbladder fundus and infundibulum was then achieved using the two flexible endoscopic graspers supported by the internal cradle. Tension on the external grasper cables stabilized the grasper retraction and provided a reasonable element of dynamic control. The gallbladder dissection

Fig. 5.7 (a) Magnetic
alligator clips; (b) retraction
of fundus and infundibulum
during SILS cholecystectomy
(Reprinted with kind
permission from Elsevier
from Galvani et al. [19])

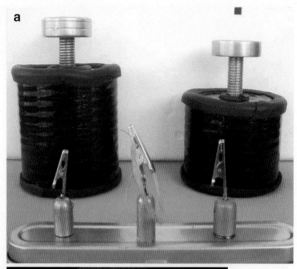

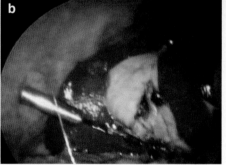

was then completed using MAGS electrocautery. While this model proved useful in performing a completely transvaginal NOTES cholecystectomy without any laparoscopic assistance, the flexible cradle grasper had limitations. Namely, the infundibulum grasper served the purpose of creating active tension, thus providing lateral and caudal retraction with expansion of Calot's triangle. However, it was often difficult to fully elevate the fundus in a cephalad direction given the relatively flexible nature of the endoscopic graspers used.

Dominguez et al. developed magnetic forceps in which an alligator clip and a magnet are attached [17, 18] (Fig. 5.7). Either one or two such retractors may be used to elevate the fundus and/or infundibulum. Relatively large external magnets are used. These techniques have been successfully used in numerous patients by Dr. Dominguez, with reportedly good results in limited-access and SILS procedures. For NOTES cholecystectomy, Dr. Dominguez's retractor has also been used in collaboration with Dr. Horgan's group, with a magnetic retractor placed transvaginally and attached to the fundus to provide excellent cephalad retraction [20].

In a somewhat unusual fashion, Ryou and Thompson described the use of magnets attached to endoclips to elevate the liver for gallbladder retraction during transcolonic cholecystectomy in a porcine model [21]. These investigators used several magnetic clips placed along the inferior edge of the liver and a very large external magnet to elevate the right anterior portion of the liver. This in turn provided reasonably good exposure of the gallbladder to facilitate dissection with flexible endoscopic instruments. After completion of the procedure, the clips were removed with apparently no major tissue trauma. While feasibility was documented for the porcine model, no human applications for this strategy have been reported.

While the use of magnetic retraction devices and strategies as described above overcomes the instrument clashing and triangulation problems associated with SILS and NOTES, there are limitations associated with their use. Even though no problems have been identified in numerous laboratory and clinical investigations, concerns regarding the potential tissue effects of magnet compression have been raised by various reviewers. Mashaud et al. examined abdominal wall tissue grossly and histologically after SILS cholecystectomy using a MAGS cautery dissector device in a porcine model [14]. The average dissection time was 36 min, after which mild skin erythema was immediately noted with a subsequent rapid resolution. In addition, there was no histological evidence of tissue necrosis or damage of skin, muscle, or peritoneum.

On the other hand, insufficient coupling strength may be problematic. Magnetic coupling across the abdominal wall is exponentially related to the distance between magnets, with magnetic attraction decreasing dramatically as separation distance increases. In an ex vivo model investigating magnetic force decay, Best et al. found that static coupling was maintained to a maximum distance of 4.78 cm [22]. Milad et al. conducted an investigation in 138 women in which they measured abdominal wall thickness in the left upper quadrant and umbilicus after insufflation using a spinal needle during gynecologic laparoscopy [23]. They found that only 1.5 % of women with a BMI greater than 40 kg/m^2 had an abdominal wall thickness greater than 4 cm. While these data do not account for potential frictional forces, current data suggest that the MAGS platform should be suitable for a significant portion of the adult population undergoing procedures such as cholecystectomy.

Liver Retraction Systems

Many advanced laparoscopic foregut procedures require retraction of the left lateral liver for visualization of the lesser curvature of the stomach or gastroesophageal junction. Traditionally, this has necessitated placement of a laparoscopic liver retractor such as a Nathanson™ (Cook Medical, Bloomington, IN), fan, paddle, or similar device through a separate 5-mm or even 10-mm incision. With the advent of SILS, several novel techniques have been developed to effectively elevate the liver without the need for an additional port.

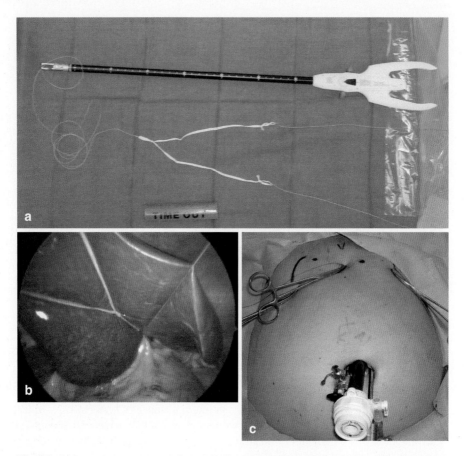

Fig. 5.8 Percutaneous suture retraction of the liver. (**a**) Endostitch™ (Covidien, Mansfield, MA) device and sutures attached to an umbilical tape; (**b**) "W" configuration of suture and umbilical tape retraction of the liver, providing exposure of hiatal hernia; (**c**) external view of suture retraction

Several groups, including ours, have described the use of a percutaneous suture to suspend the left lateral liver [24–26] (Fig. 5.8). In this technique, a suture is placed high anteriorly across the right crus of the diaphragm under the left lobe. Care must be taken to avoid injuring the inferior phrenic vein, as it usually courses quite close to this area. Care must also be taken to avoid deep bites that could penetrate the full thickness of the diaphragm and cause injury to the pericardium or heart. Fortunately, the diaphragmatic tissue at this location is sufficiently strong such that a relatively superficial bite is more than adequate to anchor the suture to the diaphragm without dislodgement. Once the diaphragm end is anchored, the ends of the suture are percutaneously retrieved through separate small stab incisions using a fascial closure device. The tails may be held under tension using hemostats externally. Two suture tails may be used such that a "V" shape configuration is con-

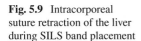

Fig. 5.9 Intracorporeal suture retraction of the liver during SILS band placement

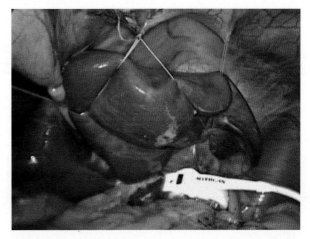

structed; in this case, the tails are usually externalized just below the costal margin in the left midclavicular line and to the left of the falciform ligament, respectively. Alternatively, three tails may be used by attaching the primary suture to an additional suture strand or even an umbilical tape such that a "W" shape configuration is constructed; in this case, the third suture strand is externalized in the right midclavicular line.

Concerns have been raised regarding suture strands cutting through the capsule or parenchyma of the liver. However, using 2-0 braided suture, we have had no such problems. The advantage of this method is its simplicity. While significant skill may be required to place the suture through the diaphragm during a SILS procedure, it is quite easy from a technical standpoint to retrieve the suture tails percutaneously. This method provides relatively good exposure, especially if three suture strands are used in a "W" fashion, such that both the lateral and medial aspects of the liver are lifted off the underlying stomach.

Similarly, Scott et al. described a purely intracorporeal suture approach [9, 26] (Fig. 5.9). In this method, a 48-in. 2-0 prolene suture on an endostitch device is used to take alternating bites between the diaphragm crura and the peritoneum in a W-shaped configuration. The initial suture is passed through a loop tied at the suture tail prior to beginning the procedure, so that the suture is anchored to the crus. The final knot is tied intracorporally as well, thus eliminating the need for any skin incisions or percutaneous retrieval.

Intracorporeal suture retraction of the liver in general has been found to be more technically challenging and tedious than percutaneous methods. This is primarily felt to be due to difficulty elevating the liver with a grasper to expose the diaphragm and maintaining tension on the suture during placement of sequential bites [26]. The percutaneous method has less of a learning curve but is not without inherent risks, such as potential bleeding from piercing abdominal wall vasculature. In addition, this technique has less cosmetic benefit compared to the completely intracorporeal method.

Uyama et al. described a modification of the suture strategy whereby the liver was retracted using a penrose drain [27]. Prior to introducing the drain into the abdomen, nylon sutures were secured at the ends and in the center of the drain. A window was made in the left triangular ligament through which the central suture was placed and pulled inferiorly to superiorly onto the ventral surface of the liver. Using an EndoClose™ (Covidien, Mansfield, MA) device, this suture was then pulled through the abdominal wall and exteriorized in the right and left subcostal areas, respectively. Interestingly, Uyama et al. reported that using the Penrose drain technique liver retraction during laparoscopic gastrectomy ($n=47$) was associated with a significantly lower postoperative transaminitis than seen with the use of a Nathanson™ retractor ($n=64$) [27]. Although the observed transaminitis was transient, there may be some clinical benefit in this method of retraction as potentially less traumatic, which may be especially beneficial in patients with baseline liver dysfunction. However, advanced skills may be required to safely create the window in the left triangular ligament and to perform this strategy.

Huang et al. developed a liver suspension tape technique by creating a device consisting of the flat portion of a Jackson–Pratt drain with 2-0 prolene sutures on a Keith needle secured on each end [28, 29]. The drain portion of the device was placed underneath the liver. One of the prolene sutures was used to pierce the lateral edge of the left liver and externalized in the left subcostal area. The second needle pierced the left lobe near the falciform and was externalized near the midline. The sutures were secured externally under tension and effectively held the liver against the anterior abdominal wall. While the liver suspension tape method as described seemed to provide excellent retraction, critics have raised concerns about potential liver injury or hemorrhage since the parenchyma is intentionally transfixed.

Given the technical difficulties associated with suture retraction, we developed a novel method of liver retraction that utilizes components of the LoneStar™ (Cooper Surgical, Trumbull, CT) retractor system [9, 26] (Fig. 5.10). The LoneStar system is typically used for anorectal, urological, and gynecological procedures. The system consists of hooks connected to rubber tubing that may be used to facilitate effacement of the anus, vagina, or other perineal tissues. The hooks are disposable, available in several sizes, and packaged separately (the cost is approximately $80 for a pack of 8); our preference is to use the 3-mm hooks (white), which are relatively small but facilitate sufficient bites of tissue. Two hooks are trimmed and sutured together to create an overall length of approximately 8 cm, functionally creating a double-armed retraction hook. Using a laparoscopic grasper to elevate the liver, one LoneStar hook is placed in the anterior right crus and its opposing hook is placed high anteriorly into the fibrous portion of the falciform ligament; this first construct serves to elevate much of the liver off the proximal stomach and provide exposure of the diaphragmatic crura (sufficient to perform a hiatal hernia repair). A second pair of LoneStar hooks are placed extending from high on the gastrohepatic ligament to a slightly more caudal location on the falciform ligament so that the retractors are parallel and the more medial aspect of the left hepatic lobe is elevated. Together these act to effectively suspend the liver and have provided excellent exposure in 18 of our patients who underwent single-incision adjustable gastric banding

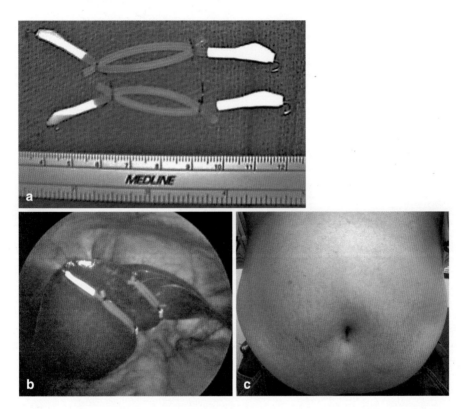

Fig. 5.10 LoneStar™ (Cooper Surgical, Trumbull, CT) retraction of the liver. (**a**) LoneStar device configured as a double-armed retraction hook; (**b**) elevation of left liver lobe using parallel LoneStar hooks; (**c**) postoperative scarless cosmesis from using this technique

procedures, with a wide variety of BMIs (up to 58 kg/m^2). Should adjustments be needed, the hooks can be relatively easily repositioned. While this approach does require advanced laparoscopic skills, it is relatively simple and reproducible from a technical standpoint. To our knowledge, the LoneStar system is not FDA-labeled for intraabdominal usage, and thus performing this technique is at the discretion of the surgeon as "off-label" usage of an FDA-approved device. Certainly, if a hook were to become lost within the abdominal cavity, there would be concerns regarding the use of a foreign body; however, this has not been our experience. Our primary problem in using the hooks is inadvertent tissue or trocar interactions. Care must be taken to avoid catching the hooks on parts of the seals of the trocar during insertion or removal; protecting the hook within a laparoscopic grasper is quite helpful to avoid this problem. Similarly, the hooks may "snag" on omentum or other intraabdominal tissues, and their manipulation must be visualized to avoid these unwanted interactions. In our experience, we have had no such complications using a very vigilant approach. The rubber segments of the retractors have been quite atraumatic on the liver parenchyma, with no injuries to the liver, as well.

Fig. 5.11 (a) LoneStar™ (Cooper Surgical) retractor attached to a laparoscopic bulldog clamp; (**b**) exposure of the gastroesophageal junction using LoneStar/bulldog clamp attached from the pars flaccid to the falciform

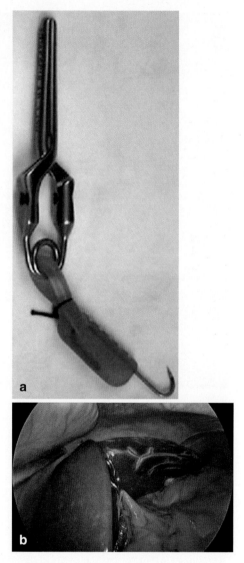

Galvani et al. also reported using the LoneStar hook retractor connected to a bulldog clamp for liver retraction during single- and dual-incision adjustable gastric band placement [19] (Fig. 5.11). This group describes attaching the bulldog clamp to the pars flaccida membrane and the LoneStar hook to the falciform ligament. From their paper, this method seems to provide reasonable exposure to the upper stomach. However, the lesser curvature of the stomach seems to become somewhat distorted anatomically as the gastric tissue near the bulldog clamp becomes quite elevated. Also, the medial aspect of the left hepatic lobe is not elevated using this technique as described.

Fig. 5.12 Endolift™ (Virtual Ports, Inc., Misgav, Israel) device

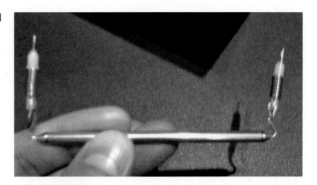

Table 5.2 Comparison of liver retraction methods

	Exposure provided	Technical difficulty	Risk of adjacent organ injury	Expense
Percutaneous suture	+	+	+	−
Intracorporeal suture	+	++	+	−
Penrose drain	+	++	+	−
Liver suspension tape	++	++	++	+
LoneStar™ (Cooper Surgical)	++	++	+	+
Endolift™ (Virtual Ports)	++	++	+	++

A relatively new device designed specifically for the purpose of liver retraction is the Endolift™ and is manufactured by the same company that makes the Endograb (Virtual Ports, Inc., Misgav, Israel) (Fig. 5.12). This device is FDA-approved and consists of dual spring graspers connected by a metal rod. Similar to the Endograb, the Endolift requires a separate reusable delivery device (5-mm laparoscopic tool). The retractor is backloaded into the introducer device and placed into the abdominal cavity. One grasper is placed on the anterior right crus and the other grasper is placed on the peritoneal surface near the falciform ligament or in the right upper quadrant. The metal rod between the two graspers is spring-loaded, adjustable (much like a shower curtain rod), and rigid, such that the liver is lifted. Per the manufacturer, one Endolift is sufficient in most cases; occasionally, a second Endolift may be necessary, especially for cases involving enlarged or redundant livers. Clinical experience with this device is currently limited, but the design seems quite robust. Costs of the device and delivery system are $250 and $700, respectively, which may be prohibitive to widespread adoption.

There are several shared benefits of these alternative methods of liver retraction beyond avoiding the placement of a separate incision and/or trocar (Table 5.2). Since all of these methods effectively use self-retaining strategies, there is no need for external retractor components, such as an iron intern or similar mechanical arms, to hold a traditional liver retractor in place. Thus, the surgeon's reliance on the operative team (scrub and OR nurse) to coordinate such retractors is eliminated, as are the cost and the need for sterilization of such components. Additionally, the OR setup is simplified, as fewer components are needed. This latter aspect deserves

Fig. 5.13 Suture retraction during dual-incision adjustable band. (**a**) Suture placement on gastric fundus and on the lesser curvature incorporating the right curs; (**b**) peritoneal suture allowing suture retraction to act as a pulley system for manipulation during the operation

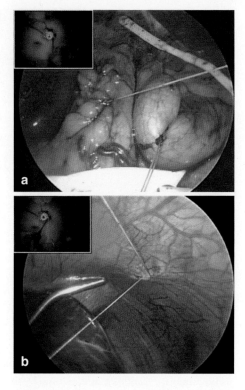

emphasis, as in many operating rooms individual pieces of such retractor systems may be missing and cause operative delays and frustration. We find it very exciting that such novel retraction systems may decrease postoperative aberrations in liver function tests as described earlier in this chapter. Certainly, a further refinement of currently available devices and techniques seems warranted, as does developing additional instrumentation.

Retraction in Other Advanced Procedures

Bariatric, foregut, and colorectal procedures are increasingly being performed via single-incision laparoscopic and NOTES approaches. As with other advancements in minimally invasive surgical procedures, several retraction systems have been adopted to facilitate these techniques.

We have developed methods for gastric retraction during single-incision adjustable gastric band placement [30–32]. Using an Endostitch (Covidien, Mansfield, MA), a suture is placed high on the gastric fundus and then externalized through the working port (Fig. 5.13). This provides exposure to the angle of His. After division of the pars flaccida, a second suture is placed on the lesser curvature incorporating

Fig. 5.14 Endograb™ (Virtual Ports, Inc., Misgav, Israel) retraction during SILS adjustable gastric band placement. Three devices are used to grasp the gastric fundus and lesser curvature to attach them to the lateral abdominal wall

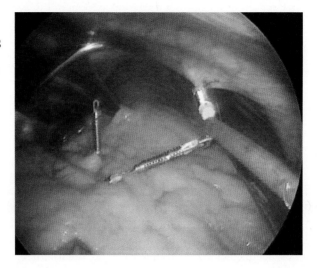

the right crus fat pad. The suture is then passed through a pretied loop at the distal end, which functionally lassoes the tissue internally. Next, the suture is passed through the peritoneum at the left costal margin in the midclavicular line, and externalized via the working port. Traction on this suture acts as a pulley system, elevating the lesser curvature anterior-laterally. This allows exposure of the base of the right crus and facilitates creation of the retrogastric tunnel under laparoscopic visualization. Other groups, such as Rosemurgy and Ross at the University of Southern Florida, have presented videos demonstrating similar suture retraction strategies to facilitate SILS Nissen fundoplication and Heller myotomy.

We have also used the Endograb device for this same purpose during single-incision adjustable gastric band placement [31] (Fig. 5.14). Three of the devices were used to grasp and retract the gastric fundus and the lesser curvature and attach them to the left lateral abdominal wall. This technique provided similar exposure to the suture method. However, we had some concerns related to the grasper design, which may not be optimized for atraumatic tissue retraction. Additionally, the expense of the Endograb device may also limit current adoption of this technique.

The use of SILS and NOTES is gaining momentum in the field of colorectal surgery as well. The use of a variety of curved and articulating instruments has been most commonly described to preserve triangulation and facilitate dissection in SILS colectomies, while a few series have described intracorporeal suture retraction of the colon and adjacent organs. Leroy et al. described a natural orifice specimen extraction (NOSE) with the transanal removal of a laparoendoscopic single-incision sigmoidectomy specimen [33]. During the operation, transparietal sutures were placed around bilateral round ligaments to suspend the uterus to the abdominal wall, providing exposure of the rectum. Mobilization of the colon was performed in a standard medial-to-lateral laparoscopic fashion. Once the rectum was divided, transparietal sutures were used to suspend the open rectum to the anterior abdominal wall, allowing passage of the sigmoid specimen.

Similarly, Bucher et al. described a single-incision right hemicolectomy using intracorporeal suture retraction [34]. In this technique, the right colon was suspended to the abdominal wall by transparietal sutures. The ileocolic pedicle was then suspended to the abdominal wall with a second transparietal suture anchored distally on the pedicle. This allowed exposure for a standard medial-to-lateral dissection to be performed using conventional laparoscopic instruments. The use of suture retraction during colonic single-incision procedures provides the benefit of a self-retaining suspension of the colon, thus freeing working instruments for dissection and other active roles. Concerns for potential intraabdominal contamination from either transluminal passage of the suture or shearing forces on the colon wall may be avoided by placing sutures in the subserosa, mesentery, or omentum.

The use of magnetic retractors has also been reported for NOTES colorectal procedures. In a porcine model, Leroy et al. used a very clever flexible plastic tube with magnets at its tip inserted transanally to elevate the sigmoid colon using an external magnet [35]. This maneuver provided sufficient exposure of the mesentery to allow for vascular division. Furthermore, magnetic coupling was used to hold the anvil of a circular stapler in position within the proximal colon to facilitate a colorectal anastomosis.

Conclusion

Single-incision laparoscopic surgery (SILS) and natural orifice translumenal endoscopic surgery (NOTES) are increasingly becoming attractive alternatives to conventional laparoscopy. The retraction techniques described in this chapter demonstrate the diversity of advancements in the field of minimally invasive surgery and the need for continued innovations in surgical techniques and technologies to preserve triangulation and surgical exposure. As the paradigm shifts toward less invasive operations, the development of feasible solutions to potential barriers and limitations in SILS and NOTES will allow a further evolution of the field and facilitate mainstream adoption.

References

1. Rattner D, Kalloo A, and the SAGES/ASGE Working Group on Natural Orifice Translumenal Endoscopic Surgery. ASGE/SAGES Working Group on natural orifice translumenal endoscopic surgery. Surg Endosc. 2006;20:329–33.
2. Gill I, Teixeira J, et al. Consensus statement of the consortium for laparoendoscopic single-site surgery. Surg Endosc. 2010;24:762–8.
3. Navarra G, Pozza E, Occhionorelli S, et al. One wound laparoscopic cholecystectomy. Br J Surg. 1997;84:695.

4. Schlager A, Khalaileh A, Mintz Y, et al. Providing more through less: current methods of retraction in SIMIS and NOTES cholecystectomy. Surg Endosc. 2009;24:1542–6.
5. Ponsky T. Single port laparoscopic cholecystectomy in adults and children: tools and techniques. J Am Coll Surg. 2009;209:e1–6.
6. Philipp S, Miedema B, Thaler K. Single-incision laparoscopic cholecystectomy using conventional instruments: early experience in comparison with the gold standard. J Am Coll Surg. 2009;209:632–7.
7. Rivas H, Varela E, Scott D. Single-incision laparoscopic cholecystectomy: initial evaluation of a large series of patients. Surg Endosc. 2010;24:1403–12.
8. Rawlings A, Hodgett S, Brunt M, et al. Single-incision laparoscopic cholecystectomy: initial experience with critical view of safety dissection and routine intraoperative cholangiography. J Am Coll Surg. 2010;211:1–7.
9. Scott D. Using Endograb and sutures instead of ports. SAGES 2011 annual meeting-minimizing MIS postgraduate course. 2011.
10. Shussman N, Schlager A, Mintz Y, et al. Single-incision laparoscopic cholecystectomy: lessons learned for success. Surg Endosc. 2011;25:404–7.
11. Horgan S, Cullen J, Ferraina P, et al. Natural orifice surgery: initial clinical experience. Surg Endosc. 2009;23:1512–8.
12. Horgan S, Mintz Y. NOTES: transvaginal cholecystectomy with assisting articulating instruments. Surg Endosc. 2009;23:1900.
13. Zornig C, Mofid H, Emmermann A, et al. Scarless cholecystectomy with combined transvaginal and transumbilical approach in a series of 20 patients. Surg Endosc. 2008;22:1427–9.
14. Mashaud L, Kabbani W, Scott D, et al. Tissue compression analysis for magnetically anchored cautery dissector during single-site laparoscopic cholecystectomy. J Gastrointest Surg. 2011;15:902–7.
15. Scott D, Tang S, Cadeddu J, et al. Completely transvaginal NOTES cholecystectomy using magnetically anchored instruments. Surg Endosc. 2007;21:2308–16.
16. Cadeddu J, Fernandez R, Scott D, et al. Novel magnetically guided intra-abdominal camera to facilitate laparoendoscopic single-site surgery: initial human experience. Surg Endosc. 2006;20:329–33.
17. Dominguez G. Colecistectomia con un trocar asistida por imanes de neodimio. Reporte de un caso. Cirugia Endoscopia. 2007;8:172–6 [in Spanish].
18. Dominguez G, Durand L, Ferraina P, et al. Retraction and triangulation with neodymium magnetic forceps for single-port laparoscopic cholecystectomy. Surg Endosc. 2009;23:1660–6.
19. Galvani C, Gallo A, Gorodner M. Single-incision and dual-incision laparoscopic adjustable gastric band: evaluation of initial experience. Surg Obes Relat Dis. 2012;8(2):194–200.
20. Horgan S, Ferraina P, Talamini M, et al. Magnetic retraction for NOTES transvaginal cholecystectomy. Surg Endosc. 2008;22:S177–85.
21. Ryou M, Thompson C. The use of magnets in natural orifice transluminal endoscopic surgery (NOTES): addressing the problem of traction and counter-traction. Endoscopy. 2009;41:143–8.
22. Best S, Bergs R, Scott D, et al. Maximizing coupling strength of magnetically anchored surgical instruments: how thick can we go? Surg Endosc. 2011;25:153–9.
23. Milad M, Terkildsen M. The spinal needle test effectively measures abdominal wall thickness before cannula placement at laparoscopy. J Am Assoc Gynecol Laparosc. 2002;9:514–8.
24. De la Torre R, Satgunam S, Scott J, et al. Transumbilical single-port laparoscopic adjustable gastric band placement with liver suture retractor. Obes Surg. 2009;12:1707–10.
25. Tacchino R, Greco F, Matera D. Laparoscopic gastric banding without visible scar: a short series with intraumbilical SILS. Obes Surg. 2010;20:236–9.
26. Oltmann S, Mashaud L, Scott D, et al. Single incision laparoscopic gastric banding: evolution towards scarless surgery during 50 consecutive cases. Surg Endosc. 2010;24:S299.
27. Shinohara T, Kanaya S, Uyama I, et al. A protective technique for retraction of the liver during laparoscopic gastrectomy for gastric adenocarcinoma: using a Penrose drain. J Gastrointest Surg. 2011;15:1043–8.

28. Huang C, Lo C, Huang S. A novel technique for liver retraction in laparoscopic bariatric surgery. Obes Surg. 2010;21:676–9.
29. Huang C, Houng J, Lee P. Single incision transumbilical laparoscopic Roux-en-Y gastric bypass: a first case report. Obes Surg. 2009;19:1711–5.
30. Oltmann S, Rivas H, Scott D, et al. Single laparoscopic surgery: case reports of SILS adjustable gastric banding. Surg Obes Relat Dis. 2009;5:362–4.
31. Scott D, Castellvi A, Rivas H, et al. Modified single incision laparoscopic (SILS) adjustable gastric band (video). Surg Endosc. 2010;24:2314.
32. Mashaud L, Eisenstein E, Scott D, et al. 605 modified single incision laparoscopic gastric band placement with intracorporeal gastric retraction. Gastroenterology. 2010;138:S857.
33. Leroy J, Diana M, Marescaux J, et al. Laparo-endoscopic single-site (LESS) with transanal natural orifice specimen extraction (NOSE) sigmoidectomy: a new step before pure colorectal natural orifices transluminal endoscopic surgery (NOTES). J Gastrointest Surg. 2011;15:1488–92.
34. Bucher P, Pugin F, Morel P. Single port access laparoscopic right hemicolectomy. Int J Colorectal Dis. 2008;23:1013–6.
35. Leroy J, Cahill A, Peretta S, et al. Single port sigmoidectomy in an experimental model with survival. Surg Innov. 2008;15:260.

Chapter 6
Exit Strategies

Melissa S. Phillips and Jeffrey L. Ponsky

Keywords Endoscopic suture • Endoscopic clip • Gastrointestinal closure • NOTES access site closure

Introduction

Natural orifice translumenal endoscopic surgery, or NOTES, has shown promise over the past few years as an alternative to standard laparoscopic surgery. It has potential promises of less pain, better cosmesis, and shortened recovery. Any new approach, however, will face challenges for generalized use. With regards to the NOTES techniques, patient safety in the face of an intentional visceral opening must be clearly documented. While research on the ideal platform for NOTES continues, adequate transvisceral closure is a necessity in the human application of this new operative technique. With little or no tolerance for a postprocedural leak from the viscerotomy, access site closure has been clearly identified as one limitation that must be overcome.

Many attempts have been made to design methods for transvisceral closure. These have ranged from the application of endoscopic clips to the performance of endoluminal suturing. Others have performed this closure with stapling devices, tacks, or viscerotomy occlusion. This manuscript will detail the current and previous approaches used for closure following NOTES, including the advantages and limitations of each.

M.S. Phillips, M.D. (✉)
Department of Surgery, University of Tennessee Health Science Center,
1930 Alcoa Hwy, Suite 240, Knoxville, TN 37920, USA
e-mail: phillips.melissa@gmail.com

J.L. Ponsky, M.D.
Department of Surgery, University Hospitals Case Medical Center,
11100 Euclid Ave LKS-5047, Cleveland, OH 44106, USA
e-mail: jponsky@yahoo.com, jeffrey.ponsky@uhhospitals.org

A. Rane et al. (eds.), *Scar-Less Surgery*,
DOI 10.1007/978-1-84800-360-6_6, © Springer-Verlag London 2013

Once a method for closure has been invented, the next step in the process is to decide how to evaluate the closure mechanism. Assessments of access site closure have been based on the application of non-NOTES literature. For example, it has been supported that the idea of a pressure-based anastomotic test following colorectal surgery can lead to a lower clinical leak rate [1, 2]. This presumption as applied to NOTES has led to the idea of both air- and fluid-based leak testing. Others have described the use of bursting pressures as a measurement for durability. A "gold standard" for the evaluation of anastomotic integrity remains to be documented, but until that time, this chapter will review the currently accepted practices for assessing closure.

A variety of modifications were made to existing endoscopic products, as well as the invention of new technologies, in an attempt to provide a safe and effective method for closure following NOTES intervention. When compared to laparoscopy, a low complication profile and low acceptable leak rate have been documented, raising the bar for the evaluation of closure techniques. Despite the numerous attempts, a single method for transvisceral closure has not demonstrated superiority above all others, providing a continued challenge for the widespread introduction of NOTES.

Challenges and Requirements for Closure

The technologies available for current endoscopic options for full-thickness closure devices before the development of NOTES were crude and limited. Endoscopic equipment has only limited degrees of freedom and lacks the ability to provide triangulation, which is a basic surgical principle. These limited technologies presented a challenge when the idea of NOTES was born because no preexisting devices were ideal for transvisceral closure without modification.

Adequate full-thickness closure can be accomplished using endoscopic approaches, but it must be developed in line with established surgical technique in order to facilitate acceptance by the surgical community [3]. Specifically, the defect must be clearly visualized to allow for an adequate assessment of closure. The closure mechanism must then incorporate tissue in a way that leads to a durable closure. It should avoid injury to surrounding viscera and should maintain a low postprocedure leak rate.

When assessing visualization, a standard endoscope provides optics that are of a quality to allow for closure. What presents more of a challenge for visualization is the inability to maintain insufflation of the lumen with a full-thickness opening through which air is lost into the abdomen. This lack of established working space can greatly impair visualization and lead to inadvertent injury of the intraabdominal contents. It may also be responsible for longer procedural times, of which the clinical significance is unknown.

Assessing appropriate tissue incorporation is an important aspect to closure devices. If the selected tissue is too thin or does not encompass the full thickness of the tissue, inadequate closure may result. The dependability to provide tissue incorporation without "small bites" that would lead to weakness in the closure is an essential aspect in accepting a new closure device for NOTES.

All transvisceral closure devices carry a risk of inadvertently incorporating surrounding viscera in the closure. This may be an asymptomatic finding or may lead to the development of clinically significant problems, such as enterocolic or rectovaginal fistula formation. When comparing four independent devices for transgastric closure in a swine model, the author [4] noted an 8 % inadvertent injury rate on necropsy, despite no implications of injury at the time of the NOTES procedure. An ideal closure device should incorporate a safety mechanism against unintended visceral injury.

Finally, security of the closure must be documented through evidence of a low leak rate and high rates of intact anastomosis in animal models. Chronic animal models assessing transvisceral closure mechanisms have shown a low but persistent leak rate, which remains a barrier to human translation [5]. All leak rates must still be compared to the current gold standard of suture gastrostomy repair, which carries a near-zero leak rate. The Natural Orifice Surgery Consortium for Assessment and Research White Paper published in 2005 with the goal of creating safety in the development of NOTES states that a "100 % reliable means of gastric closure must be developed" [6]. This group recognizes the detriment to this new technique of the potential complications and morbidity from even a low leak rate. For the benefits of NOTES to be advantageous over laparoscopic approaches, the potential complication profile of the transvisceral closure must be kept to a minimum.

Closure Types and Devices

Many techniques for transvisceral closure following NOTES have been described. Multiple authors, including Arezzo and Morino [7] and Sodergren et al. [8], have performed thorough reviews, detailing procedural specifics associated with multiple devices. For the purpose of this chapter, the generalized approaches used for closure will be detailed, but we refer you to the primary literature for specifics. Options available for closure have included endoscopic sutures, endoscopic staplers, clips, T-tags, tunnel formation, and PEG tube placement. When assessing closure devices, the Natural Orifice Surgery Consortium for Assessment and Research Working Group has developed generalized recommendations regarding the advantages and disadvantages for each type of closure technique [9]. The closure devices listed below are the commonly described techniques for the treatment of full-thickness viscerotomy following NOTES.

Direct Suture Closure

Suture closure of a transvisceral incision is feasible in the situation of transvaginal closure, requiring standard open instrumentation and suture. The skills and supplies used for this type of closure are performed frequently following accepted surgical procedures, such as a standard transvaginal hysterectomy. This approach of primary closure is safe and effective, with no reported cases of transvaginal evisceration following NOTES, although this rare complication has been described in the literature following gynecologic surgery [10]. The approach of direct suture-based closure may also be applicable to NOTES procedures performed through the rectum, as supported by the TEM literature [11], but the true safety of this approach for NOTES remains to be determined.

Laparoscopic-Assisted Closure

Many NOTES approaches are currently being performed under the assistance of laparoscopic guidance until the technical advances required for pure NOTES are accomplished. In these circumstances, visceral closure is often assisted by or performed using standard laparoscopic techniques. This may be as straightforward as a primary repair using suturing or stapling devices or may be a laparoscopic-assisted buttress, such as omental patch or oversewing of a primarily endoscopic closure. Until the endoscopic closure devices detailed below are optimized, laparoscopic (or open) surgical closure remains the gold standard in the treatment of viscerotomy.

Endoscopic Suturing Devices

Several methods for endoscopic suturing techniques have been reported. Closure with sutures is a traditional, validated way of closing a full-thickness incision, as has been evidenced in both open and laparoscopic techniques. Endoscopic suturing is valuable in that the technique for closure can be applied to most situations, allowing applicability to various anatomic sites. By modification of the suturing pattern, any size or shape of opening can be successfully closed. When compared to other devices, endoscopic suture placement may allow for greater control, determining adequate tissue incorporation and preventing damage to surrounding structures.

Endoscopic suturing, however, does have challenges. These devices may be difficult to use, and ergonomic design leaves room for improvement. Endoscopic suturing does require a higher level of skill needed for accurate and successful stitch placement when compared to clip closure devices. The cost of a single device is not low, and multiple reloads may be required for the closure of a standard transvisceral opening.

Additional improvements in endoluminal suturing devices are focusing on a more user-friendly platform with the desire of minimizing the learning curve associated with the use of these new devices. Advances in endoluminal tissue manipulation and the development of multiple stitch deployments will also help these platforms become more widely used.

Stapling Devices

Stapling devices have become a commonly used device in both open and laparoscopic surgical approaches, and, to the surgeon, it would make sense that an endoscopic stapling device would be an ideal closure for transvisceral openings. Staplers provide a validated, one-step approach to full-thickness closure that can be applied to both large and small visceral openings. The ability to perform tissue manipulation to allow for appropriate placement of the staple line, however, may limit the use of this technique. The current devices for endoscopic stapling are larger platforms and the directional manipulation is limited. There is also no optical component included, relying on an additional endoscope to provide visualization of the working space. These devices also carry a high cost and require complex engineering on the part of the designer. There are currently no commercially available, FDA-approved endoscopic stapling devices on the market.

Stapling devices continue to be an appropriate platform for NOTES closure, but the addition of maneuverability and optics to existing platforms will greatly improve the ease of use for these products. Other limitations that must be improved before widespread use include methods for tissue manipulation, allowing accurate and adequate staple line location, and smaller-diameter instruments, especially if an additional endoscope is required for visualization.

Clip Closure Devices

Clips are one of the most straightforward ways to close a full-thickness opening following NOTES. They offer a significant ease of use with a straightforward approach to deployment. Clips have been shown to produce high closure pressures but may not result in full-thickness reapproximation of divided tissue. Clips are economical for single use, but to obtain adequate closure, multiple applications may be required, increasing cost. Clips may also be disadvantageous from the perspective that they may have orientation issues for placement, especially in the setting of inadequate insufflation pressures or poor visualization. Clips are also not removable if applied to an inappropriate location. The application of endoscopic clips may be supplemented by other approaches, improving the efficacy of closure, for example, the use of omental patches or the application of preformed endoloop sutures.

Further investigations into the use of clips for transvisceral closure should focus on the durability of clip placement. Details regarding migration and dislodgement remain to be clarified. The improvement of tissue manipulation or the development of a repositionable clip would offer great advantage in the NOTES use for these endoscopic devices. Other ideas described for the development of clips would be a platform capable of multiple clip deployments and the use of a bioabsorbable clip, hypothesized to have less foreign body reaction.

T-Tag Closure Systems

T-tag–based systems are commercially available and are quick ways of reapproximating tissue. Surgeons are comfortable with the deployment of these devices, as they are used in laparoscopic gastrostomies and many other procedures. T-tags have the advantage of ease of use when compared to other closure methods. They provide a possibility for preplacement of the closure device before the viscerotomy is performed, potentially decreasing the risk of poor visualization as a limitation of closure.

The primary limitation to T-tag systems currently is the risk of injury to surrounding structures, which has been reported in up to 12.5 % of all deployments [12]. Because of the relatively blind nature of the deployment, the depth of puncture and location of firing cannot always be assessed as safe. Multiple T-tags may be required for the closure of a standard viscerotomy and, due to the uneven distribution, may have unequal force distribution over the closure. This may lead to less secure closures if T-tags are not deployed appropriately.

Future directions for the development of T-tag closure devices need improvements in deployment to assure safety. Modifications in the design that would allow for a more equal distribution of tension would also be advantageous.

Tunnel-Based Closures

As a modification of access to the peritoneum, creation a tunnel during entry may also function as a way for addressing closure of the viscerotomy. This approach can be performed using mechanical, water-based, or air-based dissection. It requires technical skill and can be time-consuming but financially adds little cost to the supplies needed for NOTES. This approach has only been described for upper gastrointestinal access approaches and is restricted in the ability to extract larger specimens, given the limited size of the tunnel created. It does, however, have the potential advantage of stabilizing the scope for the duration of the NOTES procedure. The potential infectious risks of tunnel formation compared to direct viscerotomy remain to be clarified. Future directions for tunnel-based therapies must be directed at the generalizability of this approach, reducing the time and training needed to perform this procedure.

Other Endoscopic Closure Techniques

Plugs offer the advantage of quick, easy closure but are limited by the commercially available sizes and shapes of these devices. Investigational development of absorbable occlusion devices may increase the use of this device by reducing the risk of a foreign body reaction. The use of a PEG tube for closure of gastrostomy access sites has been reported [13]. This approach uses available materials but does result in a visible scar, changing the scar-free idea of NOTES. Other mechanisms, such as the application of glues, have been mentioned but have not come to widespread use for reliable closure.

Evaluation of Adequate Transvisceral Closure

In the assessment of closure strategies, one must evaluate what is the best criterion on which to judge transvisceral closure. Multiple published studies assessing transvisceral closure have not come to a consensus as to what is the ideal method for this evaluation. Described methods include the use of air- and water-leak pressures, appearance at necropsy, fluoroscopic imaging, animal survival models, and abdominal microbiology as means of assessing quality.

When looking at the colorectal literature, intraoperative evaluation of the anastomosis through leak testing has been shown to decrease both the rate of clinical and radiographic anastomotic leak rate [2]. A similar trend has been shown in the bariatric literature [14]. It is the hope that this assessment of intraoperative anastomotic integrity will be able to decrease the rate of and/or prevent complications associated with anastomotic breakdown.

One method for assessing closure following NOTES is through the use of pressure testing. When critically evaluating the data available by authors from our institution and others [15], the idea of bursting pressures as the ideal test for anastomotic integrity falls short. In comparison of four independent transgastric closure devices by pressure testing, most specimens failed at a nonsurgical site, implying that the strength of the anastomosis created by all devices was superior to that of the native, nonsurgical tissue [4]. Because of this finding, additional methods beyond pressure measurement are required to assess adequate closure following NOTES.

Leak testing using fluid or air, as is commonly performed in colorectal and bariatric surgery, have been evaluated in the assessment of closure devices. Air-leak tests have been performed using saline submersion under laparoscopic guidance and using intraperitoneal pressure measurements as a marker for leak [12]. Fluid-leak tests have been described using methylene blue injection under visual inspection and using contrast injection under fluoroscopic assessment. As we have seen with similar leak tests in humans following other procedures, the sensitivity and specificity of these tests are not 100 %. The idea, however, behind anastomotic evaluation to decrease morbidity is an important one.

After performing a review of 46 studies describing 20 closure devices, Sodergren et al. [8] concluded that there is no standardized method for testing anastomotic integrity following NOTES in the published literature. The authors have proposed an inclusive approach for evaluating transvisceral closure in an animal model for future device development. Following the closure approach, radiographic imaging with fluoroscopy should be performed. Animals should be serially evaluated for sepsis or signs of peritonitis. Endoscopic examination of the closure area should be performed on postprocedure day 7 to assess anastomotic integrity. Euthanasia should be deferred until at least 7 days following the procedure, with a thorough evaluation at necropsy of the abdomen and closure site. Explanted closure sites should then be subjected to air- and water-leak testing, and histologic evaluation should be performed on the closure area. This approach for evaluating closure methods remains to be tested but does offer a thorough approach into the investigation of new closure devices.

In summary, NOTES offers many potential advantages, including less pain, improved cosmesis, and shortened recovery. The widespread introduction of this operative technique remains limited by reliable, safe transvisceral closure. Many attempts have been made to develop closure methods that will consistently maintain a high standard of repair with low patient morbidity. Devices continue to face challenges of providing full-thickness tissue incorporation, visualizing closure sites adequately, and avoiding inadvertent injury to surrounding structures. Options for closure have included open or laparoscopic suture closure, endoscopic suturing, clip devices, endoscopic stapling, T-tag closures, tunnel-based approaches, and others. Once designed, the platform on which to assess a NOTES closure continues to allow room for improvement. Despite the multiple publications and ideas at this time, no single approach has shown superiority in providing reliable results with low morbidity. This challenge of appropriate transvisceral closure continues to be an obstacle that must be conquered before NOTES can be introduced into widespread use.

Conflict of Interest   The authors have no relevant financial disclosures or conflicts of interest.

References

1. Davies AH, Bartolo DC, Richards AE, et al. Intra-operative air testing: an audit on rectal anastomosis. Ann R Coll Surg Engl. 1988;70:345–7.
2. Beard JD, Nicholson ML, Sayers RD, Lloyd D, Everson NW. Intraoperative air testing of colorectal anastomoses: a prospective, randomized trial. Br J Surg. 1990;77:1095–7.
3. Sclabas GM, Swain P, Swanstrom LL. Endoluminal methods for gastrotomy closure in natural orifice transenteric surgery (NOTES). Surg Innov. 2006;13(1):23–30.
4. Schomisch S. Overcoming barriers to natural orifice translumenal endoscopic surgery (NOTES). OhioLINK Electronic Theses and Dissertations Center. 2009. Available at: http://olc1.ohiolink.edu:80/record=b27746215~S0. Accessed on 20 June 2012.
5. Rattner D, Kalloo A. ASGE/SAGES Working Group on natural orifice translumenal endoscopic surgery, October 2005. Surg Endosc. 2006;20:329–33.
6. Hawes R. ASGE/SAGES Working Group on natural orifice translumenal endoscopic surgery white paper, October 2005. Gastrointest Endosc. 2006;63:199–203.
7. Arezzo A, Morino M. Endoscopic closure of gastric access in perspective NOTES: an update on techniques and technologies. Surg Endosc. 2010;24(2):298–303.
8. Sodergren MH, Coomber R, Clark J, et al. What are the elements of safe gastrotomy closure in NOTES? A systematic review. Surg Innov. 2010;17(4):318–31.

9. Natural Orifice Surgery Consortium for Assessment and Research 2009 Working Group on closure. 2009. Available at: http://www.noscar.org. Accessed 14 Mar 2011.
10. Kang WD, Kim SM, Choi HS. Vaginal evisceration after radical hysterectomy and adjuvant radiation. J Gynecol Oncol. 2009;20(1):63–4.
11. Gavagan JA, Whiteford MH, Swanstrom LL. Full-thickness intraperitoneal excision by transanal endoscopic microsurgery does not increase short-term complications. Am J Surg. 2004;187(5):630–4.
12. Dray X, Gabrielson KL, Buscaglia JM, et al. Air and fluid leak tests after NOTES procedures: a pilot study in a live porcine model. Gastrointest Endosc. 2008;68:513–9.
13. Marks J, Rosen M, McGee M, et al. A novel technique for management of endoscopic gastrotomy following natural orifice transvisceral endoscopic surgery. Surg Endosc. 2006;20:S287.
14. Shin RB. Intraoperative endoscopic test resulting in no postoperative leaks from the gastric pouch and gastrojejunal anastomosis in 366 laparoscopic Roux-en-Y gastric bypasses. Obes Surg. 2004;14(8):1067–9.
15. Ryou M, Fong DG, Pai RD, et al. Transluminal closure for NOTES: an ex vivo study comparing leak pressures of various gastrotomy and colotomy closure modalities. Endoscopy. 2008;40(5):432–6.

Chapter 7
Mini-Laparoscopic Systems

John E. Humphrey and David Canes

Keywords Laparoscopy • Minimally invasive • LESS • Mini-laparoscopy • NOTES

Introduction

The Impetus for Mini-Laparoscopic Systems

One of the driving forces behind the development of laparoscopy has always been to decrease the morbidity of a laparotomy incision. The evolution from open surgery to laparoscopy was the initial and most dramatic step in this progression. Mini-laparoscopy, whereby the size of each laparoscopic instrument was decreased to the limits of useful instrumentation, was thought to be the next natural evolution in accomplishing this goal. By developing the smallest tools possible to safely and effectively perform surgery, and if each access point creates pain and potential complications, one might limit the trauma inherent to a given operation by miniaturizing each access point.

Traditional laparoscopy utilizes laparoscopes between 5 and 10 mm in diameter, affording excellent resolution and lighting. Mini-laparoscopy refers to the transition to even smaller scopes and instruments. Mini-laparoscopic systems are those that utilize these newer instruments and their technologies to provide an environment for patients to have smaller incisions and, theoretically, less overall pain.

J.E. Humphrey, M.D. (✉) • D. Canes, M.D.
Lahey Clinic Institute of Urology, Institute of Urology,
Lahey Clinic Medical Center, Tufts University School of Medicine,
41 Mall Road, Burlington, MA 01805, USA
e-mail: john.e.humphrey@lahey.org; david.canes@lahey.org

A. Rane et al. (eds.), *Scar-Less Surgery*,
DOI 10.1007/978-1-84800-360-6_7, © Springer-Verlag London 2013

A multitude of terms have been applied in this arena, including mini-laparoscopy, micro-laparoscopy, small-diameter laparoscopy, and needlescopic surgery. The published literature is broadly inclusive as regards the actual diameter of the instruments, ranging from 1.9 to 5 mm. For the purposes of this chapter, we define mini-laparoscopy to encompass the use of instruments 3.5 mm or smaller. We exclude 5 mm since they are widely regarded as conventional pure laparoscopy. Our goals are to review the origins of mini-laparoscopy and describe its use as a standalone technique, as an adjunct to standard laparoscopy, as well as its resurgence as an adjunct to the latest scarless surgical techniques, including laparoendoscopic single-site surgery (LESS) and natural orifice translumenal endoscopic surgery (NOTES).

Early History

Gynecologic surgeons were the first to incorporate mini-laparoscopy and publish their experience. The first reports describe its use for diagnostic laparoscopy in 1991, but the results were hampered by the prevailing technology, given the low levels of light and poor resolution through the smaller laparoscopes [1]. As instrumentation and optics advanced, the technique showed more promise not only for diagnostic purposes, but also for therapeutic interventions. Bauer et al. described mini-laparoscopy use for diagnosis as well as for obtaining peritoneal access for conventional laparoscopy in patients with extensive intraabdominal adhesions [2]. A 1.9-mm laparoscope was used through a Veress needle port. Although one may argue that the resolution did not have to be profound for the purpose, the visualization through these diminutive scopes was felt to be comparable to conventional for the diagnosis and staging of endometriosis and adnexal adhesions in patients with pelvic pain [3].

The progression of mini-laparoscopy eventually led other specialties to extend its early indications. General surgeons have used mini-laparoscopy for traditionally laparoscopic cases such as cholecystectomy [4] and appendectomy [5], with comparable outcomes, including hospital stay and perioperative complications. In these retrospective reviews, perioperative outcomes were equivalent between standard and mini-laparoscopic techniques, and a trend was apparent that more mini-laparoscopic cases were converted to open surgery. Tu and Advincula [6] reviewed the rise of mini-laparoscopic systems as they relate to gynecologic surgery. They point out both the benefits and limitations of using smaller instruments. The main deterrent to smaller instruments as described above has been the limitations of the optics inherent in smaller scopes. The 5- and 10-mm endoscopes use a rod-lens system that allows the operator to see with great clarity, and include a variety of viewing angles, from the 0° lens to 30°, 45°, and 70° lenses. Smaller 2-mm scopes use semirigid and deflectable fiber optic bundles, which, although they have improved, still provide less resolution and a decreased depth of field compared to the larger lenses. Durability has also been a concern with smaller instruments, given the inherent fragility with decreasing size.

The initial experience with mini-laparoscopy (specifically 2-mm instruments) in the field of urology was reviewed by Soble and Gill in 1998 [7]. They described the use of "needlescopic" instruments in 42 procedures. At the time, certain tools were unavailable with a diameter of 2 mm, such as a clip-applier and hook-blade electrode. Not all procedures were pure mini-laparoscopy. The extirpative procedures required one 10-mm port and one 5-mm port to supplement the remaining 2-mm ports. The 5-mm port was necessary given the lack of certain 2-mm instruments at the time. The authors report that 90.5 % of the cases were successful, with three cases converted to conventional laparoscopy and one to an open procedure. The authors highlighted inferior optics (resolution, clarity, and light-carrying capacity), lack of instrument rigidity, and weaker grasping capability as inherent disadvantages. The advantages were threefold: improved cosmesis, decreased analgesic requirements, and possibly reduced hospital stay. The learning curve was steep, however, and patient selection important (the procedure converted to open was in an obese patient). Although the technology at the time was inferior to 5- and 10-mm instruments, the authors hoped that future developments would make these procedures more feasible.

Although these early results of needlescopic surgery in urology were promising, the anticipated surge was not realized. The reasons are multifactorial but may be due to the fact that standard laparoscopy was itself diffusing nationwide in its own right, and surgeons may have been reluctant to simultaneously adopt instrumentation that was harder to control, deflectable, and more difficult to obtain and maintain. More recently, even as laparoscopic techniques have become commonplace, attention has turned to other rising technical advances such as robotics and, more recently, single-site surgery. Now, with renewed interest in patient cosmesis and perioperative pain management, mini-laparoscopy has reentered the conversation.

Nomenclature

In an effort to standardize the terms used to describe NOTES and LESS within the literature, the Urologic NOTES Working Group published nomenclature for both techniques [8]. NOTES is designated as a surgical procedure utilizing a natural orifice to puncture a hollow viscera to enter an otherwise inaccessible body cavity. If there are additional ports/instruments passed transabdominally, this is designated as a hybrid NOTES procedure (if >75 % is performed via the natural orifice). However, if the natural orifice is not the main port of the procedure, it is considered a NOTES-assisted surgery.

LESS, or laparoendoscopic single-site surgery, refers to a minimally invasive operation performed through a single incision/location using conventional laparoscopic or newer instrumentation (fixed prebent or deflectable flexible laparoscopic instruments). This term was put forward to incorporate previous terms, such as E-NOTES, SILS, OPUS, SPA, VSUS, SPL, and SIL, among others. LESS was further defined in 2010 at a consensus conference, where the ancillary use of

Fig. 7.1 LESS donor
nephrectomy, whereby
(*arrow*) mini-lap site does not
detract from the overall
cosmesis

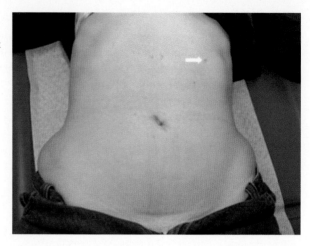

1.9-mm needle instruments was embraced, in the hopes that it would promote the
advancement of the bourgeoning field [9]. In addition to a single-site port used for
the majority of the operation, the needle instruments can be placed through a 2-mm
Veress needle port requiring only a skin puncture and no true incision. There are
several potential advantages to using mini-laparoscopic adjuncts to LESS: enhanced
patient safety, increased intraoperative dexterity, and a greater repertoire of LESS
surgery to more complex procedures. In addition, and most importantly, needlescopic instruments help to restore surgical triangulation without substantially
detracting from the overall cosmesis with LESS (Fig. 7.1). Also noted are the limitations, however, of reliability, strength, design, and lack of variety in needle instruments. Even with these difficulties, it is clear that the use of ancillary needle
instruments will continue to provide invaluable aid to surgeons performing LESS
procedures, particularly during their learning curves.

What Benefits Are Proven?

With every purported surgical advance, one must avoid the allure of technology for
technology's sake alone. Our patients must always be the focus, such that a successful
operation fits the surgical indication for a given disease process. The ultimate goal of
an operation is defined by the patient's clinical disease and the indication for performing the operation. This must be kept in mind with new technology that is geared toward
smaller incisions. Micali et al. [10] pointed out that LESS has only been shown to give
a benefit in cosmetic outcome. Functional and oncological outcomes are lacking.
Moreover, with extirpative procedures, an incision may need to be extended anyway at
the end of a case for specimen retrieval, therefore nullifying the cosmetic advantage.

One technique that has been evaluated in the urologic literature to conceal the single-site scar is LESS performed through an umbilical incision, or U-LESS (previously
coined "embryonic natural orifice transumbilical endoscopic surgery," or E-NOTES).

Fig. 7.2 MiniPort™
(Covidien, Dublin, Ireland)
for 2-mm access

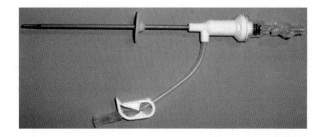

In a review article, Canes et al. [11] described the technique, instrumentation, and perioperative outcomes of U-LESS in both nonurologic and urologic procedures. An intraumbilical incision is used to place various types of ports (e.g., TriPort, Olympus, Center Valley, PA) that can accommodate one 12-mm instrument and two 5-mm instruments. The procedures completed range from extirpative (e.g., nephrectomy) to reconstructive (pyeloplasty). Live-donor nephrectomy is one procedure in which mini-laparoscopy has been used in conjunction with LESS: A needlescopic grasper was used through a 2-mm port for tissue retraction. This is an example of the use of mini-laparoscopy as an adjunct to LESS in early series. The technical challenges of LESS include triangulation, retraction, instrument crowding, and patient-related limitations. There is a real difference in technique compared with conventional laparoscopy, and therefore a steep learning curve even for fully trained laparoscopists. However, with ever-improving instrumentation, the future direction of LESS is promising. The addition of mini-laparoscopy as an adjunct to LESS has been important in easing the transition from standard laparoscopy.

Technique and Instruments

The armament of mini-laparoscopic instruments has grown since its initial use. For 2-mm instruments, the MiniSite™ MiniPort™ (Covidien, Dublin, Ireland) combines a Veress needle with an outer sheath (Fig. 7.2) that is left in place as a needlescopic port [7, 12]. As such, it serves a dual purpose. These skin punctures only need a single Steri-strip or dermal adhesive alone for closure, negating the need for suturing. An apparent cosmetic advantage to their use is therefore apparent (Fig. 7.1). Table 7.1 shows the available trocars, instruments, and scopes for mini-laparoscopy.

Applications

Pure Mini-Laparoscopy

The use of mini-laparoscopy as a standalone technique is limited in urology. However, diminutive instrumentation has had particular allure in the pediatric arena. The treatment of pediatric hydroceles by mini-laparoscopic high-ligation of the

Table 7.1 Mini-laparoscopic instrumentation

Name	Size (mm)	Manufacturer
Trocars		
ENDOPATH mini/micro trocars nonoptical	2–3	Ethicon
ENDOPATH access needle	3	Ethicon
Minisite™ MiniPort™ introducer system	2	Covidien
Instruments		
KOH ultramicro needle holder	3	Karl Storz
Pediatric laparoscopic instrument set[a]	3	Karl Storz
Reusable laparoscopic instruments	2	Covidien
Minisite™ ENDO GRASP™	2	Covidien
Minisite™ Minishears™	2	Covidien
Scopes		
0° and 30° laparoscope[a]	3	Karl Storz
0° laparoscope	3	Olympus

[a]Designed for pediatric use, therefore shorter length

processus vaginalis has been described [13]. Orchiopexy and orchiectomy for cryptorchidism has also been performed with success [14].

Adult applications have included varicocelectomy [15] and adrenalectomy [16]. For varicocelectomy, three 3.5-mm trocars were used with successful ligation of all spermatic veins and preservation of spermatic arteries and lymphatics. The authors report success with only a 0.6 % recurrence rate in 87 patients treated. An impressively large series of mini-laparoscopic adrenalectomies was performed for 112 patients with adrenal tumors of less than 5 cm. The diameter used for the working ports was 2 mm, while the tumor was extracted from an umbilical incision. The operative time was longer compared to conventional laparoscopy, but the feasibility of mini-laparoscopic adrenalectomy was demonstrated.

Nonurologic pure mini-laparoscopy has seen a broader application. As previously mentioned, gynecologists have used mini-laparoscopy for diagnostic purposes as well as pelvic pain mapping [6], and general surgeons for cholecystectomy [4] and appendectomy [5]. Pediatric laparoscopic inguinal hernia repair using three 3.5-mm trocars with corresponding telescope and instruments has also been shown to be an effective alternative to standard open herniotomy [17]. Overall, pure mini-laparoscopy has solidified its presence in the surgical community as an effective standalone technique.

Conventional Laparoscopy with Mini-Laparoscopy

Recoiling somewhat from purists, surgeons began to incorporate the selective use of mini-laparoscopic instrumentation during standard laparoscopy. Indeed, the patient can still gain cosmetic benefit from using needlescopic instruments during conventional laparoscopic procedures where applicable. In this way, 2- or 3-mm instruments replace the traditional 5-mm working ports, while still utilizing a larger 10–12-mm trocar for the endoscope and larger instruments. This combines excellent optics with improved cosmesis, without sacrificing triangulation. An example of such a technique has been described for laparoscopic adrenalectomy with selective use of needlescopic instruments [18]. A 12-mm umbilical port is used with the addition of two 2-mm working ports in the left subcostal region in order to complete the operation. The same concept can be applied to any laparoscopic procedure, and as such the combinations of standard and mini-laparoscopic instruments are limited only by surgical creativity.

Nonurologic applications of this technique have been demonstrated as well. Ventral hernia repair has been performed using both conventional and mini-laparoscopic ports [19]. A main 12-mm port is introduced as well as a variable number of working ports (2–5-mm) individualized based on the size, location, and number of hernia defects present. Similarly, total laparoscopic hysterectomy has benefited from needlescopic instruments by using a 5-mm umbilical laparoscope with 3-mm working ports [20]. The port size can safely be reduced with improvement in cosmesis and no detriment to the surgeon's technical performance.

NOTES and Mini-Laparoscopy

The use of NOTES in urology has mainly been described utilizing transvaginal access for the portal of entry. Pure NOTES transvaginal nephrectomy without any transabdominal incisions/ports is already a reality [21]. However, without assistance from an umbilical port or needle instruments, the operation is time-consuming and technically difficult. Hybrid NOTES nephrectomy was previously described [22], using two abdominal 5-mm trocars to aid in visualization and triangulation. Although this still requires abdominal incisions, it points toward the advantage in having abdominal instruments to aid in the procedure.

Mini-laparoscopic abdominal instruments have successfully bridged the gap in nonurologic NOTES procedures. The term used to describe them is "mini-laparoscopic-assisted natural orifice surgery," or MANOS [23]. Gynecological procedures such as ovarian cystectomies, oophorectomies, and salpingo-oophorectomies have been completed in this fashion. Appendectomy has also been described using the MANOS technique. The use of mini-laparoscopy with NOTES combines the cosmetic and triangulation advantage of additional mini-laparoscopic abdominal ports with the optimal insufflation, irrigation, extraction, and larger instruments utilized by the transvaginal port.

Porpiglia et al. described a similar urologic technique (not actually coined as MANOS), with transvaginal NOTES-assisted mini-laparoscopic nephrectomy [24]. They describe their experience with five patients undergoing nephrectomy with a 12-mm vaginal port and three 3.5-mm transabdominal ports. In contrast to a pure

Table 7.2 NOTES and mini-laparoscopy

Year	Author	Procedure(s) (number performed)	Access	Comments
Urologic				
2011	Porpiglia et al. [24]	Nephrectomy [5]	One 12-mm transvaginal port Three 3.5-mm abdominal ports	Simpler than pure NOTES, with less operative time and technical difficulty
Nonurologic				
2007	Tsin et al. [23]	Ovarian cystectomy, oophorectomy, salpingo-oophorecto- mies, myomectomies, appendectomies, and cholecystectomies (total = 100)	One 12-mm transvaginal port Three 3-mm abdominal ports	Describes a variety of NOTES procedures aided by mini- laparoscopy
2009	Noguera et al. [25]	Cholecystectomy [16]	One 12-mm transvaginal port One 5-mm umbilical port One 3-mm right upper quadrant port	Safe technique to bridge NOTES with laparos- copy, without abdominal wall incisions

NOTES nephrectomy, this technique offers a simpler approach with less difficulty without compromising the cosmetic benefit. Most importantly, the presence of needlescopic instruments arguably made this pioneering work possible. There will no doubt be more uses of mini-laparoscopy with NOTES in urology since these techniques are in their infancy, and such hybrid approaches add a degree of safety to these challenging procedures. Table 7.2 shows the use of mini-laparoscopy as an adjunct to NOTES procedures, in both urologic and nonurologic literature.

LESS and Mini-Laparoscopy

Many of the first reports of LESS incorporated needlescopic instrumentation as adjuncts. The use of ancillary needle instruments during LESS restores triangula- tion, improves dexterity, may enhance patient safety and cosmesis, and broadens the scope of LESS within urology. The reader should certainly not get the impression that mini-laparoscopic instrumentation is required for LESS, as surgeons have made significant strides successfully with pure LESS [26–28]. However, pure LESS with- out the use of adjunctive needlescopic instruments can be frustrating, given the poor

Table 7.3 LESS and mini-laparoscopy in urology

Year	Author	Procedure(s) (# performed)	Access	Mini-laparoscopic function	Comments
2010	Kawauchi et al. [29]	Pyeloplasty [1]	Triport at umbilicus 2-mm miniport at left subcostal area	Used for difficult dissection, left hand grasper, and placement of drain postprocedure	Insertion of 2-mm port helps to reduce operative time
2007	Raman et al. [30]	Right nephrectomy [1]	Three adjacent umbilical 5-mm trocars One 3-mm subxyphoid trocar	Used for liver retraction	Not needed during two left nephrectomies
2008	Desai et al. [12]	Pyeloplasty [1]	Umbilical triport One 2-mm needlescopic left subcostal port	Aid in retraction and triangulation for pyeloplasty suturing	Suggest use of needlescopic port facilitates triangulation during LESS
2008	Gill et al. [31]	Donor nephrectomy [4]	Umbilical triport One 2-mm needlescopic left subcostal port	Used for initial pneumoperitoneum, adds triangulation and retraction	Selective use of 2-mm instruments expands scope of single-site surgery
2008	Aron et al. [32]	Partial nephrectomy [5]	Umbilical triport One 2-mm needlescopic right lower quadrant port	Used for retraction and dissection	2-mm site heals with excellent cosmesis
2009	Ganpule et al. [33]	Donor nephrectomy [11]	Umbilical triport Extra 3- or 5-mm port	Used for retraction in 11 of 13 patients	Majority of cases benefited from extra-small grasper

(continued)

Table 7.3 (continued)

Year	Author	Procedure(s) (# performed)	Access	Mini-laparoscopic function	Comments
2009	Desai et al. [34]	Pyeloplasty [4] Ileal ureter [1] Psoas hitch [1]	Umbilical triport Variable-position left-sided needlescopic port	Used with left hand during suturing	Complex suturing for reconstruction facilitated by needlescopic instruments
2009	Desai et al. [35]	Simple nephrectomy [5] Radical nephrectomy [3] Donor nephrectomy [18] Partial nephrectomy [6] Kidney cyst excision [1] Pyeloplasty [20] Ureteral reimplant [2] Ileal ureter [3] Adrenalectomy [1]	Umbilical triport One 2-mm needlescopic port in various positions	Assist with retraction and suturing	Demonstrates wide variety in procedures
2009	Raman et al. [36]	Right nephrectomies (not reported)	Three adjacent 5-mm umbilical trocars One 3-mm subxyphoid trocar	Used for liver retraction	Only with right nephrectomy for liver retraction
2009	Tracy et al. [37]	Pyeloplasty [15]	Three adjacent 5-mm umbilical trocars One 5-mm trocar midaxillary line One 3-mm subxyphoid port (right side only)	5-mm used for suturing and drain site, 3-mm for liver retraction in right pyeloplasty	Note difficulty in performing suturing without extra port

2010	Raybourn et al. [38]	Nephrectomy [2]	Umbilical triport One 2-mm needlescopic grasper in one case One 5-mm grasper through 3-mm incision in second case	Used for retraction	Only used in 2 of 11 nephrectomies due to difficult retraction
2010	Canes et al. [39]	Donor nephrectomy [19]	Umbilical triport One 2-mm needlescopic grasper in hypochondrium	Tissue retraction and dissection	Solidifies technique previously described

Fig. 7.3 Mini-laparoscopic
adjunct for liver retraction
during LESS (Courtesy of
Jay Raman, M.D.)

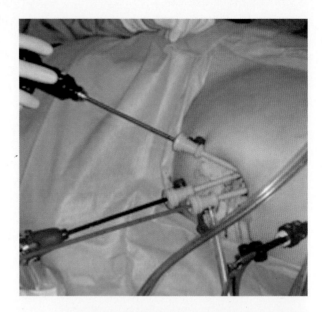

Fig. 7.4 Mini-laparoscopic
adjunct to LESS pyeloplasty

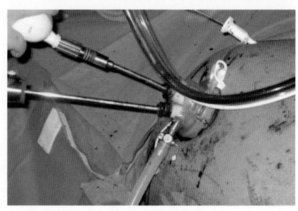

triangulation with instrument clashing and a steep learning curve. As a result, the
early LESS literature saw a resurgence in needlescopic instruments. Table 7.3 demonstrates the impact of mini-laparoscopy on LESS. Although we define mini-laparoscopy as using instruments equal to or less than 3.5 mm in diameter, we have
included those series using up to 5-mm ancillary ports for completeness.

As the table demonstrates, the number of different LESS procedures to which
mini-laparoscopic assistance has been applied is vast. The functions of the ancillary
instruments generally fall into three categories: (1) right-sided upper tract surgery,
where liver retraction is required and cannot be accomplished easily from the primary entry site (Fig. 7.3); (2) to facilitate suturing as a nondominant hand grasping
tool during complex reconstructive cases such as pyeloplasty (Fig. 7.4); and (3) as
a generic dissection or retraction tool. To put it simply, the needlescopic instruments

restore triangulation, thereby overcoming the most frustrating aspects of pure LESS. While not yet substantially patient-driven, a subset of patients does express a desire for improved cosmesis. Mini-laparoscopic-assisted LESS provides an opportunity for the surgeon to safely complete a given procedure while addressing this concern. Needlescopic surgery lay relatively dormant until the steep LESS learning curve revived its use. Depending on the trajectory of dedicated LESS instrumentation, mini-laparoscopy may continue to find a role in this regard.

Conclusion

Mini-laparoscopy began in the 1990s and was thought to be the next natural progression in the ever-increasing drive for surgery to become less invasive. In spite of its promise, its diffusion was limited and its applications remained limited to single centers based on surgical preference. Most agree that a cosmetic advantage exists for these instruments compared to standard (5-mm and larger) laparoscopic port sites. While scattered retrospective series demonstrated decreased pain and in some cases shorter convalescence for patients undergoing mini-laparoscopic surgery, such advantages have never been conclusively proven in adequately powered prospective studies.

With the emergence of LESS and NOTES and the drive for scar-free or nearly scar-free surgery, mini-laparoscopy has enjoyed a resurgence. Industry has provided new and more robust instrumentation. The adjunctive use of mini-laparoscopic systems enables the urologist to have confidence in learning and completing NOTES, and LESS procedures, and also serves as an adjunct during conventional laparoscopy. Prospective studies examining the effect of mini-laparoscopy on perioperative outcomes are needed.

References

1. Dorsey JH, Tabb CR. Mini-laparoscopy and fiber-optic lasers. Obstet Gynecol Clin North Am. 1991;18(3):613–7.
2. Bauer O, Devroey P, Wisanto A, et al. Small diameter laparoscopy using a microlaparoscope. Hum Reprod. 1995;10(6):1461–4.
3. Faber BM, Coddington III CC. Microlaparoscopy: a comparative study of diagnostic accuracy. Fertil Steril. 1997;67(5):952–4.
4. Thakur V, Schlachta CM, Jayaraman S. Minilaparoscopic versus conventional laparoscopic cholecystectomy. Ann Surg. 2011;253:244–58.
5. Sajid MS, Khan MA, Cheek E, Baig MK. Needlescopic versus laparoscopic appendectomy: a systematic review. Can J Surg. 2009;52(2):129–34.
6. Tu FF, Advincula AP. Miniaturizing the laparoscope: current applications of micro- and mini-laparoscopy. Int J Gynaecol Obstet. 2008;100:94–8.
7. Soble JJ, Gill IS. Needlescopic urology: incorporating 2-mm instruments in laparoscopic surgery. Urology. 1998;52:187–94.

8. Box G, Averch T, Cadeddu J, et al. Nomenclature of natural orifice transluminal endoscopic surgery (NOTES™) and laparoendoscopic single-site surgery (LESS) procedures in urology. J Endourol. 2008;22(11):2575–81.

9. Gill IS, Advincula AP, Aron M, et al. Consensus statement of the consortium for laparoendoscopic single-site surgery. Surg Endosc. 2010;24:762–8.

10. Micali S, Pini G, Teber D, et al. New trends in minimally invasive urological surgery. What is beyond the robot? World J Urol. 2010. doi:10.1007/s00345-010-0588-5.

11. Canes D, Desai MM, Aron M, et al. Transumbilical single-port surgery: evolution and current status. Eur Urol. 2008;54:1020–30.

12. Desai MM, Rao PP, Aron M, et al. Scarless single port transumbilical nephrectomy and pyeloplasty: first clinical report. BJU Int. 2008;101:83–8.

13. Ho C, Yang SS, Tsai Y. Minilaparoscopic high-ligation with the processus vaginalis undissected and left *in situ* is a safe, effective, and durable treatment for pediatric hydrocele. Urology. 2010;76:134–7.

14. Gill IS, Ross JH, Sung GT, Kay R. Needlescopic surgery for cryptorchidism: the initial series. J Pediatr Surg. 2000;35(10):1426–30.

15. Chung SD, Wu CC, Lin VC, et al. Minilaparoscopic varicocelectomy with preservation of testicular artery and lymphatic vessels by using intracorporeal knot-tying technique: five-year experience. World J Surg. 2011;35(8):1785–90. doi:10.1007/s00268-011-1115-6.

16. Liao CH, Lai MK, Li HY, et al. Laparoscopic adrenalectomy using needlescopic instruments for adrenal tumors less than 5 cm in 112 cases. Eur Urol. 2008;54:640–6.

17. Tsai YC, Wu CC, Ho CH, et al. Minilaparoscopic herniorrhaphy in pediatric inguinal hernia: a durable alternative treatment to standard herniotomy. J Pediatr Surg. 2011;46:708–12.

18. Liao CH, Chueh SC. Laparoscopic adrenalectomy for a 6-cm left adrenal pheochromocytoma with needlescopic instruments. J Endourol. 2008;22(9):1949–51.

19. Tagaya N, Aoki H, Mikami H, et al. The use of needlescopic instruments in laparoscopic ventral hernia repair. Surg Today. 2001;31:945–7.

20. Ghezzi F, Cromi A, Siesto G, et al. Needlescopic hysterectomy: incorporation of 3-mm instruments in total laparoscopic hysterectomy. Surg Endosc. 2008;22:2153–7.

21. Kaouk JH, Haber GP, Goel RK, et al. Pure natural orifice translumenal endoscopic surgery (NOTES): transvaginal nephrectomy. Eur Urol. 2010;57:723–6.

22. Branco AW, Filho AJ, Kondo W. Hybrid transvaginal nephrectomy. Eur Urol. 2008;53:1290–4.

23. Tsin DA, Colombero LT, Lambeck J, Manolas P. Minilaparoscopy-assisted natural orifice surgery. JSLS. 2007;11:24–9.

24. Porpiglia F, Fiori C, Morra I, Scarpa RM. Transvaginal natural orifice transluminal endoscopic surgery-assisted minilaparoscopic nephrectomy: a step towards scarless surgery. Eur Urol. 2011;60:862–6.

25. Noguera J, Dolz C, Cuadrado A, et al. Hybrid transvaginal cholecystectomy, NOTES, and minilaparoscopy: analysis of a prospective clinical series. Surg Endosc. 2009;23:876–81.

26. Irwin BH, Rao PP, Stein RJ, Desai MM. Laparoendoscopic single site surgery in urology. Urol Clin North Am. 2009;36:223–35.

27. Park YH, Park JH, Jeong CW, Kim HH. Comparison of laparoendoscopic single-site radical nephrectomy with conventional laparoscopic radical nephrectomy for localized renal-cell carcinoma. J Endourol. 2010;24(6):997–1003.

28. Andonian S, Herati AS, Atalla MA, et al. Laparoendoscopic single-site Pfannenstiel donor nephrectomy. Urology. 2010;75(1):9–12.

29. Kawauchi A, Kamoi K, Soh J, et al. Laparoendoscopic single-site urological surgery: initial experience in Japan. Int J Urol. 2010;17:289–93.

30. Raman JD, Bensalah K, Bagrodia A, et al. Laboratory and clinical development of single keyhole umbilical nephrectomy. Urology. 2007;70:1039–42.

31. Gill IS, Canes D, Aron M, et al. Single port transumbilical (E-NOTES) donor nephrectomy. J Urol. 2008;180:637–41.

32. Aron M, Canes D, Desai MM, et al. Transumbilical single-port laparoscopic partial nephrectomy. BJU Int. 2008;103:516–21.
33. Ganpule AP, Dhawan DR, Kurien A, et al. Laparoendoscopic single-site donor nephrectomy: a single-center experience. Urology. 2009;74:1238–41.
34. Desai MM, Stein R, Rao P, et al. Embryonic natural orifice transumbilical endoscopic surgery (E-NOTES) for advanced reconstruction: initial experience. Urology. 2009;73:182–7.
35. Desai MM, Berger AK, Brandina R, et al. Laparoendoscopic single-site surgery: initial hundred patients. Urology. 2009;74:805–13.
36. Raman JD, Bagrodia A, Caddedu JA. Single-incision, umbilical laparoscopic versus conventional laparoscopic nephrectomy: a comparison of perioperative outcomes and short-term measures of convalescence. Eur Urol. 2009;55:1198–206.
37. Tracy CR, Raman JD, Bagrodia A, Caddedu JA. Perioperative outcomes in patients undergoing conventional laparoscopic versus laparoendoscopic single-site pyeloplasty. Urology. 2009;74:1029–35.
38. Raybourn III JH, Rane A, Sundaram CP. Laparoendoscopic single-site surgery for nephrectomy as a feasible alternative to traditional laparoscopy. Urology. 2010;75:100–3.
39. Canes D, Berger A, Aron M, et al. Laparo-endoscopic single-site (LESS) versus standard laparoscopic left donor nephrectomy: matched-pair comparison. Eur Urol. 2010;57:95–101.

Chapter 8
Access: Transgastric

Bernard Dallemagne, Silvana Perretta, and Michele Diana

Keywords NOTES • Transgastric • Endoscopic closure • Transluminal access Gastrotomy closure

Introduction

The original idea of natural orifice translumenal endoscopic surgery was to create a port of entry into the peritoneal cavity through the gastric wall [1]. Subsequently, other routes of access were developed to surmount the challenges generated by the original concept and extend the scope of existing natural orifice accesses, such as the transvaginal or transanal route. Until then, perforation of the stomach was considered a complication of interventional endoscopy. Gauderer and Ponsky were the first to break this dogma in 1980 by developing the technique of percutaneous placement of a gastrostomy tube under endoscopic control [2]. Another currently widely accepted procedure that involves a gastric perforation, endoscopic pseudocyst drainage, dates to 1985. Likewise, pancreatic necrosectomy and pancreatic pseudocyst gastrotomy both breach the integrity of the visceral wall [3]. Finally, fine-needle aspiration, which typically involves translumenal puncture, is a routine component of endoscopic ultrasound examinations, with negligible rates of postprocedure complications. Even if some purists consider pancreatic necrosectomy via a posterior gastrotomy as the first published NOTES procedure, it is in 2004 that Kalloo et al. brought new fuel and new prospective to this approach [1].

B. Dallemagne, M.D. (✉) • S. Perretta, M.D. • M. Diana, M.D.
Department of Digestive and Endocrine Surgery
and IRCAD (Institut de Recherche contre les Cancers de l'Appareil Digestif),
University Hospital of Strasbourg,
1, Place De L'Hopital, Strasbourg 67091, France
e-mail: bernard.dallemagne@ircad.fr; silvana.perretta@ircad.fr; michelediana@virgilio.it

A. Rane et al. (eds.), *Scar-Less Surgery*,
DOI 10.1007/978-1-84800-360-6_8, © Springer-Verlag London 2013

Contrary to transgastric drainage, the aim was to penetrate into the peritoneal cavity and not in a closed cavity. This opening of the stomach into the peritoneal cavity was common for surgeons, but quite new to the endoscopists. Surgeons and endoscopists have formed collaboration to identify concerns and challenges in the development of NOTES. Guidelines for the implementation of the technique were outlined by the NOSCAR Working Group [4]. The challenges were to develop and validate techniques for creating the transgastric approach, taking into account the blind nature of the maneuver, the risks of injury to adjacent organs, the potential contamination of the peritoneal cavity, and to develop safe and reliable techniques for closing the door after the completion of intraabdominal surgery. Many experimental studies have been performed to address theses issues, but it should be recognized that this route has not yet reached a significant clinical development.

Preparation of the Stomach for Transgastric Access

In the first report issued by Kalloo et al. on transgastric natural orifice surgery, the authors prepared the stomach by lavage with 1,000 ml of antibiotic solution to reduce the risk of intraoperative contamination [1]. This methodology had been established empirically and had been repeated by other teams until the study by Narula et al. on intraoperative contamination observed at the opening of the stomach during the implementation of bypass procedures in obese patients [5]. The authors demonstrated that transgastric instrumentation does contaminate the abdominal cavity, but the pathogens are clinically insignificant due to species or bacterial load. This observation was confirmed by additional studies of patients undergoing transgastric staging of pancreatic cancer [6] or transgastric peritoneoscopy [7]. Patients on proton pump inhibitors (PPIs) had an increased bacterial load in the gastric aspirate, with no clinically significant infection. Ramamoorthy et al. confirmed the impact of PPIs on peritoneal contamination in a study demonstrating a significant increase in intraabdominal infection and bacterial contamination in pigs on PPIs therapy before open gastrotomy and intraperitoneal injection of the gastric content [8]. Several transgastric experiments with survival study were subsequently performed that did not confirm the primary hypothesis of the seminal transgastric report.

In the clinical setting, the authors did not experience any relevant infectious complications, although systematic sampling of the peritoneal cavity revealed peritoneal contamination in 2 of 11 patients. Today, the only preventive measure that is used to prevent peritoneal contamination is the cessation of PPIs 10 days before transgastric surgery.

Planning the Entry Site

The access to the peritoneal cavity starts with the planning of the entry site. Several methods of transgastric entry into the peritoneum have been described, all of which require blind puncture through the GI wall, with the inherent risk of injury to adjacent extramural structures. The surgeon has to take into account the anatomy and vascularization of the stomach [9], accessibility to the target organ [10], and the technical possibility to properly close the port after the surgical procedure.

Techniques of Gastrotomy

PEG Technique

The PEG-like approach to the peritoneal cavity, described by Kantsevoy et al., is a modification of the traditional endoscopic insertion of a percutaneous gastrostomy tube developed and introduced into the clinical practice by Gauderer and Ponsky [2, 11].

A gastroscopy is performed to identify the anterior stomach wall. Transillumination of the anterior abdominal wall allows the surgeon to exclude the interposition of any organs between the stomach and the anterior abdominal wall. Digital pressure is applied to the abdominal wall, which the endoscopist can see indent the anterior gastric wall. A small (21-gauge, 40-mm) needle is passed percutaneously into the stomach and a soft guidewire is inserted through this, grasped by an endoscopic snare or grasper, and pulled through the biopsy channel of the endoscope. A sphincterotome or a needle-knife is inserted into the gastric wall over the guidewire. A gastric incision is performed. The incision can be large (1–1.5 cm) to allow the direct passage of the endoscope, or small (0.5 cm) and dilated with an 18–20-mm through-the-scope balloon. The latter is less traumatic, splitting instead of cutting the muscular layers. This technique is unlikely to cause bleeding and may facilitate closure as the muscles tend to recoil back snugly around the scope. On balloon semideflection, the endoscope is pushed forward and passed through the gastric wall (Fig. 8.1).

The limitation of the PEG-like approach is that the gastric incision is usually located on the anterior gastric wall. This location may not be optimal for certain procedures. The PEG-like transgastric approach to the peritoneal cavity is technically simple and safe and will allow incision of the gastric wall and entrance to the peritoneal cavity without a significant risk of damage to adjacent organs.

Linear Incision with a Needle-Knife

Advancing a needle-knife through the gastric wall performs a 1-cm incision. Electrocautery is discontinued immediately upon tactile perception of full-thickness puncture. The metallic tip of the needle-knife is then retracted and the catheter pushed through the gastrotomy and used as a guide to advance the video gastroscope into the peritoneal cavity.

Fig. 8.1 Transgastric access by a PEG-like technique in an animal model

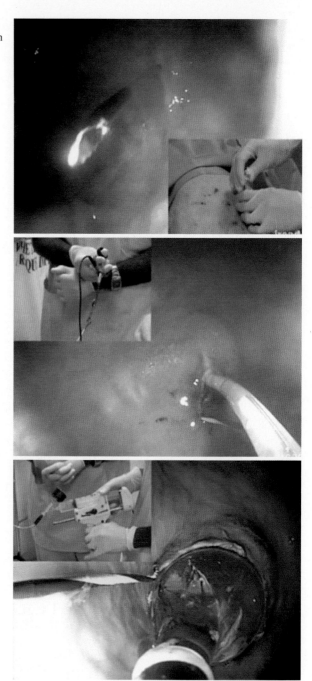

An alternative is to perform a 0.5-cm incision and, after removing the needle-knife, an esophageal dilating balloon is used to radially dilate the incision into an 18-mm circular gastrotomy. The endoscope is then advanced through this opening and into the abdominal cavity.

This technique has the theoretical advantage of being performed in different sites of the stomach. But it carries a high risk of injury to adjacent organs because it is totally blind. In their review of 73 transgastric experimental procedures on pigs, Sohn and colleagues reported that 15.5 % of the traditional transgastric needle-knife NOTES gastrotomies performed without laparoscopic visualization caused some type of intraabdominal injury [12].

In the clinical setting, this method of small gastrotomy with guided balloon dilation under laparoscopic visual control by means of a 5-mm rigid laparoscope introduced in an umbilical trocar is used by the majority of teams performing transgastric surgery [13–15]. It was successfully utilized in a series of transgastric cholecystectomies [16]. An endoscopic monopolar needle-knife was used to create a 0.5-cm gastrotomy on the anterior gastric wall in the antrum of the stomach. A guidewire was passed through the gastrotomy to guide an 18-mm balloon dilator, which expanded the gastrotomy and allowed for the passage of a double-channel gastroscope (Fig. 8.2). Neither bleeding nor injuries to adjacent organs were observed. With growing experience, some teams have started to perform the transgastric approach without laparoscopic surveillance [15].

The only technology currently available to visualize the surrounding structures when performing a transgastric approach is endoscopic ultrasound. In a study comparing anterior and posterior needle-knife gastrotomies performed with and without ultrasound control, Elmunzer et al. identified clinically significant complications, including liver laceration, spleen laceration, gallbladder puncture, pancreatic laceration, and kidney puncture in all "unsafe" approaches, while all the ultrasound-guided gastrotomies were uneventful [17].

Submucosal Flap Technique

Another seductive approach is the submucosal flap technique that was developed in a bid to control peritoneal contamination and facilitates closure of the gastrotomy (Fig. 8.3).

Moyer et al. described the self-approximating transluminal access technique (STAT) [18]. By using an injection needle, 10 ml of normal saline solution is introduced submucosally to elevate the mucosa from the underlying muscle in the posterior cardiac portion of the stomach. A 1–1.5-cm incision is then created in this submucosal cushion with a needle-knife. A grasping forceps is used to continue the dissection of the loose areolar tissue in the submucosal plane, separating the mucosa from the adjacent circular muscle layer. By using a combination of sharp and blunt dissection with the forceps, as well as blunt and pneumatic dissection with the leading edge of the endoscope, an extended submucosal tunnel (10–12 cm) is created.

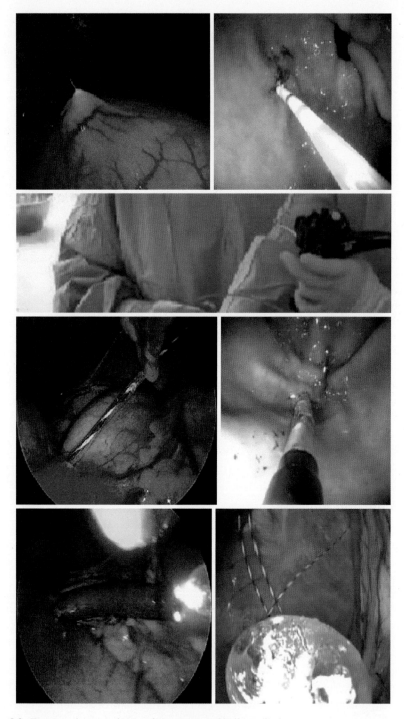

Fig. 8.2 Transgastric access by gastric puncture and balloon dilation

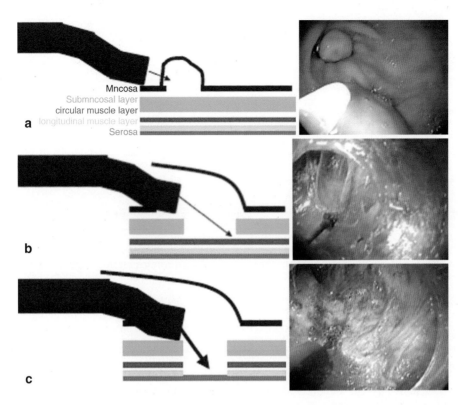

Fig. 8.3 Submucosal flap technique for transgastric access (**a**) lifting of the mucosa by injecting saline (**b**) submucosal tunel (**c**) submucosal gastrotomy

A needle-knife is used to incise the seromuscular layer at the distal end of the sub-mucosal tract. This allows the endoscope to advance from the tunnel and achieve transluminal access. At the end of the procedure, the muscosa is closed with endo-scopic clips. In a survival study, the authors achieved excellent closure of the gas-trotomy but reported abscess in the submucosal tunnel in one animal, and in the peritoneal cavity in another animal (2/5: 40 %) [19].

The submucosal tunnel is not as long in the submucosal endoscopy with mucosal flap safety valve (SEMF) technique described by Sumiyama et al. [20]. High-pressure CO_2 is injected into the submucosal layer through a standard 23-gauge injection needle to create a submucosal gas cushion (greater than 10 cm in diameter). Hydroxypropyl methylcellulose is then injected to prevent gas escape and to main-tain the cushion. A mucosal incision (10 mm) is made at one margin of the cushion with a bipolar needle-knife; a 15-mm biliary retrieval balloon is repeatedly inserted into the insufflated submucosal layer from the mucosal incision and is distended to dissect strands of connective tissue to create a space to easily insert the endoscope with the attached EMR cap. The length of the submucosal space is 65–80 mm. Opposite the mucosal entry point and within the submucosal space, the muscular layer is resected by cap EMR. The mucosal incision is closed by mucosal apposition with metal clips or T-tags. In an animal survival study, all gastrotomies were successfully created, but complications were encountered in the pig, where a posterior site was chosen [21].

Unlike Sumiyama, Pauli et al. [22] do not resect the sero-muscular wall but incise it, and Yoshizomi uses a balloon dilation of the incision [23]. Both groups reported excellent results in animal survival studies.

The issue of the retrieval of organs through this submucosal channel was recently addressed, and a study suggests STAT will tolerate the mechanical forces of peroral transgastric procedures provided the organ resected is small to moderate in size ($<8 \times 3$ cm) [24].

What Is the Best Technique?

The literature presents many techniques for gastrotomy creation, which can be classified into three main types: direct approach with a gastric linear incision with a needle-knife/sphincterotome; direct approach with a gastric wall puncture with a needle-knife and balloon dilation of the puncture and indirect approach via a submucosal tunnel. The type of approach can influence the technical difficulty of the procedure, potential complications, access to certain quadrants of the abdomen, and, of course, the quality of the closure of the gastrotomy.

Von Delius et al. compared the three types of gastrotomy creation in ex vivo stomachs [25]. The submucosal flap technique was divided into two subgroups, one with a short tunnel (4 cm), and a group with an extended tunnel (8 cm). They closed all the gastrotomies/mucosal flaps with clips and measured the operative time and the leak pressures obtained with the different technical variations. Extended submucosal tunneling required the longest operative time, showed the highest leakage pressures, and resulted in twice as strong a closure of the gastrotomy, as observed in the group with balloon dilation ($P = 0.002$).

One major question is the ideal site of gastric access for visualization of different organs in humans. Similar to the varied port placements used in laparoscopic surgery, certain gastric sites of access are likely to be better suited for visualization and manipulation of certain abdominal organs. Nikfarjam et al. addressed this problem in a series of transgastric peritoneoscopy in human [10]. The site for NOTES gastrotomy was the body in three cases, the lesser curvature in three cases, the greater curvature in one case, the fundus in one case, and the antrum in one case. The endoscope provided satisfactory navigation to and visualization of the right upper quadrant, both lower quadrants, and the anterior abdominal wall. Visualization of the left upper quadrant, particularly visualization of the spleen, was problematic and could be satisfactorily achieved in only one of nine cases (11 %). It was possible in one case where the site of gastrotomy was at the greater curvature in the midbody of the stomach. Hazey et al. reported on ten human cases where transgastic NOTES was performed as part of diagnostic endoscopy in patients with pancreatic cancer [13]. The site of gastrotomy in that series was in the anterior antral region, so that it could be incorporated into a gastrojejunostomy in cases where patients were deemed to be unresectable. In their report, four of ten patients had inadequate visualization of the right upper quadrant, whereas all ten were reported to have good visualization of the left upper quadrant. These findings differ from the previous study, possibly due to the more distal gastric access site chosen, which allows greater retroflexion of the endoscope to view the left upper quadrant while providing a straighter path to clearly visualize the right upper quadrant.

In cholecystectomy, most teams use an anterior body-antrum site for the gastrotomy that allows "comfortable" access to the gallbladder [14–16]. However, specific anatomical distortions, along with the lack of exposure provided by present methods of retraction and retroflexion, tend to distort Calot's triangle by flattening it rather than opening it up, exposing it to anatomical misinterpretation [26].

Closure of the Gastrotomy

The Natural Orifice Surgery Consortium for Assessment and Research clearly states that gastric closure is an important issue that needs thorough assessment. There is general agreement that there must be near-zero tolerance for leaks. The ideal closure should be rapid, reproducible, and safe, ideally performed under vision to avoid any injury to the adjacent organs, and should grant a full-thickness bite.

Although some authors performed experiments in survival animal models without gastric closure at all, without the development of peritonitis or sepsis, there is general agreement that a secure closure with a minimal risk of leak must be achieved to avoid major complications [27].

To date, a variety of endoscopic techniques have been described to close gastric wall incisions, including the application of endoscopic clips, endoloops, tissue anchoring systems, endoscopic suturing, stapling, and occluding devices (Table 8.1). Objective and analytic evaluation of the results is complex. The security of closure is estimated by different parameters in in vivo and ex vivo studies. In ex vivo studies, results using burst pressure as a surrogate marker of a leak-proof suture are difficult to extrapolate. Most of the survival studies were performed on a porcine model, which presents several drawbacks. Experience shows that the pig response to infection and inflammation may be unpredictable, with a frequent mismatch between the clinical outcome and the presence of peritoneal infection.

The tested devices reflect two different philosophies: The endoscopic attitude of closing the visible defect by approximating the mucosal edges with clips opposes the surgeon's tendency to reproduce the hand-sewn suture with a full-thickness closure.

EndoClips™ (Olympus Optical Co., Ltd., Tokyo, Japan)

The simple application of current endoclips enables only a single-layer mucosal approximation. In addition, their application might be difficult at times due to a tangential orientation of the tissue or because of tissue edema. Kalloo et al. used this

Table 8.1 Summary of NOTES gastrotomy closure techniques

Author	Device technique	N	Type	Burst	Leak
Voermans [28]	OTSC	16	Surv		0
Romanelli [29]	LAPS	4	Surv		0
Desilets [30]	Padlock-G™ (Aponos Medical, Kingston, NH)	4	Surv		0
Dray [31]	Resolution® clips (Boston Scientific, Natick, MA) T-tags	4 8	Surv		0
Bergman [32]	Plug No CLOSURE	12 D 11 D	Surv	77 76	0
Romanelli [33]	Padlock-G™ (Aponos Medical, Kingston, NH)	8	Ex vivo	68	
Asakuma [34]	Per-oral dual scope	6	Surv		1/6, 16 %
Park [35]	Tissue apposition system Suture laparotomy	16 16	Surv		0
Willingham [36]	Resolution® clips (Boston Scientific, Natick, MA) (T-tags in case of leak)	36	Surv		4/36, 11 %
Hucl [37]	Double endoloops	10	Surv	160	0
Sherwinter [38]	SurgASSIST® (Power Medical Interventions, Langhorne, PA) (circular stapler)	15 5	Ex vivo Surv	260	0
Pauli [22]	Directed submucosal tunneling + Resolution® clips (Boston Scientific, Natick, MA) (STAT)	14	Surv		0
Von Renteln [39]	OTSC Clips	10 10	Surv		0

Reference	Technique	n	Study		
Voermans [40]	OTSC	11	Ex vivo	233	
Desilets [41]	Hand-sewn	15	Ex vivo	206	
	LAPS	9		27.3	
	Clips	9		14	2/15, 13.3 %
Rolanda [42]	OTSC	15	Surv	83 (30–140)	
Von Renteln [43]	OTSC	18	Acute	67 (30–130)	
	Suture	18			
Hookey [44]	Queen's closure (clips + loop)	5	Surv		0
Ujiki [45]	Gastric valve (HUMAN STUDY)	10 P / 5 M	Surv		0
Moran [46]	Endoscopic suturing device	?	?	?	?
Trunzo [47]	Tissue anchors	5	Acute		
Bhat [48]	Endoscopic tacks	6	Surv		0
Dray [49]	Omentoplasty	6	Surv		1/6
Kratt [50]	OTSC	9	Acute		5/9

? - not specified

technique in the seminal report on transluminal surgery. At necropsy, intraperitoneal abscesses were found in two of five animals. Alternative methods that use current endoscopic clips were developed to obtain full-thickness gastric closure. Using
two endoscopes to provide a layer-by-layer endoscopic clip closure was proposed
by Asakuma et al., who reported minor intraperitoneal infection in two of five animals in a survival study [34]. Hwang et al. described a retracted clip-assisted gastrotomy closure technique that involves deploying three or four clips (modified by
attaching a 90-cm length of suture string to the end of each clip) along the margin
of the gastrotomy with one jaw on the serosal surface and the other jaw on the
mucosal surface. The suture strings are then threaded through an endoloop. Traction
is then applied to the strings, causing the gastric wall to tent. The endoloop is then
secured below the tip of the clips, completing a full-thickness gastrotomy closure
[51]. In Katsarelias's technique with endoloops, the incisional margins are separately grasped in their center, elevated, and looped, with care taken to include all
layers except the serosa. The two loops are then grasped and elevated, and a third
loop is applied encompassing the entire length of the incision and tied down [52].

In a study of the effectiveness of gastrotomy closure comparing the Katsarelias
technique, endoclips, and hand-sewn closure as a control, Shabbir et al. concluded
that endoclip closure endured a significantly higher median pressure before leaking
compared to that of an endoloop [53].

A new concept of endoscopic clip, the OTSC™ (over-the-scope-clip, Ovesco
Endoscopy GmbH, Tübingen, Germany) was recently adapted and tested for closure of the gastrotomy. The applicator is mounted onto the distal tip of the endoscope. A clip is installed onto the system in a bent state and can be released by a
wire, which is led through the working channel. When released from the applicator,
the shape-memory effect and the high grade of elasticity of the clip nitinol alloy
cause closure of the clip [54]. The system was tested in nonsurvival and survival
animal studies and compared favorably with surgical suture while showing higher
efficiency than current endoscopic clips [39, 40, 42, 43, 50, 55, 56].

Suturing Devices

Accurate stitch placement, control of the needle insertion depth, and knot tying are
the basic steps that still challenge any endoscopic attempt at suturing in NOTES.
Novel suturing devices and techniques have been developed, and some of them are
now commercially available and used in clinical applications. In 2003, Swain's
team proposed a method consisting of a series of double tags that are positioned
around the defect, through the wall, to be then approximated in pairs, and locked at
the same time by various locking mechanisms [57]. This uses a flexible endoscopic
hollow needle to deliver a threaded tag through tissues. Endoscopic gastrotomy
closure with T-tags is technically simpler than with clips, allows a tight leak-proof
approximation of the gastric wall opening, and can withstand higher intragastric
bursting pressure than closure achieved with the clips [58, 59]. The full-thickness

closure performed with tissue anchors was nearly ten times firmer than mucosal apposition by clips [35, 60]. Variations of the original device, combined with the endoloop technique, were subsequently developed and tested [29, 41, 48, 58, 61]. If the system's effectiveness has been well studied, there are still concerns related to the blind nature of the introduction of tags: Tissue anchors that are errantly placed beyond the serosal surface can potentially puncture critical structures that are adjacent to the closure site [62, 63]. A new method of application has been proposed: Before T-tag deployment, the gastric wall is suctioned into a specially designed transparent cap attached to the tip of the endoscope [31]. This method reduces the risk of injury but results in more mis-/displacements of the tags. A recent clinical application of the method in transgastric appendectomy led to a pneumothorax caused by a deep needle perforation [64]. However, Bergström et al. reported successful clinical treatment of perforated ulcers, gastric fistula, and bleeding using T-tags [65]. Some authors are concerned with the fact that the healing process of the gastric wall after closure with this device is not optimal. Approximation of the endoscopically delivered T-tags results in a robust plication inverting the edges of the gastric wall opening, rather than opposing the layers of the gastric wall toward each other. Dray et al. demonstrated that gastric wall healing achieved after closure with endoscopic clips was far superior to that after the T-tag closure. Overall, transmural healing was seen in 75 % of animals with clip closure compared with only 12.5 % after the T-tag closure [31].

Swanstrom et al. developed the g-Prox® needle (USGI, San Capistrano, CA) [66]. The technique consists of perforating the two margins of the defect with a 19-gauge needle in which two expandable baskets connected by a nonabsorbable suture are loaded. Once both baskets are released, pulling on one end of the suture causes approximation of the baskets, and consequently of the edges of the enterotomy. In ex vivo tests, this proved comparable for closure of gastrotomies with hand sutures [67]. In his IRB-approved trial on transgastric cholecystectomy, Swanstrom used the g-Prox to apply stay-sutures on the gastric wall before the gastric incision. For closure, traction on the suture allows the surgeon to maintain the pneumogastrium and to have good visualization for precise closure.

The Eagle Claw Endoscopic Suturing Device (ECESD) was designed and manufactured by the Apollo Group in collaboration with the Olympus Medical Systems Corp (Tokyo, Japan) [68]. The ECESD is an over-the-scope device and consists of three components: a proximal control arm, an endoscope mounting bracket, and a distal functioning tip. The tip contains the mechanism for suture delivery using two opposing jaws that move simultaneously, one to fix the target tissue and a curved needle to deliver the suture through the tissue. On opposing the jaws, the device is able to appose the tissue under direct endoscopic vision. After passing through the tissue, the needle is detached and trapped by a plastic casing. The device was tested in a comparative study of different closure modalities and compared satisfactorily with the surgical repair [69].

Other prototype devices are still in development, such as the flexible Endostitch™ (Covidien, North Haven, CT), derived from the laparoscopic device [69]. It is based on the same principle as the shuttle needle that is caught alternatively on one of the two puncture sites of the needle, while the thread is attached in the middle of it. The group of C. Thompson described a new suturing device, the Purse String Suturing (LSI Solutions, Victor, NY) [59]. This is a device consisting of a large chamber in which the tissue containing the defect to be closed is aspirated, obtaining an invagination of the tissue. Two needles are then advanced through the tissue, creating a sort of purse string, which is then closed. Comparison with the hand-sewn suture of gastrotomy was promising [59].

Currently, devices available for clinical use are the T-tags device, the g-Prox®, and the Eagle Claw.

Occluding Devices

The simplest technique to close an orifice with a flexible endoscope is to occlude it. This method does not require complex tasks in difficult positions in a deflated stomach. Cios et al. demonstrated that the application of a bioabsorbable device, the Gore Bioabsorbable Hernia Plug (W.L. Gore & Associates, Flagstaff, AZ), results in the durable closure of a gastric perforation with physiologic healing of the injury site in a survival study on dogs [70]. The same group repeated the experiment with a piece of bioabsorbable polyglycolic acid mesh (Dexon; Covidien, Mansfield, MA) inserted into the gastrotomy [32]. It was positioned so that it was protruding halfway into the stomach and halfway into the peritoneal cavity. All dogs survived without any signs of surgical complications until the necropsy 14 days after the procedure. All gastrotomies had sealed and did not leak at low filling pressures. More intriguing is the fact that the authors compared this method to another group of dogs in which the gastrotomy was left unclosed. The animals left to heal without treatment had equivalent gastric burst pressures and healed with a lesser inflammatory reaction than the dogs closed with the plug. The authors concluded that although in a canine model, gastric perforations are effectively sealed either by an endoluminal plug technique or without therapy, in humans, some type of repair will always be indicated.

Others have described pulling the omentum into the gastrotomy and clipping it in place to provide a repair conceptually similar to the Graham patch [49].

An original technique using a cardiac septal occluder has demonstrated a zero leak rate. The system was widely used for survival studies on animal models, but it was not transferable to a clinical setting due to cost issues and concerns about the long-term outcome of the intraperitoneal, nonabsorbable, part of the mechanism made with nitinol [71].

Conclusions

The Natural Orifice Surgery Consortium for Assessment and Research has identified visceral closure as one of the fundamental hurdles to the successful clinical introduction of endoscopic transluminal surgery: A 100 % reliable means of gastric closure must be developed. Peritoneal access enterotomies must clearly be shown to cause no additional morbidity over the established safety profiles of conventional transabdominal access routes, whether they are open or laparoscopic approaches [4]. Without it, ethical and patient safety concerns will confine NOTES to the animal laboratory and prevent a significant foray into mainstream clinical practice.

Conflict of Interest   The authors declare no conflict of interest and no financial or commercial disclosure.

References

1. Kalloo AN, Singh VK, Jagannath SB, et al. Flexible transgastric peritoneoscopy: a novel approach to diagnostic and therapeutic interventions in the peritoneal cavity. Gastrointest Endosc. 2004;60(1):114–7.
2. Gauderer MW, Ponsky JL, Izant Jr RJ. Gastrostomy without laparotomy: a percutaneous endoscopic technique. J Pediatr Surg. 1980;15(6):872–5.
3. Seifert H, Wehrmann T, Schmitt T, et al. Retroperitoneal endoscopic debridement for infected peripancreatic necrosis. Lancet. 2000;356(9230):653–5.
4. Rattner D, Kalloo A. ASGE/SAGES Working Group on natural orifice translumenal endoscopic surgery, October 2005. Surg Endosc. 2006;20(2):329–33.
5. Narula VK, Hazey JW, Renton DB, et al. Transgastric instrumentation and bacterial contamination of the peritoneal cavity. Surg Endosc. 2008;22(3):605–11.
6. Narula V, Happel L, Volt K, et al. Transgastric endoscopic peritoneoscopy does not require decontamination of the stomach in humans. Surg Endosc. 2009;23:1331–6.
7. Memark V, Anderson J, Nau P, et al. Transgastric endoscopic peritoneoscopy does not lead to increased risk of infectious complications. Surg Endosc. 2011;25(7):2186–91.
8. Ramamoorthy S, Lee J, Mintz Y, et al. The impact of proton-pump inhibitors on intraperitoneal sepsis: a word of caution for transgastric NOTES procedures. Surg Endosc. 2010;24(1):16–20.
9. Linke GR, Zerz A, Kapitza F, et al. Evaluation of endoscopy in localizing transgastric access for natural orifice transluminal endoscopic surgery in humans. Gastrointest Endosc. 2010;71(6):907–12.
10. Nikfarjam M, McGee MF, Trunzo JA, et al. Transgastric natural-orifice transluminal endoscopic surgery peritoneoscopy in humans: a pilot study in efficacy and gastrotomy site selection by using a hybrid technique. Gastrointest Endosc. 2010;72(2):279–83.
11. Kantsevoy SV, Jagannath SB, Niiyama H, et al. A novel safe approach to the peritoneal cavity for per-oral transgastric endoscopic procedures. Gastrointest Endosc. 2007;65(3):497–500.
12. Sohn D, Turner B, Gee D, Willingham F, Sylla P, Cizginer S, et al. Reducing the unexpectedly high rate of injuries caused by NOTES gastrotomy creation. Surgical Endoscopy. 2010;24(2):277–82.
13. Hazey JW, Narula VK, Renton DB, et al. Natural-orifice transgastric endoscopic peritoneoscopy in humans: initial clinical trial. Surg Endosc. 2008;22(1):16–20.
14. Auyang ED, Hungness ES, Vaziri K, et al. Human NOTES cholecystectomy: transgastric hybrid technique. J Gastrointest Surg. 2009;13(6):1149–50.
15. Salinas G, Saavedra L, Agurto H, et al. Early experience in human hybrid transgastric and transvaginal endoscopic cholecystectomy. Surg Endosc. 2010;24(5):1092–8.
16. Dallemagne B, Perretta S, Allemann P, et al. Transgastric hybrid cholecystectomy. Br J Surg. 2009;96(10):1162–6.
17. Elmunzer BJ, Schomisch SJ, Trunzo JA, et al. EUS in localizing safe alternate access sites for natural orifice transluminal endoscopic surgery: initial experience in a porcine model. Gastrointest Endosc. 2009;69(1):108–14.

18. Moyer MT, Pauli EM, Haluck RS, Mathew A. A self-approximating transluminal access technique for potential use in NOTES: an *ex vivo* porcine model (with video). Gastrointest Endosc. 2007;66(5):974–8.
19. Pauli EM, Moyer MT, Haluck RS, Mathew A. Self-approximating transluminal access technique for natural orifice transluminal endoscopic surgery: a porcine survival study (with video). Gastrointest Endosc. 2008;67(4):690–7.
20. Sumiyama K, Gostout CJ, Rajan E, et al. Submucosal endoscopy with mucosal flap safety valve. Gastrointest Endosc. 2007;65(4):688–94.
21. Sumiyama K, Gostout CJ, Rajan E, et al. Transgastric cholecystectomy: transgastric accessibility to the gallbladder improved with the SEMF method and a novel multibending therapeutic endoscope. Gastrointest Endosc. 2007;65(7):1028–34.
22. Pauli EM, Haluck RS, Ionescu AM, et al. Directed submucosal tunneling permits in-line endoscope positioning for transgastric natural orifice translumenal endoscopic surgery (NOTES). Surg Endosc. 2010;24:1474–81.
23. Yoshizumi F, Yasuda K, Kawaguchi K, et al. Submucosal tunneling using endoscopic submucosal dissection for peritoneal access and closure in natural orifice transluminal endoscopic surgery: a porcine survival study. Endoscopy. 2009;41(8):707–11.
24. Moyer M, Pauli E, Gopal J, et al. Durability of the self-approximating transluminal access technique (STAT) for potential use in natural orifice translumenal surgery (NOTES). Surg Endosc. 2011;25:315–22.
25. von Delius S, Gillen S, Doundoulakis E, et al. Comparison of transgastric access techniques for natural orifice transluminal endoscopic surgery. Gastrointest Endosc. 2008;65:940–7.
26. Perretta S, Dallemagne B, Donatelli G, et al. The fear of transgastric cholecystectomy: misinterpretation of the biliary anatomy. Surg Endosc. 2011;25:648.
27. Jagannath SB, Kantsevoy SV, Vaughn CA, et al. Peroral transgastric endoscopic ligation of fallopian tubes with long-term survival in a porcine model. Gastrointest Endosc. 2005;61(3):449–53.
28. Voermans R, van Berge Henegouwen M, Bemelman W, Fockens P. Hybrid NOTES transgastric cholecystectomy with reliable gastric closure: an animal survival study. Surg Endosc. 2011;25:728–36.
29. Romanelli JR, Desilets DJ, Chapman CN, et al. Loop-anchor purse-string closure of gastrotomy in NOTES procedures: survival studies in a porcine model. Surg Innov. 2010;17(4):312–7.
30. Desilets DJ, Romanelli JR, Earle DB, Chapman CN. Gastrotomy closure with the Lock-It system and the Padlock-G clip: a survival study in a porcine model. J Laparoendosc Adv Surg Tech A. 2010;20(8):671–6.
31. Dray X, Krishnamurty DM, Donatelli G, et al. Gastric wall healing after NOTES procedures: closure with endoscopic clips provides superior histological outcome compared with threaded tags closure. Gastrointest Endosc. 2010;72(2):343–50.
32. Bergman S, Fix DJ, Volt K, et al. Do gastrotomies require repair after endoscopic transgastric peritoneoscopy? A controlled study. Gastrointest Endosc. 2010;71(6):1013–7.
33. Romanelli JR, Desilets DJ, Earle DB. Natural orifice transluminal endoscopic surgery gastrotomy closure in porcine explants with the Padlock-G clip using the Lock-It system. Endoscopy. 2010;42(04):306–10.
34. Asakuma M, Perretta S, Cahill RA, et al. Peroral dual scope for natural orifice transluminal endoscopic surgery (NOTES) gastrotomy closure. Surg Innov. 2009;16(2):97–103.
35. Park PO, Bergström M, Rothstein R, et al. Endoscopic sutured closure of a gastric natural orifice transluminal endoscopic surgery access gastrotomy compared with open surgical closure in a porcine model. A randomized, multicenter controlled trial. Endoscopy. 2010;42:311–7.
36. Willingham FF, Turner BG, Gee DW, et al. Leaks and endoscopic assessment of break of integrity after NOTES gastrotomy: the LEAKING study, a prospective, randomized, controlled trial. Gastrointest Endosc. 2010;71(6):1018–24.
37. Hucl T, Benes M, Kocik M, et al. A novel double-endoloop technique for natural orifice transluminal endoscopic surgery gastric access site closure. Gastrointest Endosc. 2010;71(4):806–11.

38. Sherwinter DA, Gupta A, Cummings L, Eckstein JG. Evaluation of a modified circular stapler for use as a viscerotomy formation and closure device in natural orifice surgery. Surg Endosc. 2010;24:1456–61.
39. von Renteln D, Vassiliou MC, Rothstein RI. Randomized controlled trial comparing endoscopic clips and over-the-scope clips for closure of natural orifice transluminal endoscopic surgery gastrotomies. Endoscopy. 2009;41(12):1056–61.
40. Voermans RP, van Berge Henegouwen MI, Bemelman WA, Fockens P. Novel over-the-scope-clip system for gastrotomy closure in natural orifice transluminal endoscopic surgery (NOTES): an *ex vivo* comparison study. Endoscopy. 2009;41(12):1052–5.
41. Desilets DJ, Romanelli JR, Earle DB, et al. Loop-anchor purse-string versus endoscopic clips for gastric closure: a natural orifice transluminal endoscopic surgery comparison study using burst pressures. Gastrointest Endosc. 2009;70(6):1225–30.
42. Rolanda C, Lima E, Silva D, et al. *In vivo* assessment of gastrotomy closure with over-the-scope clips in an experimental model for varicocelectomy (with video). Gastrointest Endosc. 2009;70:1137–45.
43. von Renteln D, Schmidt A, Vassiliou MC, et al. Natural orifice transluminal endoscopic surgery gastrotomy closure with an over-the-endoscope clip: a randomized, controlled porcine study (with videos). Gastrointest Endosc. 2009;70:732–9.
44. Hookey LC, Khokhotva V, Bielawska B, et al. The Queen's closure: a novel technique for closure of endoscopic gastrotomy for natural-orifice transluminal endoscopic surgery. Endoscopy. 2009;41(2):149–53.
45. Ujiki MB, Martinec DV, Diwan TS, et al. Video: natural orifice translumenal endoscopic surgery (NOTES): creation of a gastric valve for safe and effective transgastric surgery in humans. Surg Endosc. 2010;24(1):220. Epub 2009 Jun 17.
46. Moran EA, Gostout CJ, Bingener J. Preliminary performance of a flexible cap and catheter-based endoscopic suturing system. Gastrointest Endosc. 2009;69(7):1375–83.
47. Trunzo JA, Cavazzola LT, Elmunzer BJ, et al. Facilitating gastrotomy closure during natural-orifice transluminal endoscopic surgery using tissue anchors. Endoscopy. 2009;41(6):487–92.
48. Bhat YM, Hegde S, Knaus M, et al. Transluminal endosurgery: novel use of endoscopic tacks for the closure of access sites in natural orifice transluminal endoscopic surgery (with videos). Gastrointest Endosc. 2009;69(6):1161–6.
49. Dray X, Giday SA, Buscaglia JM, et al. Omentoplasty for gastrotomy closure after natural orifice transluminal endoscopic surgery procedures (with video). Gastrointest Endosc. 2009;70(1):131–40.
50. Kratt T, Kuper M, Traub F, et al. Feasibility study for secure closure of natural orifice transluminal endoscopic surgery gastrotomies by using over-the-scope clips. Gastrointest Endosc. 2008;68(5):993–6.
51. Hwang JH, Soares RV, Lee S-S, et al. Assessment of a simple, novel endoluminal method for gastrotomy closure in NOTES. Gastrointest Endosc. DDW Abstract Issue 2009, Dig Dis Wkly 2009;69(5):AB305–6.
52. Katsarelias D. Endoloop application as an alternative method for gastrotomy closure in experimental transgastric surgery. Surg Endosc. 2007;21(10):1862–5.
53. Shabbir A, Liang S, Lomanto D, et al. Closure of gastrotomy in natural orifice transluminal endoscopic surgery: a feasibility study using an *ex vivo* model comparing endoloop with endoclip. Dig Endosc. 2011;23(2):130–4.
54. Kirschniak A, Kratt T, Stüker D, et al. A new endoscopic over-the-scope clip system for treatment of lesions and bleeding in the GI tract: first clinical experiences. Gastrointest Endosc. 2007;66(1):162–7.
55. Arezzo A, Kratt T, Schurr MO, Morino M. Laparoscopic-assisted transgastric cholecystectomy and secure endoscopic closure of the transgastric defect in a survival porcine model. Endoscopy. 2009;41:767–72.
56. Von Renteln D, Schmidt AR, Rudolph HU, et al. Endoscopic closure of the transgastric NOTES® access by means of an over the scope clip system (OTSC). A randomized controlled porcine study. Gastrointest Endosc. DDW Abstract Issue 2009, Dig Dis Wkly 2009;69(5):AB165.

57. Fritscher-Ravens A, Mosse CA, Mukherjee D, et al. Transluminal endosurgery: single lumen access anastomotic device for flexible endoscopy. Gastrointest Endosc. 2003;58(4):585–91.
58. Seaman DL, Gostout CJ, de la Mora Levy JG, Knipschield MA. Tissue anchors for transmural gut-wall apposition. Gastrointest Endosc. 2006;64(4):577–81.
59. Ryou M, Pai R, Sauer J, et al. Evaluating an optimal gastric closure method for transgastric surgery. Surg Endosc. 2007;21(4):677–80.
60. Ikeda K, Fritscher-Ravens A, Mosse CA, et al. Endoscopic full-thickness resection with sutured closure in a porcine model. Gastrointest Endosc. 2005;62(1):122–9.
61. Sumiyama K, Gostout CJ, Rajan E, et al. Endoscopic full-thickness closure of large gastric perforations by use of tissue anchors. Gastrointest Endosc. 2007;65(1):134–9.
62. Dray X, Gabrielson KL, Buscaglia JM, et al. Air and fluid leak tests after NOTES procedures: a pilot study in a live porcine model (with videos). Gastrointest Endosc. 2008;68:513–9.
63. Kantsevoy SV. Endoscopic full-thickness resection: new minimally invasive therapeutic alternative for GI-tract lesions. Gastrointest Endosc. 2006;64(1):90–1.
64. Park PO, Bergström M. Transgastric peritoneoscopy and appendectomy: thoughts on our first experience in humans. Endoscopy. 2010;42(01):81–4.
65. Bergström M, Swain P, Park PO. Early clinical experience with a new flexible endoscopic suturing method for natural orifice transluminal endoscopic surgery and intraluminal endosurgery (with videos). Gastrointest Endosc. 2008;67(3):528–33.
66. Swanstrom L, Whiteford M, Khajanchee Y. Developing essential tools to enable transgastric surgery. Surg Endosc. 2008;22(3):600–4.
67. Sclabas GM, Swain P, Swanstrom LL. Endoluminal methods for gastrotomy closure in natural orifice transenteric surgery (NOTES). Surg Innov. 2006;13(1):23–30.
68. Pham BV, Raju GS, Ahmed I, et al. Immediate endoscopic closure of colon perforation by using a prototype endoscopic suturing device: feasibility and outcome in a porcine model (with video). Gastrointest Endosc. 2006;64(1):113–9.
69. Voermans RP, Worm AM, van Berge Henegouwen MI, et al. *In vitro* comparison and evaluation of seven gastric closure modalities for natural orifice transluminal endoscopic surgery (NOTES). Endoscopy. 2008;40(7):595–601.
70. Cios T, Reavis K, Renton D, et al. Gastrotomy closure using bioabsorbable plugs in a canine model. Surg Endosc. 2008;22(4):961–6.
71. Perretta S, Sereno S, Forgione A, et al. A new method to close the gastrotomy by using a cardiac septal occluder: long-term survival study in a porcine model. Gastrointest Endosc. 2007;66(4):809–13.

Chapter 9
Access: Transcolonic

Nitin Kumar and Christopher C. Thompson

Keywords Transcolonic • NOTES • Transvesical • Transvaginal • Transgastric
Colotomy • Colonic perforation

Introduction

Natural orifice translumenal endoscopic surgery (NOTES) has developed fairly rapidly over the past decade. Multiple access points have been evaluated, and their relative advantages and disadvantages continue to be elucidated as applied to an
ever-expanding array of NOTES-like procedures. The evolution of transcolonic
access to the peritoneal cavity and its future will be discussed herein.

The Precedence of Transcolonic Access

Transanal endoscopic microsurgery (TEM) laid the foundation for NOTES procedures using transcolonic access. Developed by Buess and colleagues in the early
1980s, it was originally used for transanal resection of rectosigmoid tumors below
the peritoneal reflection; more recently, it has been used to resect upper rectal tumors

N. Kumar, M.D. (✉)
Department of Gastroenterology, Harvard Medical School, Brigham and Women's Hospital,
400 Brookline Avenue, Apt 12C, Boston, MA 02215, USA
e-mail: nkumar2@partners.org

C.C. Thompson, M.D., M.Sc., FACG, FASGE
Division of Gastroenterology, Brigham and Women's Hospital,
75 Francis Street, Boston, MA 02115, USA
e-mail: christopher_thompson@hms.harvard.edu

A. Rane et al. (eds.), *Scar-Less Surgery*,
DOI 10.1007/978-1-84800-360-6_9, © Springer-Verlag London 2013

and for circumferential sleeve resection [1–3]. In 2004, it was reported in a study of 34 patients that inadvertent entry into the peritoneum during TEM did not require conversion to open laparotomy for closure and did not result in excess postoperative complications, including infection [3]. However, the finding that over 90 % of colonoscopic perforations result in peritonitis suggests that specialized procedures for transcolonic access will be required before transcolonic NOTES can be applied widely.

The development of NOTES began using transgastric access; Kalloo reported peritoneoscopy in 2004 [4]. As more studies were completed, some limitations of the transgastric approach became apparent. In 2005, our group found that upper abdominal organs were not consistently identified via transgastric entry; the gallbladder, for example, was adequately visualized only 55 % of the time, and engaging it was even more difficult [5]. Further attempts at transgastric cholecystectomy by the Swanstrom group in retroflexed position using stabilized-platform ShapeLock™ technology (USGI Medical, San Clemente, CA) were only successful in one of three animals, with poor visualization and insufficient exposure of biliary anatomy cited [6]. The Swain group, despite using two endoscopes or laparoscopic assistance in a nonsurvival study, had a similar difficulty [7]. Transgastric NOTES procedures in the lower abdomen and pelvis, however, were more successful. Transgastric tubal ligation and hysterectomy were reported in survival porcine models, as a surrogate for appendectomy [8, 9]. Transgastric oophorectomy and tubectomy were successfully performed [10]. These procedures benefitted from having a straight path from the transgastric access point.

The Evolution of Transcolonic Access

It was hypothesized that such an *en face* view of upper abdominal organs could be achieved via transcolonic entry into the peritoneum. Earlier survival studies investigated peritoneal access, closure methods, and infectious complications. As the importance of effective closure in the prevention of postoperative complications became clear, several studies focusing on closure methods were performed. Other studies directly compared transcolonic access with transgastric access and laparoscopy. Finally, innovative procedures using transcolonic access have been developed. Notable studies in these areas will be reviewed here in turn.

Access Studies

In 2006, Pai et al. reported the first series of transcolonic cholecystectomy [11]. A survival porcine study comprising five pigs was performed. Pigs were deprived of food for 48 h preoperatively. Preoperative IV cefazolin was given; colonic preparation was done with sterile water enemas, endoscopic cleaning, instillation of cefazolin suspension, and lavage and external cleaning with Betadine. A needle-knife (Microvasive, Boston Scientific, Natick, MA) and double-channel endoscope were used to create a subcentimeter colotomy in the anti-mesenteric colon wall (identified by external palpation over the ventral abdomen) 15–20 cm from the anal verge. While the needle-knife was retracted, its sheath was advanced into the peritoneal cavity to guide the endoscope. Colotomy creation was assisted by application of pressure with the endoscope; unlike many transgastric protocols, balloon dilation was not needed. With the *en face* view, visualization and engagement of the gallbladder were readily achieved; cholecystectomy was successful in all five cases. The average time from entrance into the peritoneal cavity to removal of the gallbladder from the anal orifice was 68 min. Endoloops (Endoloop®; Olympus, Tokyo, Japan) or endoclips (QuikClips™; Olympus, Tokyo, Japan) were used for colostomy closure. The complete closure of the colostomy was not possible in one pig, resulting in peritonitis; the remaining four pigs remained healthy for 2 weeks postoperatively. Microscopic evaluation of the colotomy site revealed ulceration and necrosis; submucosal and/or serosal microabscesses were found in all pigs, and one pig had necrotizing granulomas. No adjacent organ injury was found on necropsy.

Fong et al. subsequently reported transcolonic peritoneoscopy in six pigs [12]. Again, all pigs were given preoperative IV cefazolin. Preparation was with multiple tap water enemas, cefazolin suspension, and povidone-iodine lavage with external scrub. A colotomy was created with a needle-knife in two pigs and with a prototype incision and closure device (LSI Solutions, Victor, NY) in four pigs. A Veress needle was used to maintain pneumoperitoneum. Once in the peritoneal cavity, the group reported visualization of the stomach, liver, gallbladder, spleen, small bowel, colon, and peritoneal surfaces within 3 min in all pigs. However, due to limited retraction ability, visualization near the dome and hilum of the liver, lesser curvature of the stomach, and bilateral lower quadrants was limited. When retroflexed, the colotomy was visible, but the bladder was sometimes not seen, and the ovaries, fallopian tubes, and uterine structures were consistently not seen. Retroperitoneal structures were also not visible. Upon return into the colon, the colotomy was found to be markedly extended in cases without the LSI device (which placed a purse-string suture prior to peritoneal entry). Colotomy closure with endoclips and endoloops was found to be challenging; once the endoscope was back in the colon, colonic distention, and hence visualization, was difficult to maintain. Closure with the LSI device, in contrast, was easily performed within 2 min. Postoperative cephalexin was given for 3 days. All pigs were healthy for 2 weeks postoperatively; necropsy at that time revealed no evidence of visceral injury or suppurative peritonitis. There was no evidence of microscopic peritonitis. At the closure site, however, microscopic abscesses, microscopic mucosal ulcerations, and serositis were found. Most pigs also had incision-related colovesicular and salpingocolonic adhesions.

The LSI device was further evaluated in a transcolonic NOTES survival study by Ryou et al. [13]. Using similar methods as the prior study, Ryou and colleagues were able to achieve access in less than 3 min and closure in less than 1 min. All animals were healthy for the 2-week postoperative survival period. The findings affirmed those of the prior study: There was no evidence of organ injury, bleeding, suppurative peritonitis, or microscopic peritonitis. Three of four pigs had salpingocolonic and colovesicular adhesions to the incision site.

Fong et al. reported feasibility of hernia repair mesh fixation to the peritoneal cavity [14]. Preparation methods similar to their prior study were used. T-tags were placed at the colotomy site and a 2–3-mm colotomy was made with a needle-knife. The mesh was loaded onto the delivery device and advanced into the peritoneum over a wire. An external magnet assembly was used to manipulate the mesh transcutaneously, and transfascial suture T-tags were used to secure the mesh to the ventral wall successfully in all five pigs. Colotomy closure was performed by threading the previously placed T-tag sutures through the endoloop prior to loop closure. All three survival pigs thrived for 14 days.

Wilhelm et al. evaluated and reported a transcolonic access method designed to decrease potential for infection: innovative, safe, and sterile sigmoid access (ISSA) [15]. Eight pigs (three acute, five survival) were prepared with preoperative IV ampicillin and sulbactam, tap water enemas and sterile irrigation, and instillation of mucosal disinfection solution. Fluidoperitoneum was induced with taurolidin, a decontaminant used for the prevention of peritonitis, via a Veress needle. Endoluminal ultrasound was used to verify pelvic ascites and to locate bowel and major vessels. A modified TEM device (Storz, Tuttlingen, Germany) was used to apply a purse-string suture around the future entry point at the ventral rectosigmoid junction; an endoscopic guide was used to perforate the entry point and advanced into the peritoneal cavity. The guide, which was attached to an airtight valve, was used to introduce a sterilized endoscope. After peritoneoscopy of both upper quadrants for at least 30 min, the endoscope and guide tube were withdrawn and the purse-string suture closed. A linear stapler was used to secure closure. Oral enrofloxacin was given for 2 days postoperatively. The average time was 9.3 min for the incision process and 7.8 min for withdrawal of the scope and closure of the entry site. Identification of the liver, spleen, and stomach was possible in moments, and direct access to the gallbladder was possible within 2 min. All animals did well during the 10-day survival period. On necropsy, there were no signs of infection or peritonitis; peritoneal cultures were negative, and there were no intramural microabscesses. There were no significant peritoneal adhesions.

Dubcenco et al. subsequently reported using an inflatable balloon to occlude the colonic lumen proximal to the colotomy in order to both improve the procedural sterility and prevent loss of pneumoperitoneum due to escape of air through the colonic incision [16]. Five acute study and ten survival pigs were prepared with 1 gal of Pedialyte orally, oral Fleet Phospho-soda, and IV cefazolin and metronidazole. Two acute study pigs were prepared with tap water enemas and underwent peritoneoscopy via a 10-mm needle-knife colostomy after the balloon was in place. After the withdrawal of the endoscope from the peritoneal cavity, fecal contents arrived from the proximal colon and contaminated the incision site. As significant colonic distention obscured the view and fecal contents contaminated the incision area, the procedure was refined for the remaining three acute study and ten survival pigs. These animals were prepared with tap water enemas, subsequent sterile water in the survival animals, and 10 % povidone-iodine solution external scrub. The soft latex balloon was endoscopically placed at 20 cm and inflated with air to seal the lumen; the colon distal to the balloon was irrigated with 10 % povidone-iodine solution. Colotomy, peritoneoscopy, and closure were performed as before. Survival pigs were given oral ciprofloxacin and metronidazole for 3 days postoperatively, and a regular diet was resumed within hours of surgery. The stomach, liver, gallbladder, spleen, small bowel, colon, and urinary bladder were identified in all animals. Closure with endoclips was successful in one of two pigs without using the balloon as the colonic lumen was often collapsed; with the balloon, endoclip closure was successful in all 13 pigs in a mean of 15.6 min, half of which was used reloading clips. All ten survival pigs did well postoperatively for 2 weeks; necropsy at that time found minimal intraabdominal adhesions in four of ten pigs and no incidental visceral injury. There were no microscopic abscesses. Microscopic mucosal ulceration and granulation tissue were present in the area of endoclips when present.

Closure Studies

Many of the above access method studies used endoclips for colotomy closure. Although these appose superficial layers, leaving serosal margins apart, Pai et al., Fong DG et al., and Dubcenco et al. reported successful closure with this technique [11, 12, 16]. Pai et al. and Fong et al. also used endoloops in the above studies; one pig undergoing endoloop closure in the Pai study developed peritonitis and was found to have a 4-mm defect at necropsy.

Early studies of endoclips for the closure of colonic perforation were performed by Raju et al. [17]. In 2005, Raju and colleagues reported a pilot survival study of four pigs prepared with Visicol and IV enrofloxacin and then subjected to 1–2-cm longitudinal perforation made with needle-knife 25 cm from the anal verge. One, two, three, and four clips were used to close the perforations in the four pigs, respectively (an additional acute study pig had a 5-cm incision closed with six endoclips and then was euthanized immediately). IV enrofloxacin was given for 7 days postoperatively, and a regular diet was introduced on day 3. Necropsy in the acute study pig revealed mucosal but not muscular or serosal apposition; there was no peritoneal contamination. At 7 days, necropsy of the survival animals revealed fecal material in the perforated segment of colon but no fecal soiling in the peritoneum or pericolic abscess. Thin fibrinous material was noted throughout the peritoneal cavity.

A subsequent study by Raju et al. in four acute and four survival pigs investigated the closure of larger perforations [18]. Preparation was similar to the preceding pilot study with the addition of Fleet's Phospho-soda enema as the last step of the preparation. A 5-cm longitudinal needle-knife incision was made 25 cm from the anus, and the endoscope was passed into the peritoneum for confirmation. Closure was achieved with Resolution® clips (Microvasive, Boston Scientific, Natick, MA) placed every 5 mm in acute study pigs and every 5–10 mm in survival pigs. Six of eight pigs had successful perforation closure; one had prolapse of adjacent viscera through a gaping perforation and another had severe bleeding at the cautery site. The two acute study pigs with successful closure had no evidence of leak on methylene blue leak test. Necropsy at 2 weeks in the four survival pigs did not reveal evidence of peritoneal fecal soiling or pericolic abscess; scant fibrinous material was seen in the two pigs given 1 week of postoperative enrofloxacin but not in the pigs given 2 weeks. There was no leak on methylene blue leak test. Bacterial culture of fluid from the paracolic gutter was positive in all four pigs.

Ryou et al. used an enhanced endoloop colotomy closure method in a five-pig study of NOTES distal pancreatectomy [19]. Three to four transmural T-tags were placed around the planned colotomy site. After the distal pancreatectomy was complete, the colotomy was closed using an endoloop-over-forceps method with concurrent pull on the T-tags to evert the incisional margins prior to closing the endoloop. Both survival pigs did well for 2 weeks, at which time necropsy revealed well-healed incisions and no evidence of peritonitis. Colovesicular and uterovesicular adhesions were present in both pigs and colouterine adhesions in one.

Mathews et al. studied early healing after closure with endoloops and endoclips [20]. Robust granulation tissue formation during this proliferative phase of healing is needed for healing and scarring of the perforation site. Eight pigs were prepared with preoperative IV cefazolin, sterile water enemas and suctioning, instillation of cefazolin suspension and then Betadine, and external Betadine scrub. The colotomy was created 15–20 cm from the anal verge followed by a 20-min peritoneoscopy. Endoloop closure was performed by using a grasper to pull the edges of the incision through the center of an endoloop and advancing the loop to enclose the entire incision before closure and release. Endoloop closure was used in five pigs; endoclips were also used in two pigs when endoloop closure was inadequate, and endoclips alone were used in one pig. Free access to food and water was provided postoperatively. Oral cephalexin was given for 3 days. Necropsy at 7 days revealed normally healing serosa and good apposition in all cases; one animal had transmural necrosis, and another had necrotic adventitia beneath transmural ulceration. All endoloop closures demonstrated continuity of granulation tissue; one pig closed with adjunctive endoclip did not, and neither did the pig with endoclip-only closure. Endoloop–endoclip combination closures often entered the access site, preventing leak-proof closure.

Several studies of transcolonic closure have been performed using novel and purpose-specific devices. Raju et al. used the InScope® MultiClip Applier (Ethicon EndoSurgery, Cincinnati, OH), which can rotate and fire multiple clips during one insertion, to compare two- and four-clip closure with nonclosure of a 2-cm colon perforation [21]. Seventeen pigs (four control, seven for two-clip closure, and six for four-clip closure) were prepared with Visicol tablets, Fleet's Phospho-soda enema, and IV enrofloxacin. A longitudinal perforation was created approximately 20 cm from the anal verge with needle-knife puncture followed by insulated tip-knife extension to 2 cm. In the two-clip group, clips were placed about 5 mm from each end of the perforation; in the four-clip group, clips were placed at 5-mm intervals. Closure was successful in 12 of 13 pigs. Clips were placed in the two- and four-clip groups in a median time of 2 and 3 min, respectively. Enrofloxacin was given daily for the 2-week survival period. Three of four control pigs developed clinical signs of peritonitis, confirmed by finding of fibrinous peritonitis; all four pigs had adhesions. Three pigs had positive peritoneal bacterial cultures. The methylene blue dye leak test revealed leak in one control animal. None of the pigs undergoing closure demonstrated clinical signs of peritonitis during the survival period; on necropsy, there was no peritoneal soiling or pericolic abscess. Two pigs had fibrinous peritonitis, and three had adhesions; there was no dye leak on leak testing. Peritoneal cultures were contaminated in two pigs, positive with mixed flora in six pigs, and negative in four pigs.

Raju et al. then compared the InScope MultiClip Applier with the Tissue Approximation Device (TAD; Ethicon EndoSurgery, Cincinnati, OH) for the closure of larger perforations, whose edges tend to evert into the peritoneal cavity [22]. The TAD comprises a polypropylene thread attached to a T-tag, a needle catheter, and a thread-locking-cutting device. After preparation with Visicol tablets, a 4-cm incision was created 20 cm from the anal verge using a needle-knife for puncture and an insulated tip-knife for extension. The MultiClip Applier was used to place four clips at 1-cm intervals; it successfully closed five of six perforations, with fibrinous peritonitis in two of the five pigs at the end of the 2-week survival period. Microbiologic cultures were positive for mixed flora in three of five pigs. The TAD achieved perforation closure in four of four pigs; two of four had fibrinous peritonitis at the end of the survival period, and cultures were positive for enteric flora in two or four pigs. There was no histologic difference in inflammation or tissue repair between the clip and suture groups. In the suture closure group, fibrinous peritonitis only developed in the two pigs in which closure took over 30 min; one of these pigs also developed abdominal wall peritoneal abscess and the other developed transient peritonitis.

Fong et al. and Ryou et al. used the LSI purse-string suture closure device in the survival studies discussed above [13, 14]. Unlike endoclip closures, which were time-consuming and technically difficult, the LSI closure was performed quickly and with fewer technical demands. Closures made with the LSI device have compared favorably with both clips and hand-sewn suture in ex vivo leak testing [23]. The device has a flexible shaft and uses vacuum pressure to draw tissue into its hollow tip; two parallel needles create a purse-string suture, and a central blade creates a 2.5-mm transmural incision. After the procedure is completed and the endoscope withdrawn into the colon, the purse string is secured with a titanium clip applied by a separate device.

Pham et al. reported use of the EagleClaw™ Endoscopic Suturing Device (ECESD, Apollo Group) for colotomy closure in ten pigs [24]. Preparation was with Visicol tablets and IV ciprofloxacin. A 15–20-mm colotomy was created with a needle-knife 25 cm from the anus (pancreatic injury occurred at 35 cm). The colotomy was sutured with the ECESD, which required removal of the device through the overtube and reloading outside the pig for each suture. Closure was successful in eight of ten pigs in less than 10 min per closure. Necropsy at 7 days revealed no peritonitis or peritoneal abscess, but fibrinous material was present throughout the peritoneal cavity in two pigs.

Raju et al. compared endoscopic closure with surgical closure [25]. Pigs were prepared with Visicol tablets and Fleets Phospho-soda enema. Endoscopic cleaning of stool from the distal colon was performed en route to the perforation site without cleaning the endoscope prior to perforation; a 4-cm perforation was made 20 cm from the anus using a needle-knife for perforation and insulated tip-knife for extension. Pigs were then randomized to endoscopic or surgical closure. Endoscopic closure was performed using the Tissue Apposition System (Ethicon EndoSurgery, Cincinnati, OH), which comprises a 3.0 polypropylene thread attached to a metal T-tag, a needle catheter with a stylet, and a thread-locking-cutting device. The device was used to create needle puncture of one edge of the perforation and release the first T-tag, place another T-tag on the opposing edge, tie the sutures, and cut the suture; T-tags were inserted every 5–10 mm to close the perforation. As the system did not need to be removed to reload suture, continuous suction of colonic contents prevented leakage into the peritoneum. The InScope MultiClip applier, described above, was used to apply clips where needed. Surgical closure was performed via midline laparotomy; 4-0 resorbable monofilament suture was used to close the perforation site and 2-0 running resorbable monofilament was used to close the abdominal fascia. The peritoneum was not closed, as suture closure has been shown to increase adhesions. Enrofloxacin was given daily during the 2-week survival period, and a regular diet was introduced on the third day. Fifty-four pigs were randomized (an additional pig was excluded due to small bowel injury during needle-knife perforation), 27 to each group. Surgical closure was successful in all 27 pigs. Endoscopic closure was successful in 26 of 27 pigs; sutures alone were used in 12; clips were also used in 15. One pig failed to recover, and repeat endoscopic closure was attempted within 6 h; the pig did not eat normally until day 11. Four surgical closure pigs were euthanized prior to the end of the 2-week survival period, three due to bowel obstruction from dense adhesions and one after bladder rupture resulting from accidental urethral ligation during abdominal closure. Three endoscopic closure pigs were euthanized due to bowel necrosis caused by T-tag insertion into the mesentery, fecal peritonitis due to slippage of endoclips, and torsion of the colon, respectively. Necropsy at 2 weeks revealed mild fibrinous deposits in 3 of 23 surgical closure pigs and severe deposits in 2 of 23 pigs; in the endoscopic closure pigs, there were mild fibrinous deposits in 7 of 23 pigs. Pericolonic abscess was noted in 3 of 23 endoscopic closure pigs vs. 4 of 23 surgical closure pigs. Both the endoscopic and surgical closure pigs showed local adhesions in 18 of 23 pigs; adhesions distant from the colotomy were found in 6 of 23 endoscopic closure pigs (severe in 2 pigs) and 13 of 23 surgical closure pigs (severe in 10 pigs). Of 186 T-tags inserted, 5 were inserted into adjacent viscera, intestine, mesentery, and fat. Dye leak test was done in 21 endoscopic closure pigs and was negative in all; 1 of 23 surgical closure pigs demonstrated a leak through a suture abscess. This large, randomized multicenter study showed that endoscopic and surgical closure of colonic perforation were comparably effective.

Raju et al. evaluated transverse (opening the clip in the 3–9 o'clock position in relation to the defect) and longitudinal (opening the clip in the 6–12 o'clock position) endoclip closure methods for circular colonic perforations [26]. Pigs were prepared with oral electrolyte solution, Visicol tablets, and Fleet's Phospho-soda enemas. A band-ligator resector (Duette™; Cook Endoscopy, Winston-Salem, NC) and snare were used to create a full-thickness colonic resection (mean size 1.7 ± 0.075 cm) 20 cm from the anus. Ten closures were performed with endoclips (Resolution clips; Boston Scientific, Natick, MA) in nine pigs; a 10th pig underwent five perforations used to measure perforation sizes. Injury to adjacent viscera was found in 8 of 15 resections, precluding survival study. Of the three transverse closures, two were failures as their edges could not be apposed. The third succeeded only after a thread was attached to the clip and pulled to bring the wound edges together. After the methylene blue leak test was positive, a 2-mm residual defect was confirmed. All seven attempts at longitudinal closure were successful; one pig failed the leak test and was found to have a 2-mm residual defect, as the overlapping wound edges obscured the defect during closure. Longitudinal closure was found to be technically easier than transverse closure.

Comparative Studies

Voermans et al. compared transcolonic access with laparoscopy for staging peritoneoscopy [27]. Having already found that transgastric peritoneoscopy was inferior to laparoscopy due to limited visualization of the liver, the group theorized that the direct approach from the lower abdomen might result in better visualization. A total of 33 2.5-mm beads were laparoscopically placed into six pigs. They were attached to the peritoneum in likely targets of metastatic disease. Needle-knife puncture 15–20 cm from the anal verge was followed by dilation with an 18-mm CRE balloon (Boston Scientific, Natick, MA). Each pig then underwent transcolonic peritoneoscopy. Beads were touched to count for identification. While laparoscopy identified 95 % of beads in an identical porcine model, transcolonic peritoneoscopy identified 76 %. While all beads on the peritoneum and diaphragm were identified, only 61 % of beads on the liver surface were identified. An earlier study by the same group using similar methods to compare transgastric peritoneoscopy with laparoscopy found that transgastric peritoneoscopy detected 63 % of beads (and only 38 % of beads placed on the liver) [28].

Voermans et al. directly compared transgastric with transcolonic peritoneoscopy combined with intraperitoneal endoscopic ultrasound (EUS) [29]. Twelve pigs underwent bowel preparation with multiple enemas to clean the distal colon. Transgastric entry into the peritoneum was created by application of two T-tags into the anterior gastric wall followed by a needle-knife puncture and dilation with an 18-mm CRE balloon. Transcolonic access was performed 15–20 cm from the anal verge; two T-tags were placed at the incision site, and a puncture was created with a needle-knife. The target locations included the left and right peritoneal upper quadrants (two structures), left and right hemidiaphragms (two structures), liver and hepatoduodenal ligament (five structures), and the omentum, anterior stomach, and duodenal curve (three structures). One point was given for the visualization of each target and a second for touching the target with a biopsy forceps; the maximum score for the 12 locations was 24 points. The echoendoscope was introduced over a guidewire placed at the end of the peritoneoscopy. Closure was achieved with a cinch to tie the T-tag sutures together. There were no complications during access. Transgastric peritoneoscopy resulted in 20–24 points (median 23); transcolonic peritoneoscopy resulted in the maximum 24 points in all pigs. While the entire liver and hepatoduodenal surface was visualized and touched during transcolonic peritoneoscopy, this was only achieved in three of six transgastric procedures. The hepatoduodenal ligament, right inferior part of the liver, and both of these, respectively, were not visualized in these three cases. One point was awarded for visualization of each target area with EUS. Using transgastric access resulted in 8–12 points (median 11), while using transcolonic access resulted in scores of 8–12 points (median 12). The entire liver was visualized with EUS in four of six pigs. In the remaining two pigs, transgastric EUS visualized 50 % and 66 %, respectively, while transcolonic EUS visualized 66 % and 83 %, respectively. Both transgastric and transcolonic peritoneoscopy took a median 10 min, while transgastric EUS took a median 9 min and transcolonic EUS took a median 7 min.

Voermans et al. also compared transgastric, transcolonic, and laparoscopic peritoneoscopy in a human cadaver model for staging [30]. Six cadavers (four female) underwent peritoneoscopy using each modality for 30 min in random order. A total of 34 2.5-mm beads were randomly sewn to likely metastatic targets for upper gastrointestinal, hepatic, biliary, and pancreatic malignancy. Touching beads with biopsy forceps simulated biopsy. Laparoscopic peritoneoscopy was performed using a 10-mm 0° laparoscope (EndoEye™; Olympus Medical Systems Europe, Hamburg, Germany) via umbilical trocar and a Veress needle to induce pneumoperitoneum (12 mmHg). NOTES procedures were performed with pneumoperitoneum (8 mmHg) induced using a Veress needle. A needle-knife and an 18-mm CRE balloon were used for access via the anterior gastric or colonic wall (in one cadaver with extensive adhesions and residual stool, access was achieved via the retroperitoneal cavity). Peritoneoscopy was performed with a double-channel endoscope and standard accessories. Laparoscopy detected 97 % of beads, missing one in the left upper quadrant. Transgastric peritoneoscopy detected 76 % of beads, and transcolonic peritoneoscopy detected 85 % (only transcolonic peritoneoscopy was within the 15 % margin of equivalence). All beads at the diaphragm and superior surface of the liver were detected by transgastric and transcolonic peritoneoscopy, while transgastric peritoneoscopy detected eight of ten peritoneal beads and transcolonic peritoneoscopy detected nine of ten. The yield was significantly lower at the inferior surface of the liver and hepatoduodenal ligament, where transgastric peritoneoscopy found 33 % of beads and transcolonic peritoneoscopy yielded 56 %. Excluding the inferior surface of the liver would have resulted in the non-inferiority of both NOTES access modalities (transgastric yield 92 %, transcolonic yield 96 %).

Innovative Studies

Ryou et al. reported distal pancreatectomy using transcolonic and transvaginal access simultaneously. Five pigs were given 1 g of cefazolin preoperatively and prepared with water enemas, endoscopic irrigation, and instillation of cefazolin suspension followed by povidone-iodine suspension [19]. A needle-knife colotomy was made 10–15 cm from the anal verge, the endoscope was inserted, and a Veress needle was used to create a pneumoperitoneum. The animal was rotated from supine to prone to enhance the retroperitoneal exposure. The distal pancreas was dissected from the retroperitoneum using a sclerosing needle and electrocautery. An endoscope and a needle-knife were used to create a posterior colpotomy, through which a linear stapler was inserted. Once the distal pancreas was resected using the stapler, the specimen was retrieved transcolonically using a 2.8-cm Roth net. Endoloop and T-tag sutures were used for the colotomy closure. The transvaginal access site was not closed. There were no complications during peritoneal access. Two pigs were used for survival study; after 2 weeks, necropsy did not reveal gross infection or hemorrhage, and transcolonic and transvaginal access sites had healed completely. Both pigs had colovesicular and uterovesicular adhesions, and one had colouterine adhesions.

Eshuis et al. reported natural orifice specimen extraction (NOSE) in ten patients undergoing laparoscopic ileocolonic resection for Crohn's disease; this procedure obviates the need to widen a laparoscopic port incision for specimen extraction, potentially reducing pain, wound infection rate, and the risk of incisional hernia [31]. Patients underwent preoperative bowel preparation and were given 24 h of intravenous antibiotics prior to the procedure. After laparoscopic bowel division, the colonoscope was advanced to the cross-stapled colon. Once a side-to-side anastomosis was created, the colonoscope was inserted through the remaining gap in the anastomosis and the specimen was grasped with a 3-cm endoscopic snare. The laparoscopist assisted passage of the specimen through the anastomosis and held the bowel to prevent invagination as the endoscopist pulled the specimen through the colon and extracted it transanally. Specimen removal was successful in eight of ten cases; in the other two patients, large inflammatory masses (7 and 8 cm in diameter) were discovered intraoperatively. The median resection length was 25.5 cm; the median operating time was 208 min (significantly longer than 30 comparable laparoscopically assisted procedures), and the postoperative stay was 5 days. One patient developed an abscess in the pouch of Douglas requiring laparoscopic drainage and also pain of unknown origin requiring readmission; another developed a small abscess at the umbilical port, and a third developed a fever of unknown origin. Infectious complications were significantly more frequent in the transcolonic extraction group than in 30 similar laparoscopically assisted cases (3/10 vs. 1/30, $p = 0.042$).

Alternative Inferior Access Points

Transvaginal and transvesical entries into the peritoneum for NOTES have been investigated. Like transcolonic access, these provide an *en face* view of the organs of the upper abdomen.

Transvaginal access into the peritoneum has an extensive history, starting with culdoscopy in the 1940s and succeeded by transvaginal hydrolaparoscopy [19]. More recently, Tsin reported posterior colpotomy to extract large specimens, such as uterine myomas, ovarian cysts, gallbladders, appendixes, and even an intact nephrectomy specimen [32–34]. Palanivelu et al. reported seven total laparoscopic proctocolectomies with transvaginal specimen extraction [35]. Although large specimens can be extracted, the closure of ports up to 12 mm can often be accomplished safely with just a single suture [36]. Furthermore, the closure can be accomplished by external suturing [37]. Rigid instruments can be inserted transvaginally if needed, and there is evidence that these may be easier to use and more effective in many cases. In fact, many of the current human trials rely on rigid instrumentation via this route. The primary relative disadvantage of this approach is its inapplicability in males.

Transvesical access has been used alone or in combination with transgastric access for peritoneoscopy, cholecystectomy, liver biopsy, and nephrectomy [4, 7, 8, 38]. It has advantages relative to transcolonic access in natural sterility and in anterior position in the pelvis, allowing peritoneal access above the bowel loops. Lima et al. reported that closure of a 5-mm hole in the bladder is not necessary if the bladder can drain. This group also demonstrated successful closure using endoscopic suturing with T-fasteners in a 15-pig survival model. However, the narrow diameter of the urethra limits the potential size of instruments used and specimens extracted.

Advantages of Transcolonic Access

The transcolonic approach presents several advantages over the transgastric, transvaginal, and transvesicular accesses. As demonstrated in the above studies, the visualization and stable engagement of upper abdominal organs such as the stomach, liver, gallbladder, spleen, small bowel, and peritoneal surfaces are quickly and easily achieved within minutes of the transcolonic access. Transcolonic access provides an *en face* view of the upper abdominal organs, while the transgastric approach often requires retroflexion. The direct approach avoids the loss of visual orientation, distal force transmission, and accurate haptic feedback that occurs with acute endoscope tip angulation and retroflexion. Furthermore, larger specimens can traverse the colon and anus than the esophagus for removal. While the anus is routinely dilated to 40 mm prior to the use of the rigid rectoscope, the esophagus is not routinely dilated beyond 20 mm. The larger diameter of the colon also averts traction of multiple instruments on each other, which occurs more easily in the esophagus. If the colotomy is made near the anus, rigid surgical instruments can be used for rescue procedures at the incision site, avoiding laparotomy; this is not an option when gastrotomy is used for access. Finally, unlike transvaginal access, the transcolonic approach can be used in men and women.

Disadvantages of Transcolonic Access

The studies above have similarly demonstrated some disadvantages of transcolonic access for NOTES. Sterility, and the complications resulting from the introduction of bacteria and fecal material into the peritoneal space, is an important concern; many studies have demonstrated subsequent peritonitis or the development of adhesions. It has been inferred that development of adhesions is secondary to subclinical peritonitis, although other possible etiologies include wound healing, injury to adjacent structures, and inflammatory response to antibiotic or cleansing solutions used during preparation [39]. Perhaps improved bowel preparation, sterilization of instruments, and use of occlusive balloons or sterile conduits would decrease or prevent these sequelae of colotomy. Additionally, several of the above studies noted injury to adjacent viscerae. Wilhelm et al. instilled a fluidoperitoneum to create a buffer around the colon [15]. Endoscopic ultrasound, which has been studied extensively for guidance of transgastric access, holds the potential to direct safe colotomy. Shearing of the colonic wall at the colotomy site is a possibility. This may be prevented by using an overtube or guide sheath [39]. Finally, secure colotomy closure represents a challenge; a safe, consistently effective closure method will have to be demonstrated before transcolonic NOTES can be applied widely in humans.

Conclusion

Transcolonic access to the peritoneum holds the potential for direct access to upper abdominal organs during NOTES procedures. Although other inferior access sites share this advantage, only transvaginal access can be used for the removal of large specimens, and this access point is hindered by the exclusion of men as procedural candidates. However, some challenges must be surmounted before transcolonic access to the peritoneum can be applied widely—notably, issues of sterility and secure closure. As the studies discussed herein have demonstrated, novel techniques are being evaluated to address these issues.

References

1. Cataldo PA. Transanal endoscopic microsurgery. Surg Clin North Am. 2006;86:915–25.
2. Whiteford MH, Denk PM, Swanstrom LL. Feasibility of radical sigmoid colectomy performed as natural orifice translumenal endoscopic surgery (NOTES) using transanal endoscopic microsurgery. Surg Endosc. 2007;21:1870–4.

3. Gavagan JA, Whiteford MH, Swanstrom LL. Full-thickness intraperitoneal excision by transanal endoscopic microsurgery does not increase short-term complications. Am J Surg. 2004;187:630–4.
4. Kalloo AN, Singh VK, Sanjay B, et al. Flexible transgastric peritoneoscopy: a novel approach to diagnosis and therapeutic intervention in the peritoneal cavity. Gastrointest Endosc. 2004;60:114–7.
5. Wagh MS, Merrifield BF, Thompson CC. Endoscopic transgastric abdominal exploration and organ resection: initial experience in a porcine model. Clin Gastroenterol Hepatol. 2005;9: 892–6.
6. Swanstrom LL, Kozarek R, Pasricha PJ, et al. Development of a new access device for transgastric surgery. J Gastrointest Surg. 2005;9:1129–37.
7. Park PO, Bergstrom M, Ikeda K, et al. Experimental studies of transgastric gallbladder surgery: cholecystectomy and cholecystogastric anastomosis. Gastrointest Endosc. 2005;61:601–6.
8. Jagannath SB, Kantsevoy SV, Vaugh CA, et al. Peroral transgastric endoscopic ligation of fallopian tubes with long-term survival in a porcine model. Gastrointest Endosc. 2005;61(3): 449–53.
9. Merrifield BF, Wagh MS, Thompson CC. Peroral transgastric organ resection: a feasibility study in pigs. Gastrointest Endosc. 2006;63(4):693–7.
10. Wagh MS, Merrifield BF, Thompson CC. Survival studies after endoscopic transgastric oophorectomy and tubectomy in a porcine model. Gastrointest Endosc. 2006;63(3):473–8.
11. Pai RD, Fong DG, Bundga ME, et al. Transcolonic endoscopic cholecystectomy: a NOTES survival study in a porcine model (with video). Gastrointest Endosc. 2006;64(3):428–34.
12. Fong DG, Pai RD, Thompson CC, et al. Transcolonic endoscopic abdominal exploration: a NOTES survival study in a porcine model. Gastrointest Endosc. 2007;65:312–8.
13. Ryou M, Fong DG, Pai RD, et al. Evaluation of a novel access and closure device for NOTES applications: a transcolonic survival study in the porcine model (with video). Gastrointest Endosc. 2007;67:964–9.
14. Fong DG, Ryou M, Pai RD, et al. Transcolonic ventral wall hernia mesh fixation in a porcine model. Endoscopy. 2007;39:865–9.
15. Wilhelm D, Meining A, von Delius S, et al. An innovative, safe and sterile sigmoid access (ISSA) for NOTES. Endoscopy. 2007;39:401–6.
16. Dubcenco E, Grantcharov T, Streutker CJ, et al. The development of a novel intracolonic occlusion balloon for transcolonic natural orifice transluminal endoscopic surgery: description of the technique and early experience in a porcine model (with videos). Gastrointest Endosc. 2008;64:760–6.
17. Raju GS, Pham B, Xiao SY, et al. A pilot study of endoscopic closure of colonic perforations with endoclips in a swine model. Gastrointest Endosc. 2005;62:791–5.
18. Raju GS, Ahmed I, Brining D, et al. Endoluminal closure of large perforations of colon with clips in a porcine model (with video). Gastrointest Endosc. 2006;64:640–6.
19. Ryou M, Fong DG, Pai RD, et al. Dual–port distal pancreatectomy using a prototype endoscope and endoscopic stapler: a natural orifice transluminal endoscopic surgery (NOTES) survival study in a porcine model. Endoscopy. 2007;39:881–7.
20. Mathews JC, Chin MS, Fernandez-Esparrach G, et al. Early healing of transcolonic and transgastric natural orifice transluminal endoscopic surgery access sites. J Am Coll Surg. 2010;210:480–90.
21. Raju GS, Ahmed I, Xiao SY, et al. Controlled trial of immediate endoluminal closure of colon perforations in a porcine model by use of a novel clip device (with videos). Gastrointest Endosc. 2006;64:989–97.
22. Raju GS, Shibukawa G, Ahmed I, et al. Endoluminal suturing may overcome the limitations of clip closure of a gaping wide colon perforation (with videos). Gastrointest Endosc. 2006;65:906–11.
23. Ryou M, Pai R, Sauer J, et al. Evaluating an optimal gastric closure method for transgastric surgery. Surg Endosc. 2007;21(4):677–80.

24. Pham B, Raju GS, Ahmed I, et al. Immediate endoscopic closure of colon perforation by using a prototype endoscopic suturing device: feasibility and outcome in a porcine model (with video). Gastrointest Endosc. 2006;64:113–9.

25. Raju GS, Fritscher-Ravens A, Rothstein RI, et al. Endoscopic closure of colon perforation compared to surgery in a porcine model: a randomized controlled trial (with videos). Gastrointest Endosc. 2008;64:324–32.

26. Raju GS, Ahmed I, Shibukawa G, et al. Endoluminal clip closure of a circular full-thickness colon resection in a porcine model (with videos). Gastrointest Endosc. 2007;65:503–9.

27. Voermans RP, Faigel DO, van Berge Henegouwen MI, et al. Comparison of transcolonic NOTES and laparoscopic peritoneoscopy for the detection of peritoneal metastases. Endoscopy. 2010;42:904–9.

28. Voermans RP, Sheppard B, van Berge Henegouwen MI, et al. Comparison of transgastric NOTES and laparoscopic peritoneoscopy for detection of peritoneal metastases. Ann Surg. 2009;250:255–9.

29. Voermans RP, van Berge Henegouwen MI, Bemelman WA, et al. Feasibility of transgastric and transcolonic natural orifice transluminal endoscopic surgery peritoneoscopy combined with intraperitoneal EUS. Gastrointest Endosc. 2009;69:e61–7.

30. Voermans RP, van Berge Henegouwen MI, de Cuba E, et al. Randomized, blinded comparison of transgastric, transcolonic, and laparoscopic peritoneoscopy for the detection of peritoneal metastases in a human cadaver model. Gastrointest Endosc. 2010;72:1027–33.

31. Eshuis EJ, Voermans RP, Stokkers PCF, et al. Laparoscopic resection with transcolonic specimen extraction for ileocaecal Crohn's disease. Br J Surg. 2010;97:569–74.

32. Tsin DA. Culdolaparoscopy: a preliminary report. JSLS. 2001;5:69–71.

33. Tsin DA, Colombero LT, Mahmood D, et al. Operative culdolaparoscopy: a novel approach combining operative culdoscopy with minilaparoscopy. J Am Assoc Gynecol Laparosc. 2001;8:438–41.

34. Tsin DA. Vaginal extraction of the intact specimen following laparoscopic radical nephrectomy. J Urol. 2002;188:1110.

35. Palanivelu C, Rangarajan M, Jategaonkar PA, Anand NV. An innovative technique for colorectal specimen retrieval: a new era of "natural orifice specimen extraction" (NOSE). Dis Colon Rectum. 2008;51:1120–4.

36. Tsin DA, Sequeria RJ, Giannikas G. Culdolaparoscopic cholecystectomy during vaginal hysterectomy. JSLS. 2003;7:171–2.

37. Lima E, Rolanda C, Autorino R, Correia-Pinto J. Experimental foundation for natural orifice transluminal endoscopic surgery and hybrid natural orifice transluminal endoscopic surgery. BJU Int. 2010;106:913–8.

38. Lima E, Rolanda C, Pêgo JM, et al. Third generation nephrectomy by natural orifice transluminal endoscopic surgery. J Urol. 2007;178:2648–54.

39. Ryou M, Thompson CC. Techniques for transanal access to the peritoneal cavity. Gastrointest Endosc Clin N Am. 2008;18(2):245–60.

Chapter 10
Access: Transvaginal

Maria J. Ribal Caparros and Antonio Alcaraz Asensio

Keywords No-scar surgery • Minimally invasive surgery • NOTES surgery Transvaginal access • Hybrid NOTES • Transvaginal NOTES-assisted laparoscopic nephrectomy

Introduction

Endoscopic surgery through natural orifices, known as NOTES (natural orifice translumenal endoscopic surgery), is an emerging surgical modality that uses endoscopic instruments through hollow viscera to enter the peritoneal cavity and allow surgical procedures without incisions. Fundamentally, the entrances are the mouth, anus, vagina, and urethra. Any surgical procedure involves the manipulation, repair, or removal of certain tissues and organs. Two decades ago we saw the progression from the traditional open surgery to laparoscopic surgery. The minimal abdominal incision was a significant improvement in postoperative recovery, analgesic requirements, hospital stay, recovery of routine activity, and the possibility of hernias. With improved technologies and the development of new techniques, the concept of scarless surgery has emerged in an attempt to treat certain diseases, obviating the need for incisions to access the peritoneal cavity, resulting in a direct benefit to patients, offering an improvement in quality of life and an advantage over conventional laparoscopy. Laparoendoscopic single-site surgery (LESS) and natural orifice translumenal endoscopic surgery (NOTES) are evolutions of laparoscopy, but they are complementary techniques that should be included in this new concept.

M.J. Ribal, M.D., Ph.D. (✉) • A. Alcaraz, M.D., Ph.D.
Department of Urology, Hospital Clinic, University of Barcelona,
Villarroel 170, Barcelona 08036, Spain
e-mail: mjribal@clinic.ub.es; aalcaraz@clinic.ub.es

A. Rane et al. (eds.), *Scar-Less Surgery*,
DOI 10.1007/978-1-84800-360-6_10, © Springer-Verlag London 2013

With the development of NOTES, the philosophy of surgery has dramatically changed, a change that had already begun with the development of laparoscopy. Translumenal surgery has the potential to break the classical concept of surgery, and although its role is still to be determined and it may not become a break as important as that achieved by laparoscopy in place of open surgery, it is likely that NOTES involves a major revolution and a push for the improvement of endoscopic techniques [1].

Advantages and Disadvantages of NOTES

The NOTES procedure may provide additional benefits when compared with current minimally invasive procedures. The potential advantages include no skin incisions, an improved cosmetic result, reduced postoperative pain, a diminished risk of postoperative hernias, and earlier recovery [2].

In spite of all this, it should not be forgotten that translumenal surgery is still under development, which is a reason why its application in humans must be carried out by groups with prior experience in animal models and under the ethical approval of the relevant hospitals. Although the studies published on its application in clinical practice have shown favorable results, previous and simultaneous studies in animal models report complications such as peritonitis in transgastric access; therefore, patients must be adequately informed of the risks associated with this type of surgery.

Pure NOTES instruments have been criticized for their flexibility, the impossibility of retracting large organs, such as the kidney, the incongruence of the flexible material to be used in the abdominal cavity, and the limited port access for good hemostatic devices [3]. Another disadvantage is that the endoscope's camera rotates with the rotation of the instruments, misleading the surgeon and moving the surgical field outside the visual space. Ureteroscopes and gastroscopes were designed primarily as diagnostic tools and are far from being ideal for use in NOTES. Difficulty in using the instruments occurs not only for formal surgery, but especially when intraoperative complications arise during NOTES procedures, such as bleeding. The last disadvantage is the need for internal organ closure after any NOTES procedure. Once the surgery is finished, the hole in the viscera has to be closed, and we still have not developed a technique that guarantees a complete and safe suture of the stomach, bladder, or colon.

Attempts to overcome the current limitations of the technique have given rise to the concept of hybrid NOTES, which is performed with the assistance of transabdominal ports for the use of conventional laparoscopy equipment. Hybrid NOTES allows perforation of the organ under direct vision, minimizing the possibility of injury to adjacent tissues. Moreover, the hybrid approach dramatically improves spatial orientation, allowing the use of laparoscopic cameras specially designed to overcome the limitations of endoscopic material. Retraction and tissue dissection improve with the assistance of transabdominal ports for instrumentation and allow triangulation.

It has been defined that a combination of a NOTES procedure with abdominal trocars for assistance must be divided into assisted NOTES or hybrid NOTES depending on whether the visceral access is used for intrumentalization or camera viewing [4]. Some authors, and we are among them, are defending the current, minimally invasive, hybrid approach over pure NOTES without laparoscopic assistance. In our opinion, to talk about hybrid or assisted NOTES is an artificial debate. What really matters is to achieve good results in a safe manner with the fewest assistant trocars possible. Hybrid or assisted NOTES is a new, safe approach that overcomes the current technical problems while maintaining most of the advantages of NOTES.

Transvaginal Access

The use of natural orifices in the field of laparoscopic surgery started with their use for the extraction of a surgical sample. Within the ambit of urology, Breda et al. [5] were the first to describe the extraction of a nephrectomy sample after laparoscopic surgery through the vagina. In 2002, Gill et al. published their first series on laparoscopic nephrectomy with vaginal extraction of the sample [6]. Ten women with an average age of 67 were subjected to radical laparoscopic nephrectomies for renal tumors with posterior colpotomy to extract the sample. In the paper, the authors indicate that this approach for extraction has become the standard for women undergoing ablative renal surgery [6].

Gettman et al. [7] published the first experimental application of NOTES in 2002, when they carried out the first transvaginal nephrectomy in a porcine model using rigid and flexible laparoscopes and the ports of access were modified Amplatz dilators. Clayman's group reported in 2007 on their initial experience regarding transvaginal nephrectomy by NOTES, which was an experimental surgery in pigs. They used a 12-mm trocar in the median line transvaginally with a multichannel platform that allowed a bimanual manipulation [8]. Thus arose the idea of using the vagina as a working port and not just as a route for the extraction of surgical samples.

The transvaginal approach seems to adapt perfectly to the wishes of cosmetic improvement and the absence of scarring that are sought after with the development of NOTES, as well as permitting the extraction of surgical samples of considerable size, which makes it particularly attractive as an approach route in ablative and even oncological surgery.

In fact, many of the animal models developed for NOTES are based on transgastric access, yet a large part of the studies published in humans use the transvaginal route. One of the main factors for the development of NOTES is the secure closure of the transluminal access. The transvaginal access has been considered superior to the transgastric or transcolonic accesses from the moment that it could be carried out via conventional surgical techniques. In the gynecological literature, innumerable patients have been subjected to the opening of the vagina to the peritoneal cavity for a wide variety of procedures with a very low complication rate. Also, of all the accesses, the vagina is the one that allows the easiest extraction of surgical samples, especially those of a large size, as in nephrectomies. Similarly, it allows the use of rigid instruments and the maintenance of the target organ in direct line with the point of access, improving the questions related to spatial orientation. Nevertheless, in spite of the low rate of infection reported in the gynecological literature, it must be taken into consideration that the transvaginal NOTES technique involves the instrumentalization of the peritoneal cavity through the vagina, which could signify a higher peritoneal contamination and a consequent increase in the rate of infections, data that, given the lack of follow-up, should be contrasted. Also, it is necessary to explore the effect of the technique on sexual function. And, in spite of all its advantages, the transvaginal access is only available to 50 % of the population to treat due to a question of sex, and within the female population any prior pelvic or gynecological surgery may contraindicate this access, which may possibly imply that the access is only viable for around 30 % of the population to treat [8].

Transvaginal NOTES in Urological Surgery: From Assisted and Hybrid NOTES to Pure NOTES

Transvaginal Nephrectomy Assisted with Two Laparoscopic Ports

In 2007, Branco et al. reported the first hybrid transvaginal nephrectomy in a 23-year-old woman who presented with right flank pain and recurrent urinary tract infection due to a nonfunctional right kidney. The pneumoperitoneum was achieved by a Veress needle placed in the umbilicus, and afterward a 5-mm laparoscopic port was positioned in the same site. The gas was helpful for the vaginal access since it filled and distended the cul-de-sac. The vaginal walls were retracted and the cervix was anteriorly pulled to expose the posterior fornix. The vaginal mucosa in the posterior cul-de-sac was opened by a longitudinal 1.5-cm incision and the abdominal cavity was entered. They used the double-channel flexible endoscope (Karl Storz Endoskope, Tuttlingen, Germany). The flexible tip of the device was turned 180° to face the vaginal dome and rule out any possible bleeding and visceral injury. The patient was then placed in a 45° left lateral position, and her chest and lower limbs were secured to the table. The abdominal cavity was carefully inspected, and one additional 5-mm trocar was placed just below the xyphoid. Dissection was performed under endoscopic view, with the help of endoscopic instruments, following the steps of a regular laparoscopic nephrectomy. The total procedure time was 170 min and the estimated blood loss was 350 cc. The patient had an uneventful postoperative course and was discharged 12 h after the procedure [9].

Our group in Barcelona published the first hybrid transvaginal nephrectomy for renal cancer, also placing two abdominal trocars; these were a 12-mm one at the level of the right flank, 4 cm from the navel, and a 5-mm trocar in the right flank.

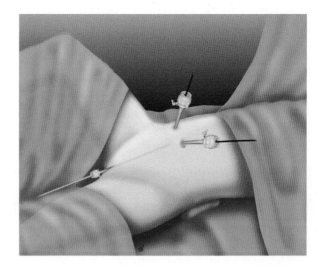

Fig. 10.1 Position of the patient for NOTES-assisted transvaginal nephrectomy (Reprinted with permission from Elsevier from Alcaraz et al. [9])

The transvaginal access was achieved using an obesity trocar of 12 mm wherein we introduced a 10-mm camera with a deflectable tip, thus solving, in part, the previously described limitations [3]. Later, the group published the first series reported (14 cases) of assisted transvaginal NOTES nephrectomies in renal cancer, proving the safety and reproducibility of the technique [9]. So far, it has been successfully completed in 18 cases.

The surgical technique is performed under general anesthesia; the patient is placed in a semilumbotomy position with separated legs to allow vaginal access (Fig. 10.1). The pneumoperitoneum is achieved by a 12-mm trocar/port placed laterally 5 cm from the umbilicus under direct vision. The intraabdominal pressure is maintained at 12 mmHg. A normal laparoscopic optic of 0° is placed into the abdominal cavity under direct vision, and an additional 5-mm trocar is placed in the flank. Finally, an obese special port is placed through the vagina into the abdominal cavity, perforating the vaginal wall in the posterior cul-de-sac under direct vision. Through the 5-mm abdominal trocar, a conventional grasper is placed to retract the uterus and facilitate visualization of the vaginal posterior wall to avoid sigmoid lesions. The trocar is guided through the vagina using a conventional vaginal valve.

A deflectable optic (Deflectable-Tip EndoEYE™; Olympus, Tokyo, Japan) is introduced into the peritoneal cavity. Dissection is performed following the steps of a regular laparoscopic transabdominal nephrectomy using instruments placed in the abdominal trocars, under direct vision achieved by a deflectable camera, placed through the vaginal trocar. The line of Toldt is incised and the colon is mobilized until the psoas muscle become visible. The ureter is dissected and sectioned using the LigaSure™ device (Valleylab, Tyco Healthcare, Boulder, CO). The renal hilum is reached by dissection of the lower pole through the cranial direction. The renal artery is ligated with Hem-o-lok® clips (Weck Closure Systems, Research Triangle Park, NC) and sectioned. Ligation of the renal vein is done by the same device.

The posterior wall and the upper pole are dissected, preserving the adrenal gland. The surgical specimen is freed and an organ bag is introduced through the trocar placed at the vagina after retrieving the deflectable optic. The kidney is placed inside the organ bag, and the specimen is removed under direct vision with an optic in the abdominal trocar through an extended incision at the posterior wall of the vagina. The vaginal wound is closed under direct vision using conventional instruments. A running 2-0 absorbable suture is used.

Transvaginal Nephrectomy with Three Abdominal Ports

The good acceptance and satisfaction of women undergoing transvaginal surgery led our group to believe that this approach would also be promising for other indications, such as live kidney donors in females. The surgical approach was then modified and three assistant abdominal ports were used.

In this modified transvaginal NOTES-assisted technique, the donor is placed in the right lateral decubitus (45°) with modified lithotomy position under general anesthesia (Fig. 10.2). A single dose of 500 mg of metronidazole and 1 g of intravenous cefoxitine is administered during the anesthetic induction. A pneumoperitoneum is achieved by a 10-mm trocar placed in the umbilicus site under direct vision. A second 10-mm trocar port is placed in the left iliac fossa and a 5-mm port next to the ribs. Finally, a 12-mm bariatric surgery trocar is placed through the vagina, perforating the posterior cul-de-sac under direct vision to avoid any intestinal lesion. Whatever transvaginal technique is used, it is very important to place this trocar in the midline to avoid uterine vessel injury. Retracting the uterus with a grasper through the 5-mm port facilitates this maneuver. Dissection is performed following the steps of a regular laparoscopic transabdominal nephrectomy using instruments through the vagina and the abdominal wall. After ureteral section, we proceed with the lower pole lifting, which is essential to facilitate vascular pedicle dissection with a forceps placed through the vaginal trocar. Once the kidney and vascular pedicle are totally dissected, an EndoCatch™ (Covidien Surgical, Dublin, Ireland) device is placed through the vaginal trocar incision. The organ is wrapped inside the bag, permitting us to apply a gentle traction with the metallic ring of the bag, to offer a good exposure of the pedicle for safe clipping and posterior section. Two Hem-o-Lok clips are placed in the proximal ends of the artery and vein before transection. The kidney is removed inside the bag through the digitally extended incision in the vagina. Then the assistant removes the kidney from the bag, avoiding any contact with its external side to prevent contamination with vaginal bacteria. Finally, the kidney is carefully transferred to a back table for perfusion. The closure of the vaginal incision is done transvaginally and includes the entire thickness of the vaginal wall. The final surgical maneuver is the removal of the trocars after checking for correct hemostasis of the vascular pedicle and vaginal incision. For postoperative pain control, an intravenously administered combination of dexketoprofen and paracetamol is used during the first 24–48 h, with the administration of morphine on demand.

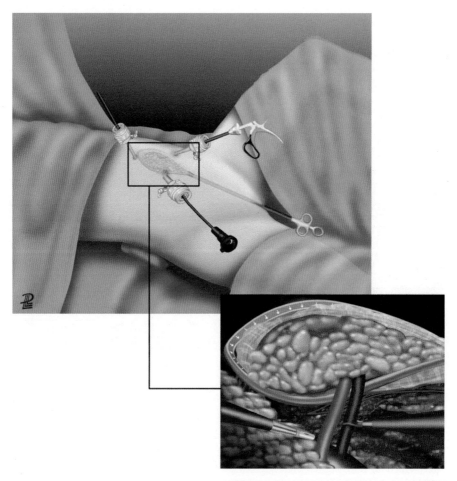

Fig. 10.2 Position of the patient and trocars for NOTES-assisted transvaginal living-donor nephrectomy (Reprinted with permission from Elsevier from Alcaraz et al. [11])

From July 2009 to June 2011, 30 women underwent transvaginal NOTES-assisted living donor nephrectomy (LDN) in our center. We compared the prospectively collected clinical data of 20 donors with those of a contemporaneous matched pair of conventional LLDNs (40 donors). The variables evaluated for donors were procedure length, blood loss, warm ischemia time (WIT), complications, hospital stay, and first-month creatinine nadir. In the transvaginal LDN group, sexual function was assessed with the Female Sexual Function Index questionnaire before and after surgery. The variables evaluated for recipients were complications, graft function, and creatinine evolution. The procedure was completed in all cases. The operative variables were similar for both groups except for the WIT, which was longer in the transvaginal LDN group ($p < 0.001$) without consequences for graft functioning. One transvaginal LDN case had postoperative bleeding requiring immediate open surgery. All transvaginal LDN donors reported unaltered sexual function after surgery and satisfaction with the results. All recipients had immediate urine output, and all had a functioning graft at last follow-up except for one recipient of the transvaginal LDN group who required transplantectomy. Despite promising results, randomized controlled studies with longer follow-up are warranted to further elucidate the potential of this novel technique [11].

Along the same line of more than two abdominal trocars for assistance during transvaginal NOTES procedure, Porpiglia et al. described their first experience with transvaginal natural orifice translumenal endoscopic surgery-assisted mini-laparoscopic nephrectomy (mLN) [12]. The patient is positioned in a semilumbotomy position with legs separated to allow for vaginal access. A 3.5-mm port is placed at the umbilicus for a 30° laparoscope; two 3.5-mm ports are placed in the flank in the same location as for a standard transperitoneal nephrectomy; and a 12-mm port is placed through the vagina, perforating the vaginal wall. Kidney dissection is performed following the steps of a traditional nephrectomy. The renal pedicle is dissected and secured with Hem-o-Lok clips through the vaginal access port. The specimen is then extracted through an extended incision in the posterior wall of the vagina. They have treated five patients. The average operative time was 120 min, blood loss was 160 ml, and no complications were recorded. Their initial experience suggests that transvaginal NOTES-assisted mLN is feasible and appears to be safe. It is simpler than a pure NOTES procedure and ensures excellent cosmetic results.

Hospital Clinic of Barcelona Experience

Over the last 4 years at the Department of Urology, Hospital Clinic, Barcelona, we have performed 48 transvaginal NOTES-assisted laparoscopic nephrectomies. All the procedures were performed with the approval of the Ethics Committee. Between March 2008 and June 2011, 18 female patients underwent transvaginal NOTES-assisted laparoscopic nephrectomy for T1-T3aN0M0 renal cancer ($n=13$), lithiasis ($n=2$), or renal atrophy ($n=3$) in our hospital. Furthermore, 30 patients donated their kidney using the application of NOTES in live-donor laparoscopic nephrectomy [13].

The mean age of the women was 53.9 years (range: 34–78 years). Thirty-two left and 16 right nephrectomies were performed. The mean operative time was 120 min (range: 80–270 min) and the mean estimated blood loss was 161 ml (range: 30–400 ml). One patient required a blood transfusion after surgery. The mean time of analgesia was 18.4 h (range: 0–72 h). The mean hospital stay was 4 days (3.6 days if we exclude from the analysis the patient with the major complication). Major complications occurred in two patients. In one patient, who had previous abdominal and pelvic surgery, a colon injury occurred. This patient underwent surgery and a temporary colostomy was performed. The patient has already undergone reconstruction. Another patient required surgical revision in the early postoperative time due to bleeding.

Clinical Indications for Hybrid NOTES Transvaginal Surgery

The NOTES procedure constitutes one of the newest innovations in surgical techniques, with very few studies having been published to date. Since the first procedure, and with the accumulating experience in the Hospital Clinic of Barcelona, the selection criteria are increasing. The procedure is currently offered to any woman with a renal tumor who is a candidate for radical nephrectomy and to those female patients who are candidates for live-donor nephrectomy.

In our own series, we have experienced two major complications, one in the radical nephrectomy series and another in the live-donor series. The first was a colon injury that appeared on the second postoperative day in a patient who had undergone previous abdominal pelvic surgery and who required surgery and a temporary colostomy. The second was a transvaginal live donor who presented with an acute hemorrhage that required surgical revision in the early postoperative time. This bleeding was due to a uterine vessel injury that occurred during transvaginal trocar insertion and was not noticed during surgery, although the whole operative field had been examined carefully after the kidney removal.

Considering our own experience, patients must be examined before surgery to determine the suitability of the vagina for specimen retrieval and surgical procedure. Those patients with a high BMI or those with a narrow vagina must be excluded. Also, the uterine vessels must be assessed with a computed tomography scan prior to surgery to rule out varicose malformations. Finally, those patients with prior pelvic surgery can be considered poor candidates for transvaginal access.

A concern of the vaginal nephrectomy approach is the possibility of sexual dysfunction after surgery. However, current literature on this topic, mainly in the gynecology field, suggests that sexual dysfunction is a rare event after vaginal surgery. Currently, all our patients complete a validated questionnaire for assessing sexual function before surgery as well as 4 months after. Preliminary results on the Female Sexual Function Index (FSFI) show no differences after transvaginal nephrectomy [11].

In our opinion, hybrid transvaginal NOTES is a feasible and reliable technique and must be considered in the female population suitable for kidney surgery. Nevertheless, further analyses and well-conducted prospective studies are warranted.

Transvaginal Nephrectomy with One Port

In 2009, Sotelo et al. reported a modification to the technique previously described in cadavers [14], on this occasion applied to a patient with a renal tumor at the level of the inferior pole. Here they only used two accesses, navel and vaginal, with a three-channel trocar (TriPort™; Advanced Surgical Concepts, Bray, Ireland) and

Fig. 10.3 Position of the trocars for the technique of NOTES with one-port assistance (Reprinted with permission from Clavijo et al. [15])

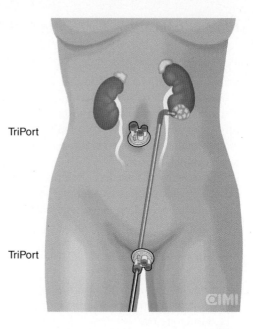

TriPort

TriPort

using a 5-mm camera with a deflectable tip (Fig. 10.3). This was the first approach where no extra-umbilical accesses were used [16], which was the main difference from the approaches described by Branco and Alcaraz.

Later, Kaouk et al. carried out a modification to the technique where they performed a right nephrectomy using a 5-mm abdominal trocar at the level of the navel and the vaginal access was via a GelPort® (Applied Medical, Rancho Santa Margarita, CA), wherein they introduced two 5-mm trocars, one 12-mm trocar, and a 5-mm deflectable optic. They described a renal dissection and retraction, exclusively through the vagina; the 5-mm trocar was placed only for the visualization and placement of the transvaginal trocar given the antecedents in the patient of prior major pelvic surgery [17].

Pure Transvaginal Nephrectomy

Kaouk et al. [18] recently reported the successful completion of the first "pure" NOTES transvaginal nephrectomy in a 58-year-old woman who presented with an atrophic right kidney. A blunt-tipped trocar was introduced transvaginally into the peritoneal cavity and a pneumoperitoneum was established. The abdominal cavity was explored transvaginally with a standard flexible video gastroscope. They used the GelPort device across the vaginal incision. Two 10-mm standard trocars and one 5-mm standard trocar were placed across the GelPort, and a 5-mm deflecting laparoscope (Olympus Surgical, Orangeburg, NJ) and 45-cm articulating graspers and scissors (Novare Surgical, Cupertino, CA) were used. The GelPort device was exchanged for the multichannel TriPort during the procedure; before finishing the surgery, the GelPort was reinserted again. An endovascular stapler was used for the section of the renal vein and renal artery. The kidney was placed into a bag and retrieved through the vaginal incision. The operative time was 420 min. The estimated blood loss was 50 ml, and there was no perioperative complication. No other pure NOTES procedures have been reported.

Transvaginal Access in General Surgery

In a recent technical review of NOTES, 432 NOTES surgical procedures were recorded and analyzed. Of interest, the majority of them were transvaginal procedures, accounting for 84 % of all NOTES procedures, followed in frequency by transgastric (13 %), transesophageal (4 %), and transrectal (0.5 %) procedures. It is important to point out that 90 % of the analyzed cases were performed in a hybrid fashion with transabdominal laparoscopic assistance. From all the approaches analyzed, transrectal and transesophageal were the ones that more frequently have utilized pure NOTES (50 % and 100 %). In the literature, the procedure more frequently reported in NOTES is cholecystectomy, accounting for 84 % of cases, followed by appendectomy [19].

The largest series published in the literature regarding transvaginal cholecystectomy involved 115 female patients. The mean age was 52.4 years and the mean operating time was 60.6 min. All the cases were performed with the assistance of one or two abdominal trocars. The pneumoperitoneum was achieved by using a Veress needle; afterward a 5-mm rigid trocar was placed and a 5-mm 30° laparoscope (EndoEye) was used for abdominal cavity inspection. The colpotomy was done, and access to the space of Douglas was achieved with a blunt extra-long 10-mm trocar. Once the 10-mm trocar was safely inserted under vision with laparoscopic control, a long bent grasper was introduced through the posterior vault adjacent to the blunt 10-mm trocar. Closure of the colpotomy was not considered mandatory.

In 8.6 % of the cases, they converted to standard laparoscopy, and in 1.6 to an open procedure. The complications following transvaginal access included one vaginal bleeding, one perforation of the urinary bladder, and one superficial lesion of the rectum. In one case, the hepatic duct had to be stented due to leakage after the procedure via endoscopic retrograde cholangiography. In a postoperative questionnaire, 95 % of patients indicated that they would recommend this procedure to other patients [20].

Conclusions

The implementation of new minimally invasive techniques is essential to optimize surgery outcomes and improve patients' recovery. Even though pure NOTES seems to be the ultimate step in this direction, technological improvements are needed before it can be accepted as a real option in clinical practice, while hybrid NOTES has already proved its feasibility. In our opinion, hybrid vs. assisted is an artificial debate. What really matters is achieving good results in a safe manner using the fewest assistant trocars possible. Whatever name we call the technique, the use of assistant trocars can make the technique much easier and reproducible, allowing the prevalence of a minimally invasive, virtually scarless technique.

NOTES techniques have been shown to be feasible in many urologic procedures, with results equivalent to conventional laparoscopy. Despite that, however, we still do not have evidence that it can overcome laparoscopic surgery; prospective trials are required to further elucidate this question.

Editorial Comment

Despite being one of the potential orifices of access for NOTES, the transvaginal route remains the dominant route for performing clinical NOTES procedures. Most clinical transvaginal procedures across surgical disciplines have also utilized transabdominal assistance although "pure" transvaginal approaches have been reported anecdotally. Until problems with other access routes in terms of entry and, more importantly, closure are resolved, it is likely that the transvaginal route will keep interest sustained in clinical NOTES surgery.

References

1. Cahill RA, Marescaux J. Natural orifice transluminal endoscopic surgery (N.O.T.E.S.) for oncologic disease. Surg Oncol. 2009;18(2):91–3.
2. Swain P. Nephrectomy and natural orifice translumenal endoscopy (NOTES): transvaginal, transgastric, transrectal, and transvesical approaches. J Endourol. 2008;22(4):811–8.
3. Ribal Caparrós MJ, Peri Cusí L, Molina Cabeza A, García Larrosa A, Carmona F, Alcaraz Asensio A. First report on hybrid transvaginal nephrectomy for renal cancer. Actas Urol Esp. 2009;33(3):280–3.
4. Box G, Averch T, Cadeddu J, Cherullo E, Clayman R, Desai M. Nomenclature of natural orifice translumenal endoscopic surgery (NOTES ™) and laparoendoscopic single-site surgery (LESS) procedures in urology. J Endourol. 2008;22(11):2575–82.
5. Breda G, Silvestre P, Giunta A. Laparoscopic nephrectomy with vaginal delivery of the intact kidney. Eur Urol. 1993;24:116–7.
6. Gill IS, Cherullo EE, Meraney AM, Borsuk F, Murphy DP, Falcone T. Vaginal extraction of the intact specimen following laparoscopic radical nephrectomy. JURO. 2002;167(1):238–41.
7. Gettman MT, Lotan Y, Napper CA, Cadeddu JA. Transvaginal laparoscopic nephrectomy: development and feasibility in the porcine model. Urology. 2002;59(3):446–50.
8. Clayman RV, Box GN, Abraham JBA, Lee HJ, Deane LA, Sargent ER, et al. Rapid communication: transvaginal single-port NOTES nephrectomy: initial laboratory experience. J Endourol. 2007;21(6):640–4.
9. Branco AW, Branco Filho AJ, Kondo W, Noda RW, Kawahara N, Camargo AAH. Hybrid transvaginal nephrectomy. Eur Urol. 2008;53:1290–4.

10. Alcaraz A, Peri L, Molina A, Goicoechea I, García E, Izquierdo L, et al. Feasibility of transvaginal NOTES-assisted laparoscopic nephrectomy. Eur Urol. 2010;57(2):233–7.
11. Alcaraz A, Musquera M, Peri L, Izquierdo L, García-Cruz E, Huguet J. Feasibility of transvaginal natural orifice transluminal endoscopic surgeryâ€"assisted living donor nephrectomy: is kidney vaginal delivery the approach of the future? Eur urol Eur Assoc Urol. 2011;22:1–9.
12. Porpiglia F, Fiori C, Morra I, Scarpa RM. Transvaginal natural orifice transluminal endoscopic surgeryâ€"assisted minilaparoscopic nephrectomy: a step towards scarless surgery. Eur Urol Eur Assoc Urol. 2010;13:1–5.
13. Alcaraz A, Peri L, Izquierdo L, Musquera M, Serapiao R, Pachón D. Transvaginal NOTES and LESS: are they the future in kidney surgery? Eur Urol Suppl Eur Assoc Urol. 2011;10(3):e58–63.
14. Aron M, Berger AK, Stein RJ, Kamoi K, Brandina R, Canes D, et al. Transvaginal nephrectomy with a multichannel laparoscopic port: a cadaver study. BJU Int. 2009;103(11):1537–41.
15. Clavijo R, Ribal MJ, Sotelo R, Fernández G, Alcaraz A. NOTES, hybrid NOTES, NOTES-assisted kidney surgery: what has been achieved so far? Arch Esp Urol. 2012;65(3):399–406.
16. Sotelo R, de Andrade R, Fernandez GF, Ramirez D, Di Grazia E, Carmona O. NOTES hybrid transvaginal radical nephrectomy for tumor: stepwise progression toward a first successful clinical case. Eur Urol Eur Assoc Urol. 2009;28:1–7.
17. Kaouk JH, White WM, Goel RK, Brethauer S, Crouzet S, Rackley RR. NOTES transvaginal nephrectomy: first human experience. Urology. 2009;74(1):5–8.
18. Kaouk JH, Haber GP, Goel RK, Crouzet S, Brethauer S, Firoozi F. Pure natural orifice translumenal endoscopic surgery (NOTES) transvaginal nephrectomy. Eur Urol Eur Assoc Urol. 2010;57(4):723–6.
19. Auyang ED, Santos BF, Enter DH, Hungness ES, Soper NJ. Natural orifice translumenal endoscopic surgery (NOTES®): a technical review. Surg Endosc. 2011;25(10):3135–48.
20. Federlein M, Borchert D, Müller V, Atas Y, Fritze F, Burghardt J. Transvaginal video-assisted cholecystectomy in clinical practice. Surg Endosc. 2010;24(10):2444–52.

Chapter 11
Access: Transvesical

Estevao Lima and Jorge Correia-Pinto

Keywords Tranvesical • NOTES • Minimally invasive • Scarless surgery

Introduction

In the last decades of the twentieth century, there was a major revolution with the advent of laparoscopy, breaking with the traditional concept of open surgery of "large incision, great surgeon" [1]. With the initial application of laparoscopy, surgeons have recognized that this approach reduced the postoperative morbidity and was quickly accepted as the gold standard technique for an increasing number of

E. Lima, M.D., Ph.D.
Department of Urology, Hospital Braga, University of Minho,
Sete Fontes – Sao Victor, Braga 4710-243, Portugal

Life and Health Sciences Research Institute,
School of Health Sciences, University of Minho,
Braga 4710-243, Portugal

ICVS/3Bs – PT Government Associate Laboratory, Braga/Guimarães,
Braga 4710-243, Portugal
e-mail: estevaolima@ecsaude.uminho.pt

J. Correia-Pinto, M.D., Ph.D. (⊠)
Department of Pediatric Surgery, Hospital Braga,
Braga 4710-057, Portugal

Surgical Sciences Research Doman, Life and Health Sciences Research Institute,
School of Health Sciences, University of Minho,
Campus de Gualtar, Braga 4710-057, Portugal
ICVS/3Bs – PT Government Associate Laboratory, Braga/Guimarães,
Braga 4710-057, Portugal
e-mail: jcp@ecsaude.uminho.pt

A. Rane et al. (eds.), *Scar-Less Surgery*,
DOI 10.1007/978-1-84800-360-6_11, © Springer-Verlag London 2013

procedures. Indeed, the laparoscopic small incisions in the abdominal wall reduce postoperative pain by shortening the time of hospitalization and convalescence, with an improved aesthetic scar [2]. Despite the laparoscopic advance, it has been a long time since humans began dreaming of performing surgery without scars. A transvisceral port to achieve the abdominal cavity could be the key to this challenge. Inspired by this possibility, Reddy and Rao in 2004 in India [3] performed a transgastric appendectomy in humans, and Kalloo et al. in the United States [4] described a peritoneoscopy with liver biopsies by a transgastric approach in a porcine model. This was the birth of NOTES (natural orifice translumenal endoscopic surgery), a new era in surgery, performed with no scars and therefore without their complications, such as wound infections, adhesions, postoperative ileus, and possibly less postoperative pain [5].

Historical Perspective of Transluminal Ports

Since the last century, surgeries have been performed via the natural orifices: urologists via urethral access, and gastroenterologists via oral and anal routes, but without exceeding the luminal barrier. It is the translumenal concept that is new in the conceptualization of NOTES; the transvaginal, transgastric, transvesical, and transcolonic ports have emerged as new approaches. The transvaginal approach was the first to be used as an entrance to the peritoneal cavity, in 1901, by Dimitri Ott, who performed a ventroscopy [5]. Later, in 1928, Decker and Cherry performed the same procedure, naming it a culdoscopy [5]. Although these dates go back to the early 1900s and gynecology has been using a transvaginal port for pelvic surgery, this access was not explored as a pathway to the abdominal cavity until 2002, when Gettman et al. described a transvaginal nephrectomy in a porcine model [6]. In 2004, Kalloo et al. carried out the first transgastric approach into the peritoneal cavity, performing liver biopsies and peritoneoscopies in the same model [4]. Since this experience and given its relevance to surgery's history, a large number of research teams have developed and explored the applications of these techniques; subsequently, many other procedures have been tried via the transgastric port [7]. Given the complications that this approach presents, Lima et al., in 2006, conceived a lower access port, the transvesical pathway, that could solve some of the limitations associated with the isolated transgastric port [8]. Thereby, the authors explored the peritoneal cavity by a transvesical port, demonstrating the feasibility of this access. After these experiments and faced with these results, Lima et al., using the same port, acceded the thoracic cavity, expanding the intervention area of NOTES into the thorax [9].

Also in 2006, Pai et al. used the transcolonic port to perform cholecystectomy, but their limitations overlapped those of the transgastric port considering the digestive tract and its characteristics [10]. Given the results of Lima et al., Rolanda et al. in 2007 associated the transvesical port to the transgastric one in order to overcome the limitations of this port with the first one, performing a pure NOTES cholecystectomy using a combined-approach concept [11].

Table 11.1 Procedures performed via the transvesical port

Peritoneoscopy and liver biopsies	Lima et al. [8]
Thoracoscopy and lung biopsies	Lima et al. [9]
Cholecystectomy combined with transgastric port	Rolanda et al. [11]
Nephrectomy combined with transgastric port	Lima et al. [13]
Peritoneoscopy after radical prostatectomy in humans	Gettman et al. [12]
Transvesical port closure	Lima et al. [15]
Transvesical and transumbilical port closure	Metzelder et al. [16]
Partial cystectomy	Sawyer et al. [14]
Liver biopsies and ileocecal appendix manipulation in cadavers	Branco et al. [17]
Varicocelectomy	Osório et al. [18]
Pure transvesical nephrectomy with abdominal morcellation of specimen	Lima et al. [24]

Transvesical Port: Technique Access

In 2006, Lima et al. were the first to suggest the bladder as a portal for NOTES [8]. Unlike other ports, this organ seemed to be instantaneously approachable with standard urological tools. The placement of the transvesical port is based on the Seldinger principle. Currently, an ureteroscope is introduced through the urethra into the bladder with pneumodistension, emptying urine from the bladder and distending it with CO_2. The vesicotomy site is carefully selected on the bladder dome. A mucosal incision is made with scissors introduced through the working channel of the ureteroscope. Subsequently, a 5-Fr open-ended ureteral catheter is pushed forward through the incision into the peritoneal cavity. A 0.035-in. flexible-tip guidewire is then inserted into the peritoneal cavity through the lumen of the ureteral catheter. Guided by the flexible-tip guidewire, the vesical hole is enlarged with a dilator of a ureteroscope sheath enveloped by a flexible 5.5-mm overtube. A ureteroscope is introduced into the peritoneal cavity through the overtube and allows the creation of a pressure-controlled CO_2 pneumoperitoneum.

In 2007, Gettman and Blute described transvesical peritoneoscopy in human-attempted before a robot-assisted radical prostatectomy using a flexible ureterorenoscope [12]. They used the same technical mode of a transvesical approach in a porcine model with a few modifications (e.g., instead of a ureteral catheter, the authors used a balloon dilator).

Transvesical Experimental Procedures

The first documented case of surpassing the bladder wall to perform simple intraperitoneal procedures was carried out and reported by Lima et al. [8] (Table 11.1). The authors introduced a transurethral and transvesical ureteroscope into the peritoneal cavity, and subsequently, liver biopsy and division of the falciform ligament were performed. Postoperatively, the survival animals were left with a catheter for

4 days, after which necroscopy revealed completely healed cystotomy sites and no evidence of peritoneal complications.

Given the unexpected good results from the first study using a transvesical port, Lima et al. felt encouraged to test the possibility to reach even the thoracic cavity [9]. A ureteroscope was introduced into the peritoneum through the transvesical port and was subsequently advanced into the thoracic cavity. The insufflation was achieved through the ureteroscope, and lung biopsies and inspection of the pleural cavity and lung surface were performed with success. A Foley catheter was left in the bladder for 4 days, and the postmortem examination 15 days after surgery revealed complete healing of the vesical and diaphragmatic incision. Although the authors had been able to perform only limited thoracoscopy and lung biopsies, it definitely extended the intervention field of NOTES from the peritoneal to thoracic cavity as well.

Some critics always questioned the feasibility and reproducibility of the transvesical port in humans, particularly regarding the use of rigid instruments. This was the aim for Branco et al. to test the access and feasibility of peritoneoscopy by using a rigid ureteroscope in two human male cadavers. This research group concluded that peritoneoscopy, liver biopsy, and ileocecal appendix manipulation using a rigid ureteroscope through a transvesical port is feasible in a cadaver model [17].

Cholecystectomy is one of the most challenging isolated transgastric approaches. Using two endoscopes, or a single endoscope conjugated with a transabdominal trocar, Park et al. [19] and Swanstrom et al. [20] experienced significant difficulties performing cholecystectomy using shape-lock technology. These authors reported difficulties related to controlling the pneumoperitoneum and obtaining a stable platform for anatomy exposure, organ retraction, secure grasping, and adequate triangulation of instruments. Rolanda et al. [11] introduced the concept of combined approaches by natural orifice using a combined transgastric and transvesical approach for cholecystectomy. This step confirmed the advantage of the transvesical port and initiated the multiple ports of entry concept in NOTES. This concept may provide advantage over the single port, such as monitoring the creation of a second port through the first one, being most likely to successfully close the otomy, and finally, but perhaps the main advantage, has increased triangulation and traction.

In a nonsurvival study, Lima et al. expanded the concept of combined transgastric and transvesical approaches performing nephrectomy in female pigs [13]. Under ureteroscope visualization through a 5-mm transvesical port, researchers controlled the orally introduced flexible gastroscope by the gastrotomy into the peritoneal cavity (Fig. 11.1). Right or left nephrectomy was carried out using instruments introduced by devices that worked in the renal hilum, alternating intervention on dissection or retraction procedures. In all animals, both kidneys were visualized, and the renal vessels and ureter were reasonably individualized and ligated separately with ultrasonic scissors introduced through the transvesical port (Fig. 11.2). In two early cases, mild hemorrhage occurred after ultrasonic ligation. Thus, complete renal release and mobilization to the stomach were achieved in all animals, but the gastrotomy site could not be closed. The authors also reported that additional improvements are needed with better devices and instruments.

Fig. 11.1 Image of the stomach provide by the ureteroscope introduced by the transvesical port

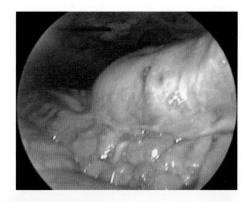

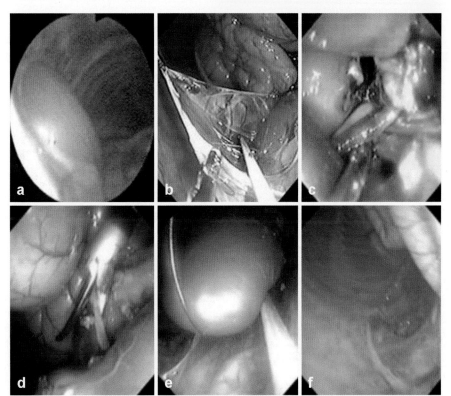

Fig. 11.2 Nephrectomy by combined transvesical and transgastric ports: (**a**) image of right kidney provide by the ureteroscope; (**b**) dissection of the posterior parietal peritoneum; (**c**) dissection of the renal vessels; (**d**) ligation of renal vessels with ultrasonic scissors introduced by the transvesical port; (**e**) snare moves the released kidney forward; (**f**) kidney removal from renal bed

After these successful upper abdominal procedures, the Minho Research Group felt that this approach might be best not only to perform simple procedures in the structure of the upper abdomen and chest, but also to carry out maneuvers in the pelvis and lower abdomen [18]. Indeed, they assessed the feasibility and the safety of a bilateral varicocelectomy through a transvesical approach using a combination of flexible cystoscope and thulium laser energy in six survival porcine models.

Recently, Sawyer et al. described a partial cystectomy by intravesical transurethral techniques in a porcine model [14]. An endoscopic loop device was advanced through one port of the multichannel cystoscope. Through the second port, a flexible-toothed grasping device was advanced through the loop to grasp the targeted area of the bladder wall. Then the grasper was slowly withdrawn while maintaining a grip on the "pseudotumor" through the loop. A full-thickness bladder segment was then excised using cutting current. At the end of the procedure, the specimen was removed en bloc with the cystoscope, and the bladder wall defect was reapproximated with endoscopic clips. The authors reported that further investigation in chronic models will be required to determine the potential for safe adaptation to human beings.

In a human case, Gettman et al. performed a transvesical peritoneoscopy using a ureteroscope prior to performing a robot-assisted radical prostatectomy [12]. There were neither intraoperative nor early postoperative complications. At discharge and at 2-month follow-up no bowel dysfunction, no pain control problems and no evidence of urine leakage from the bladder were observed.

Safety of the Transvesical Port

The first purpose had been determining the safety of the transvesical approach in terms of possible peritoneal contamination. Recent works showed elevated risks of infection-related complications in animals undergoing transintestinal (colonic, gastric) incision and peritoneal contamination after transgastric incision in humans during laparoscopic procedure [5]. Nevertheless, Lima et al. demonstrated that closure of a 5-mm bladder hole is not absolutely necessary if bladder drainage is ensured [8]. McGee examined the resultant microbial contamination of the human peritoneum after transvesical incision, confirming this as a clean portal of entry. This research group examined the resultant microbial contamination of the human peritoneum after transvesical incision during 60 robot-assisted laparoscopic prostatectomy (RALP) procedures [21]. With an average time from transvesical incision to vescicourethral anastomosis of 118 min, peritoneal contamination was seen in 5 of 60 (8.3 %) patients. Additionally, the organism resembled bacteria native to the prostate or seminal fluid because of prostate manipulation and resection during RALP. This study confirmed that transvesical incision would effectively be a clean portal of entry for NOTES.

Transvesical Port Closure

In 2006, Lima et al. described the transvesical approach to the peritoneal cavity, noting that closure of a 5-mm bladder hole is not absolutely necessary if bladder drainage is ensured. The development of an effective closure device might enable

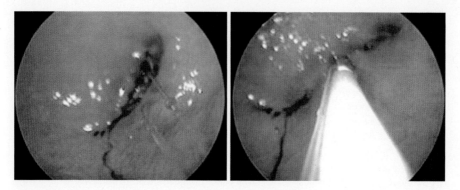

Fig. 11.3 Closure of bladder perforation with a pair of threads for a subsequent locking

the widespread adoption of transvesical port in NOTES. This was the rationale for this research group to report the usefulness of T-fasteners with a locking cinch system [15]. They demonstrated the feasibility and safety of endoscopic closure of vesical perforations with an endoscopic suturing kit (T-fasteners with a locking cinch) in a survival porcine model. Three steps were involved in the endoscopic closure of the perforation: (1) With the animals in the Trendelenburg position, the needle punctured the edge of the perforation (the 19-gauge needle was loaded with the metal T-tag attached to a 3.0 violet Monocryl 90-cm thread and was advanced through the working channel of the cystoscope and placed through the full thickness of one edge of the bladder wall). By advancing the stylet, the T-tag and thread were released from the needle and left in the exterior part of the bladder; (2) needle puncture of the opposite edge of the perforation, followed by release of the T-tag, which was performed in a similar way; and (3) knot tying was then accomplished, followed by suture cutting with a lock-and-cut combination device, which was advanced to tie the threads together (Fig. 11.3). The defect was closed by pulling the threads on either side of the incision together until they were snug against the lock, and then by closing the lock and subsequently cutting the threads with the combination thread-locking and suture-cutting device. This resulted in a secure closure of the perforation. No catheter was left in the bladder. All animals were evaluated daily; the postmortem examination 15 days after surgery revealed complete healing of the bladder wall incision. The authors concluded that these findings provided immediate support for clinical application of this method to close bladder perforations both in the management of bladder rupture and as a transvesical port in NOTES procedures.

More recently, Metzelder et al. described another method for the closure of bladder perforations in a porcine model. Five female piglets underwent right-sided transurethral nephroureterectomy using a hybrid technique with one 15-mm trocar placed umbilically and one 3-mm trocar placed transvesically. Hilar dissection was performed with a 5-mm ligasure vessel-sealing device. After umbilical retrieval of the resected kidney, the urinary bladder was closed by an endoloop via an umbilical "two-in-one system" with the assistance of a 2-mm transurethrally placed endoscopic clamp [16].

Table 11.2 Comparison among the transluminal ports

Transluminal port/features	Transvesical	Transvaginal	Transcolonic	Transgastric
Available in both genders	Yes	No	Yes	Yes
Possibility of using rigid instruments	Yes	Yes	Yes	No
Sterility	Yes	No	No	No
Limited size of access	Yes	No	No	No
Capability of closure	—[a]	Easy	—[b]	—[b]
Specimen retrieval	Yes	Yes	Yes	—[c]
Access to the abdominal cavity	Inferior, anterior	—	Inferior, posterior	Superior

[a]If the otomy is up to 5 mm and with adequate bladder drainage, it is not necessary to close it up
[b]Lack of an effective closure mechanism
[c]Depends on the size of the specimen: small pieces can be extracted as opposed to larger pieces

Transvesical port for abdominal morcellation of specimen

The morcellation was thought as a method to overcome the limitation of the size for removing specimens, regardless of the diameter of the port accessed. One of the limitations of the transvesical port was specimen retrieval, conditioned by the size of the urethra. Recently using this concept, Lima et al reported pure transvesical nephrectomy with kidney morcellation within the abdominal cavity [23]. In six pigs, after a pure transvesical nephrectomy, the peritoneal cavity was emptied of CO_2 and replaced with saline solution. Before emptying CO_2, the kidney was fixed to the abdominal wall with a fixing needle, created specifically for this purpose. Later, was introduced, through the working channel of the telescope, the morcellator (Piranha-wolf morcellator®) in the peritoneal cavity and the kidney morcellation began under saline solution. The morcellation proved to be effective, allowing excision of the entire kidney rapidly (median time: 15 minutes, range 10 to 20 minutes). This study showed, for the first time, the feasibility of morcellation of abdominal organs through a natural orifice, in porcine model.

Advantage and Limitations of Transvesical Port in Comparison with Other Ports

Considering the natural orifices that allow NOTES, in order to know which will be the best port or the most suited to a particular procedure, some aspects should be considered: ease of access, ease and safety of the otomy closure, potential infectious complications related to the closure, maximum diameter and type of instruments that the orifices can tolerate, and if it allows specimen retrieval (Table 11.2).

The transgastric port has many limitations, such as the lack of sterility of the digestive tract, being a long route—which implicates the use of flexible

instruments—and the potential infectious and iatrogenic complications. Some limitations are associated with gastroscopes, particularly the lack of triangulation and traction, the need to work in retroflexion with inverted images, and the difficulty in controlling the pneumoperitoneum. The closure of the gastrotomy is also an important limitation [22]. In order to overcome these problems, some solutions were launched, such as the design of new gastroscopes and transgastric instruments and the combination of transgastric access with a transabdominal port (hybrid NOTES) or with another natural orifice (combined pure NOTES) [23]. Despite these attempts, the application in humans depends on an effective gastrotomy closure method that still does not exist.

In the transvaginal approach, the advantages include the possibility of using rigid instruments and direct visualization of upper abdominal structures, without retroflexion and therefore with less difficulty in spatial orientation. Furthermore, it has an easy method to access the peritoneal cavity through a simple incision at the Douglas pouch. It is considered a good way for specimen retrieval, given its diameter, and the port with the safest otomy closure to date. Nonetheless, being available only in women is the limiting key factor. Other limitations are related to the patient's personal history (previous vaginal or pelvic surgery) that may not enable NOTES to be performed. Still without a full understanding, but that should be taken into account in future studies, are the effects on sexual function and quality of life of female patients [23].

The transcolonic port allows the introduction of rigid instruments and direct visualization of the upper abdomen organs, is present in both sexes, and allows the use of larger-diameter instruments and specimen retrieval due to the rectum's complacency. However, it presents a high risk of infection because it is not sterile and the transvisceral incision closure is not yet effective. It would take a colonic preparation and lumen sterilization to consider its implementation in humans [10].

The transvesical port broke down some of the most feared complications in urology: the perforation of the bladder wall that is requested by NOTES to access the abdominal cavity. However, in 2006, Lima et al. saw this port as an advantageous pathway, considering the following facts (Table 11.3): (1) The bladder and its content are naturally sterile; (2) the bladder and the lower urinary tract allow the passage of rigid instruments, which facilitates the structure's retraction; (3) it is a pathway present in both sexes; (4) it is the most anterior anatomical position in the sagittal plane, allowing access to the upper abdominal organs above the bowel loops, reducing the risk of damaging other organs, unlike the transvaginal and transcolonic ports, in which the surgeon works through the bowel loops [23]. With practice arose other advantages, among which are worth mentioning the simplicity of cystotomy closure (which may not be necessary if the otomy is less than 5 mm with an adequate bladder drainage), the ease and speed with which the pneumoperitoneum is achieved and controlled, and the diminished complexity of spatial orientation given the direct visualization of the upper abdomen organs. The disadvantage is related to the diameter of the urethra, which limits the size of the instruments used and the intact specimen retrieval.

Table 11.3 Advantages and disadvantage of the transvesical port

Advantages

Naturally sterile

Located in most anterior portion of the pelvic cavity, allowing peritoneal access above the bowel loops

Providing an *en face* orientation of the upper abdominal organs, allowing better visualization and the ability to work straightforwardly

Visualization of all the intraperitoneal structures with a direct line of sight

The possibility to introduce rigid instruments by the working channels of the scopes, enhancing the possibility to retract and grasping structures

Allows one to easily and quickly control and maintain the pneumoperitoneum with a standard instrument

The ability to be performed in both genders

Easy endoscopic closure technique of the cystostomy tract although spontaneous healing is possible

Easy spatial orientation

Disadvantage

The diameter of the urethra limits the size of the devices and the intact specimen retrieval at the end of the procedures

Table 11.4 Possible indications for transvesical port

Diagnostic procedures

Peritoneoscopy

Cancer staging

Endometriosis staging

Exploration intraabdominal testes

Ovarian pathologies

Interventional simple procedures

Intraabdominal orchidectomy

Oophorectomy

Tubal ligation

Diaphragmatic pacemakers

Accessory port for complex intraabdominal procedures

Nephrectomy

Cholecystectomy

Splenectomy

Potential Surgical Applications of the Transvesical Port

The transvesical port, because of its advantages (in particular, being naturally sterile and anatomically the most anterior access to the abdominal cavity, allowing the access to the upper abdominal organs above bowel loops), is appealing for both urological and nonurological procedures. Thus, the transvesical port can potentially be applied to several procedures such as peritoneoscopy, cancer staging, intraabdominal testes search, intraabdominal orchidectomy, varicocelectomy, ovarian pathologies treatment, nephrectomy, cholecystectomy, and procedures in the diaphragm (Table 11.4).

Editorial Comment

Dr. Lima and colleagues pioneered the transvesical (transurethral) route as an option for performing NOTES. While the bladder, like the vagina, may be a forgiving route of entry compared to the bowel, the relatively small caliber of the urethra, especially in males, and nonfamiliarity with nonurologist surgeons may limit its clinical usefulness. However, the transvesical route should be considered a potential access route, especially in women.

References

1. Harrell AG, Heniford T. Minimally invasive abdominal surgery: *Lux et veritas* past, present, and future. Am J Surg. 2005;190:239–43.
2. Autorino R, Cadeddu JA, Desai MM, et al. Laparoendoscopic single-site and natural orifice transluminal endoscopic surgery in urology: a critical analysis of the literature. Eur Urol. 2011;59(1):26.
3. Rattner D, Kalloo A. ASGE/SAGES Working Group on natural orifice translumenal endoscopic surgery. Surg Endosc. 2006;20:329–33.
4. Kalloo AN, Singh VK, Jagannath SB, et al. Flexible transgastric peritoneoscopy: a novel approach to diagnostic and therapeutic interventions in the peritoneal cavity. Gastrointest Endosc. 2004;60:114–7.
5. Lima E, Rolanda C, Autorino R, Correia-Pinto J. Experimental foundation for NOTES and hybrid NOTES. BJU Int. 2010;6:913–8.
6. Gettman MT, Lotan Y, Napper CA, Cadeddu JA. Transvaginal laparoscopic nephrectomy: development and feasibility in the porcine model. Urology. 2002;59:446–50.
7. Autorino R, Stein RJ, Lima E, et al. Current status and future perspectives in laparoendoscopic single-site and natural orifice transluminal endoscopic urological surgery. Int J Urol. 2010; 17:410–31.
8. Lima E, Rolanda C, Pêgo JM, et al. Transvesical endoscopic peritoneoscopy: a novel 5 mm port for intra-abdominal scarless surgery. J Urol. 2006;176:802–5.
9. Lima E, Henriques-Coelho T, Rolanda C, et al. Transvesical thoracoscopy: a natural orifice transluminal endoscopic approach for thoracic surgery. Surg Endosc. 2007;21:854–8.
10. Pai RD, Fong DG, Bundga ME, et al. Transcolonic endoscopic cholecystectomy: a NOTES survival study in a porcine model (with video). Gastrointest Endosc. 2006;64:428–34.
11. Rolanda C, Lima E, Pêgo JM, et al. Third-generation cholecystectomy by natural orifices: transgastric and transvesical combined approach (with video). Gastrointest Endosc. 2007;65: 111–7.
12. Gettman MT, Blute ML. Transvesical peritoneoscopy: initial clinical evaluation of the bladder as a portal for natural orifice translumenal endoscopic surgery. Mayo Clin Proc. 2007;82: 843–5.
13. Lima E, Rolanda C, Pêgo JM, et al. Third-generation nephrectomy by natural orifice transluminal endoscopic surgery. J Urol. 2007;178:2648–54.
14. Sawyer MD, Cherullo EE, Elmunzer BJ, et al. Pure natural orifice translumenal endoscopic surgery partial cystectomy: intravesical transurethral and extravesical transgastric techniques in a porcine model. Urology. 2009;74:1049–53.
15. Lima E, Rolanda C, Osório L, et al. Endoscopic closure of transmural bladder wall perforations. Eur Urol. 2009;56:151–8.

16. Metzelder M, Vieten G, Gosemann JH, et al. Endoloop closure of the urinary bladder is safe and efficient in female piglets undergoing transurethral NOTES nephrectomy. Eur J Pediatr Surg. 2009;19:362–5.
17. Branco F, Pini F, Osório L, et al. Transvesical peritoneoscopy with rigid scope: feasibility study in human male cadaver. Surg Endosc. 2011;25(6):2015–9.
18. Osório L, Silva D, Autorino R, Damiano R, Correia-Pinto J, Lima E. Pure NOTES transvesical venous ligation: translational animal model of varicocelectomy. Urology 2011;78:1082–6.
19. Park PO, Bergstrom M, Ikeda K, et al. Experimental studies of transgastric gallbladder surgery: cholecystectomy and cholecystogastric anastomosis (videos). Gastrointest Endosc. 2005;61:601–6.
20. Swanstrom LL, Kozarek R, Pasricha PJ, et al. Development of a new access device for transgastric surgery. J Gastrointest Surg. 2005;9:1129–37.
21. McGee SM, Routh JC, Pereira CW, Gettman MT. Minimal contamination of the human peritoneum after transvesical incision. J Endourol. 2009;23:659–63.
22. Rolanda C, Lima E, Silva D, et al. *In vivo* assessment of gastrotomy closure by over-the-scope-clips in an experimental model for varicocelectomy. Gastrointest Endosc. 2009;70:1137–45.
23. Lima E, Rolanda C, Correia-Pinto J. NOTES performed using multiple ports of entry: current experience and potential implications for urologic applications. J Endourol. 2009;23:756–64.
24. Lima E, Branco F, Parente J, Autorino R, Correia-Pinto J. Transvesical natural orifice transluminal endoscopic surgery (NOTES) nephrectomy with kidney morcellation: a proof of concept study. BJU Int 2012;109:1533–7.

Chapter 12
Access: Transumbilical

Abhay Rane and Riccardo Autorino

Keywords Access • Laproendoscopic single-site surgery • LESS • Transumbilical Scarless • Single port • Technique

Introduction

Laparoscopic surgery typically uses a variable number of ports for a given procedure to provide triangulation between instruments, allowing the surgeon adequate intracorporeal working space for dissection and tissue manipulation [1]. While laparoscopic surgery has evolved to be the reference standard for a number of extirpative and reconstructive procedures and is generally safe and effective, complications related to port placement have also been well recognized in laparoscopy [2].

Several urological groups initially used a variety of terms to describe the technique if it used a single-port or single-site access, now defined as LESS (laparoendoscopic single-site) [3–6]. LESS appears to offer the patient the potential benefits of decreased abdominal wall trauma, enhanced cosmesis, quicker recovery, and increased patient satisfaction [7].

A. Rane, M.D.
Department of Urology, East Surrey Hospital,
Canada Avenue, Redhill, Surrey RH1 5RH, UK
e-mail: a.rane@btinternet.com

R. Autorino, M.D., Ph.D., FEBU (⊠)
Urology Clinic, Second University of Naples,
Piazza Miraglia, Naples 80138, Italy

Center for Laparoscopic and Robotic Surgery, Glickman Urological and Kidney Institute,
Cleveland Clinic, 9500 Euclid Avenue Q10, Cleveland, OH 44195, USA
e-mail: autorir@ccf.org, ricautor@tin.it

A. Rane et al. (eds.), *Scar-Less Surgery*,
DOI 10.1007/978-1-84800-360-6_12, © Springer-Verlag London 2013

Table 12.1 Umbilical LESS: nomenclature

Current terminology	Previous terminology
Umbilical laparoendoscopic single-site surgery (U-LESS) [5]	One-port umbilical surgery (OPUS) [9]
	Keyhole umbilical surgery [10]
	Natural orifice transumbilical surgery (NOTUS) [11]
	Transumbilical endoscopic surgery (TUES) [12]
	Embryonic natural orifice transumbilical endoscopic surgery (E-NOTES) [13]

Fig. 12.1 Access techniques in laparoendoscopic single-site surgery (LESS): single-port and single-site

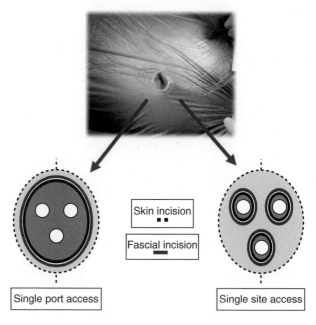

Despite being regarded by some as an evolution of standard laparoscopic surgery, LESS defies the most basic tenets of laparoscopy, including the triangulation of working instruments and external spacing to decrease intra- and extracorporeal clashing.

It may be postulated that when this access site is the umbilicus, which is a natural scar, the cosmetic outcome will be optimal. According to the current nomenclature, transumbilical LESS is more specifically defined as *umbilical* LESS (U-LESS), which includes a variety of previous definitions used by those who pioneered the technique [5, 8–13] (Table 12.1). Transumbilical LESS access can be obtained (Fig. 12.1).

- By performing a single skin and fascial incision through which a single multi-channel access platform is placed (*single-port technique*) [9]
- By placing several low-profile ports through separate fascial incisions (*single-site technique*) [10]

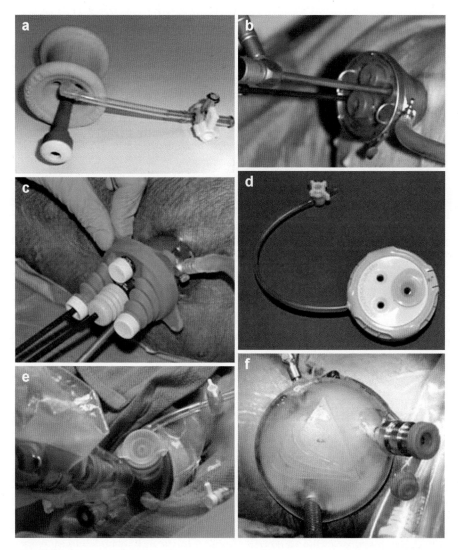

Fig. 12.2 Most commonly used purpose-built platforms for single-port surgery. (**a**) SILS port; (**b**) Endocone; (**c**) X-CONE; (**d**) single site laparoscopy (*SSL*) access system; (**e**) TriPort and QuadPort; (**f**) GelPOINT

Technique and Devices

Single-Port Umbilical Access

Access devices for single-port surgery can be broadly categorized into two categories: industry-designed platforms and homemade ones [14, 15]. The clinical use of several commercially available access devices has been reported so far (Fig. 12.2), each with its own specific feature. All devices utilize the principles of an open Hassan technique for insertion, and therefore carry the advantages of safe access under vision. The length of the incision may vary depending on the procedure to be carried out.

One of the first purpose-built devices described for single-port surgery [16, 17], the Uni-X™ Single Port System (Pnavel Systems, Inc., Morganville, NJ), was a 20-mm port with three separate flexible instrumentation channels and a portal for gas insufflation. Once sited into the abdomen, the port was anchored in place using fascial sutures. Despite being shown to be effective in the early clinical experience with urologic LESS, this device is no longer available.

At around the same time, another company (Advanced Surgical Concepts, Wicklow, Ireland) developed a different platform, known as the r-Port™. The device had a body wall retractor component and a valve component composed of an elastomeric material allowing instrument passage. Later versions (TriPort™) contained one 12-mm valve, two 5-mm valves, and two additional valves for insufflation and smoke evacuation. The device can be inserted in incisions from 12 to 25 mm in length, and the self-adjusting design allows usage in patients with varying abdominal wall thicknesses (up to 10 cm). The presence of valves as opposed to trocars helps to diminish the external clashing of instruments. In the latest version of this product (TriPort), currently marketed by Olympus Medical, there is a fourth 5-mm lipseal valve, enabling the insertion of an additional instrument. Rane et al. reported the first clinical use of the r-Port [9]. Later on, investigators from the Cleveland Clinic also described the successful use of this device for a variety of urologic indications [18, 19].

Except for its larger diameter, the QuadPort™ (Olympus Medical, Center Valley, PA) is designed according to the same principle as the TriPort. It can be used for incision lengths between 25 and 60 mm. Its larger diameter makes it more suitable for the removal of biopsy samples and organs. This version has four lipseal valves (one 5-mm valve, two 10-mm valves, and a 15-mm valve).

The GelPOINT™ (Applied Medical, Rancho Santa Margarita, CA) features a GelSeal™ gel platform for port placement, an Alexis™ (Applied Medical, Rancho Santa Margarita, CA) wound retractor for fixation to the abdominal wall, self-retaining, low-profile trocars, and a built-in valve for insufflation.

Although similar to the GelPort™ (Applied Medical, Rancho Santa Margarita, CA), which is popular in hand-assisted laparoscopic surgery, the GelPOINT has several important distinctions. It is smaller and does not contain a perforation within the gel cap. An insufflation port is located on the side of the device, and a suture attached to the wound protection apparatus allows for easier platform removal. The claimed potential advantages include adaptation to different trocar configurations, a larger outer working profile providing less external clashing, and the ability to accommodate different abdominal wall thicknesses. Recently, Gimenez et al. reported their initial experience with LESS donor nephrectomy by using a single-access GelPOINT™ device inserted into the abdomen through a 4–5-cm periumbilical incision [20]. No extra-umbilical incisions were needed, and the authors stated that the device provided more space for triangulation.

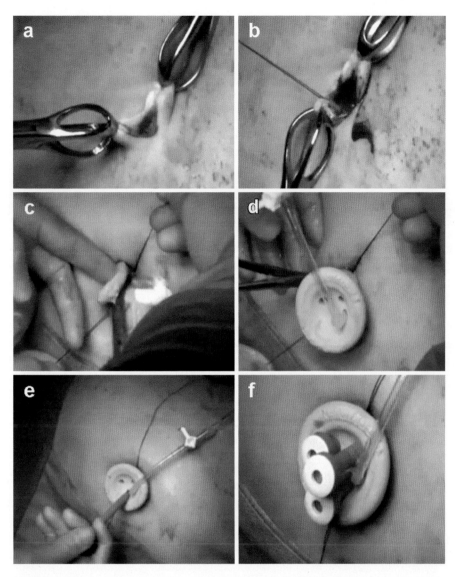

Fig. 12.3 Insertion technique for SILS port. (**a**) intraumbilical skin incision of approximately 20 mm; (**b**) blunt dissection through the fascia and peritoneum by standard Hasson; (**c**) insertion of the lower half of the SILS port device into the incision digitally, or with the help of an appropriately sized surgical clamp placed at the base of the SILS port device; (**d**) insertion of cannulae provided with the SILS port device; (**e**) removal of the obturators, (**f**) leaving the cannulae and SILS port device in place

The SILS™ (Covidien, Gosport, UK) is a foam port that, once inserted into the abdominal wall, conforms to the incision size to prevent gas leakage. The insertion requires an incision of at least 2 cm. Pre-sited spaces within the foam can accommodate either 5- or 12-mm trocars (Fig. 12.3). This allows considerable flexibility in the trocar arrangement without resulting in a loss of pneumoperitoneum. A number of centers have reported their experience with LESS using the SILS port. Burgos et al. [21] described their initial experience with the SILS port in performing laparoscopic prostatectomy. Due to its foam design, the use of this port in obese patients is somewhat difficult as a consequence of increased abdominal wall thickness [22].

The X-CONE™ (Karl Storz, Tuttlingen, Germany) is a metal conical structure consisting of two half-cones to which a plastic cap is attached. Four instrument ports and an insufflation port are available. The port is inserted using a modified Hasson approach. Each half of the cone is inserted independently and then joined together; subsequently, the plastic cap is attached. An important advantage of this platform compared to the other commercially available ports is that the platform is reusable. The use of this device has been described in urology in both the preclinical [23] and clinical settings [24, 25].

The Single Site Laparoscopy (SSL) Access System (Ethicon Endo-Surgery, Cincinnati, OH) consists of a fixed-length wound retractor (available in 2 or 4 cm), a retractor attachment ring, and a low-profile seal cap. The cap includes access for two 5-mm and one 15-mm instruments. Due to the design of the seal, trocar placement is not required. Furthermore, the seal cap is capable of rotating 360°, theoretically allowing the reorientation of instruments throughout the procedure. The seal cap is removable, allowing easier specimen removal. The use of this system for a urologic procedure has not been reported yet in the literature.

The costs associated with single-site surgery may represent a significant issue in some countries. A few centers that perform LESS have chosen to work with homemade single ports that are made from readily available material in the operating room. Tai et al. [26] described their homemade single port consisting of an Alexis™ wound retractor and a surgical glove. The wound retractor is inserted into the abdomen and a surgical glove is secured to the flange. The tips of the fingers of the glove are removed, and standard laparoscopic trocars are sited and secured to the resultant orifice with a purse-string suture. Two to three additional trocars can be placed depending on the procedure to be performed. Choi et al. [27] reported their extensive experience using a similar homemade single port consisting of an Alexis wound retractor and a size 7.5 surgical glove. Three to four ports of varying sizes were secured to the fingers of the glove. They performed 171 consecutive LESS surgeries, 73 of them robotically, all with this homemade single-port device. The disadvantages of their system included ballooning of the surgical glove with increasing operative time. In addition, while a good range of motion was present, the external collision of trocars occurred.

Single-Site Umbilical Access

Even though numerous access platforms for urologic LESS exist, many groups prefer to make a single skin incision and make separate entry points through the fascia for port placement. In this case, low-profile, small-diameter head trocars, such as the AnchorPort™ (Surgiquest, Orange, CT) (Fig. 12.4), Pediport™ (Covidien,

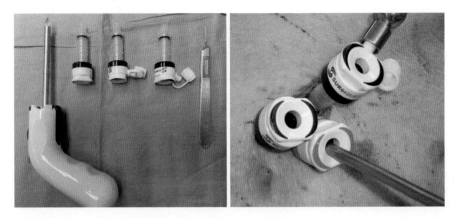

Fig. 12.4 Low-profile 5-mm ports (Surgiquest™, Milford, CT)

Mansfield, MA), or Hunt™ (Apple Medical, Marlborough, MA), can be used through separate stab incisions clustered within the umbilical ring.

In early 2007, Raman et al. first reported their initial experience with "keyhole" nephrectomy in pigs and humans using a single incision to introduce three adjacent trocars (one 10-mm and two 5-mm) [10]. From the same group, Tracy et al. [28] performed LESS pyeloplasty through a single 2.5-cm incision, siting three 5-mm trocars therein. At the time of suturing, the most caudal port was replaced by a 10.5-mm trocar. The same group also reported similar configurations for nephrectomy. At the time of hilar dissection and control, the central 5-mm port was exchanged for a 12-mm port to accommodate the endovascular stapler [29].

Derweesh et al. [30] recently described their slightly different access technique for performing radical nephrectomy and partial nephrectomy. A 3–4-cm periumbilical skin incision was made and deepened down to the abdominal fascia. An extralong (150-mm length) trocar then was inserted at the most cranial aspect of the incision. Subsequently, after the establishment of a pneumoperitoneum, a nonshielded low-profile (65-mm length) trocar was inserted 1.0–1.5 cm caudal to the initial port. This was followed by the insertion of a 12-mm standard-length (100 mm) trocar at the most caudal aspect of the incision 1.0–1.5 cm caudal to the low-profile port.

Nozaki et al. have described their umbilical access technique to perform LESS adrenalectomy [31]. They everted the umbilicus and made a longitudinal skin incision within the umbilicus in the midline, within the cicatrix. Then a wider area of subcutaneous tissue was dissected to accommodate the placement of three 5-mm trocars through the longitudinal umbilical skin incision.

Robotic Single-Site Access

Early clinical experience with the application of the currently available da Vinci robotic system (Intuitive Surgical, Sunnyvale, CA) to LESS has been encouraging, as some of the constraints encountered during conventional LESS may be overcome using robotic technology [32].

Kaouk et al. reported the first successful series of single-port robotic procedures in humans in 2009 [33]. The authors noted less challenging intracorporeal dissecting and suturing using robotic instrumentation compared to standard LESS. In another study, the same group reported robotic LESS using a GelPort as the access platform [22]. A 12-mm port for the camera was placed through the GelPort followed by two 8-mm robotic ports, and an additional 12-mm port was sited for assistance. They claimed that using the GelPort as an access platform provided adequate spacing and flexibility of port placement. More recently, the same group from the Cleveland Clinic described the techniques and outcomes for robotic LESS radical prostatectomy [34] and nephrectomy [35].

For radical prostatectomy, access was gained by creating a 3–4.5-cm intraumbilical incision and releasing the umbilicus from the rectus fascia. A 2-cm incision was sited through the linea alba. An 8-mm robotic port was placed at the most caudal portion of the incision on the right side and directed as far laterally as possible. This was repeated on the opposite side with a 5-mm pediatric or standard 8-mm robotic port. A SILS port was inserted through the fascial incision into the abdomen (Fig. 12.5). The patient was positioned in steep Trendelenburg, and the da Vinci S® or Si® (Intuitive Surgical, Sunnyvale, CA) system was docked. The robotic 12-mm scope was introduced through the SILS port, and a 5-mm channel remained free to utilize for suction or for delivering sutures [34].

For the radical nephrectomy, the patient was positioned in the modified flank position at approximately 60° and the incision sited, intraumbilically, 2 cm above and 1 cm below the umbilicus. The abdomen was entered in the midline using an open Hasson technique. When the SILS port was used, the fascial incision was enlarged enough to accommodate two fingers. The robotic trocars were placed inside the skin incision at the apices of the incision; these were tunneled into the abdomen atop two fingers and directed lateral to the midline. The SILS port was inserted with the abdomen insufflated. When the GelPort or GelPOINT port was used, the fascial incision was enlarged and the device deployed in the standard fashion. The robotic trocars were inserted at the most cephalad and caudal aspects of the device, while the camera trocar was placed at the most medial and central portion (Fig. 12.5). Either the da Vinci S or daVinci Si system (in a three-arm approach) was then positioned over the patient's shoulder, with the camera oriented in line with the kidney, and docked. The 12-mm robotic scope was introduced, with a 30 lens directed downward, and either a 5-mm channel in the SILS port or an additional 12-mm port added through the GelPort or GelPOINT port remained free for assistance [35].

Drawbacks

Besides port availability, which can account for the use of one port over the others, potential problems one may encounter during LESS umbilical access include [36].

- Patients with a high BMI
- Adhesions from previous surgery

Fig. 12.5 Port placement for robotic laparoendoscopic single-site surgery procedures. (**a**) SILS port for radical prostatectomy; (**b**) GelPOINT for radical nephrectomy (Both courtesy of Prof. Jihad H. Kaouk, Cleveland Clinic)

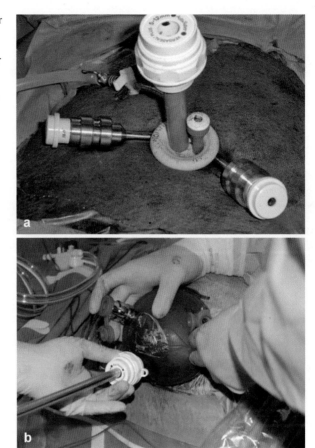

- Difficulty in reaching all areas of the peritoneal cavity from the umbilicus because of insufficient instrument length
- CO_2 insufflation leak
- Risk of hernia

Conclusions

Transumbilical access for LESS surgery offers the most desirable cosmetic outcome by minimizing *visible* postoperative scars.

Editorial Comment

Transumbilical single-site surgery or LESS has rapidly emerged as a readily applicable alternative to NOTES in contemporary clinical practice. The various technologies being developed for NOTES are readily applied transumbilically to perform varieties of clinical procedures across surgical disciplines. Additionally, as most NOTES procedures require transabdominal assistance, typically through the umbilicus, the trend may very well have shifted from NOTES to LESS.

References

1. Frede T, Stock C, Renner C, et al. Geometry of laparoscopic suturing and knotting techniques. J Endourol. 1999;13(3):191–8.
2. Pemberton RJ, Tolley DA, van Velthoven RF. Prevention and management of complications in urological laparoscopic port site placement. Eur Urol. 2006;50:958–68.
3. Tracy CR, Raman JD, Cadeddu JA, Rane A. Laparoendoscopic single-site surgery in urology: where have we been and where are we heading? Nat Clin Pract Urol. 2008;5(10):561–8.
4. Gill IS, Advincula AP, Aron M, et al. Consensus statement of the consortium for laparoendoscopic single-site surgery. Surg Endosc. 2010;24(4):762–8.
5. Box G, Averch T, Cadeddu J, et al. Nomenclature of natural orifice translumenal endoscopic surgery (NOTES) and laparoendoscopic single-site surgery (LESS) procedures in urology. J Endourol. 2008;22(11):2575–81.
6. Kommu SS, Chakravarti A, Luscombe CJ, et al. Laparoendoscopic single-site surgery (LESS) and NOTES; standardised platforms in nomenclature. BJU Int. 2009;103(5):701.
7. Autorino R, Cadeddu JA, Desai MM, et al. Laparoendoscopic single site and natural orifice transluminal endoscopic surgery in urology: a critical analysis of the literature. Eur Urol. 2011;59:26–45.
8. Sooriakumaran P, Kommu S, Rane A. NOTES, SILS and OPUS. Battle of the acronyms for the future of laparoscopic urology. Int J Clin Pract. 2008;62:988.
9. Rane A, Rao P, Rao P. Single-port-access nephrectomy and other laparoscopic urologic procedures using a novel laparoscopic port (r-Port). Urology. 2008;72(2):260–3.
10. Raman JD, Bensalah K, Bagrodia A, et al. Laboratory and clinical development of single keyhole umbilical nephrectomy. Urology. 2007;70:1039–42.
11. Cuesta MA, Berends F, Veenhof AA. The "invisible cholecystectomy": a transumbilical laparoscopic operation without a scar. Surg Endosc. 2008;22(5):1211–3.
12. Zhu JF. Scarless endoscopic surgery. NOTES TUES. Surg Endosc. 2007;21:1898–9.
13. Desai MM, Stein R, Rao P, et al. Embryonic natural orifice transumbilical endoscopic surgery (E-NOTES) for advanced reconstruction: initial experience. Urology. 2009;73(1):182–7.
14. Kommu SS, Rane A. Devices for laparoendoscopic single-site surgery in urology. Expert Rev Med Devices. 2009;6(1):95–103.
15. Khanna R, White MA, Autorino R, et al. Selection of a port for use in laparoendoscopic single-site surgery. Curr Urol Rep. 2011;12(2):94–9.
16. Kaouk JH, Haber GP, Goel RK, et al. Single-port laparoscopic surgery in urology: initial experience. Urology. 2008;71(1):3–6.
17. Goel RK, Kaouk JH. Single port access renal cryoablation (SPARC): a new approach. Eur Urol. 2008;53(6):1204–9.
18. Desai MM, et al. Scarless single port transumbilical nephrectomy and pyeloplasty: first clinical report. BJU Int. 2008;101:83–8.
19. Desai MM, Berger AK, Brandina R, et al. Laparoendoscopic single-site surgery: initial hundred patients. Urology. 2009;74:805–12.
20. Gimenez E, Leeser DB, Wysock JS, et al. Laparoendoscopic single site live donor nephrectomy: initial experience. J Urol. 2010;184(5):2049–55.

21. Burgos JB, Flores JA, de la Vega JS, et al. Early experience in laparoscopic radical prostatec-tomy using the laparoscopic device for umbilical access SILS port. Actas Urol Esp. 2010;34(6): 495–9.
22. Stein RJ, White WM, Goel RK, et al. Robotic laparoendoscopic single-site surgery using GelPort as the access platform. Eur Urol. 2010;57(1):132–6.
23. Autorino R, Kim FJ, Rane A, et al. Low-cost reusable instrumentation for laparoendoscopic single-site nephrectomy: assessment in a porcine model. J Endourol. 2011;25(3):419–24.
24. Greco F, Wagner S, Hoda MR, et al. Single-portal access laparoscopic radical nephrectomy for renal cell carcinoma in transplant patients: the first experience. Eur Urol. 2010;59(6):1060–4.
25. Cindolo L, Autorino R, Scoffone C, et al. Laparoendoscopic single-site (LESS) adrenalectomy and partial nephrectomy: current Italian experience with two challenging surgical procedures. Surg Technol Int. 2010;20:240–4.
26. Tai HC, Lin CD, Wu CC, et al. Homemade transumbilical port: an alternative access for laparoendoscopic single-site surgery (LESS). Surg Endosc. 2010;24(3):705–8.
27. Choi KH, Ham WS, Rha KH, et al. Laparoendoscopic single-site surgeries: a single-center experience of 171 consecutive cases. Korean J Urol. 2011;52(1):31.
28. Tracy CR, Raman JD, Bagrodia A, Cadeddu JA. Perioperative outcomes in patients undergoing conventional laparoscopic versus laparoendoscopic single-site pyeloplasty. Urology. 2009;74: 1029–35.
29. Raman JD, Bagrodia A, Cadeddu JA. Single-incision, umbilical laparoscopic versus conven-tional laparoscopic nephrectomy: a comparison of perioperative outcomes and short-term measures of convalescence. Eur Urol. 2009;55(5):1198–206.
30. Derweesh IH, Silberstein JL, Bazzi W, et al. Laparo-endoscopic single-site surgery for radical and cytoreductive nephrectomy, renal vein thrombectomy, and partial nephrectomy: a prospec-tive pilot evaluation. Diagn Ther Endosc. 2010;2010:107482.
31. Nozaki T, Ichimatsu K, Watanabe A, et al. Longitudinal incision of the umbilicus for laparoen-doscopic single site adrenalectomy: a particular intraumbilical technique. Surg Laparosc Endosc Percutan Tech. 2010;20(6):e185–8.
32. Rane A, Autorino R. Robotic natural orifice translumenal endoscopic surgery and laparoendo-scopic single-site surgery: current status. Curr Opin Urol. 2011;21(1):71–7.
33. Kaouk JH, Goel RK, Haber GP, et al. Robotic single-port transumbilical surgery in humans: initial report. BJU Int. 2008;103:366.
34. White MA, Haber GP, Autorino R, et al. Robotic laparoendoscopic single-site radical prostate-ctomy: technique and early outcomes. Eur Urol. 2010;58(4):544–5.
35. White MA, Autorino R, Spana G, et al. Robotic laparoendoscopic single-site radical nephrec-tomy: surgical technique and comparative outcomes. Eur Urol. 2011;59(5):815–22.
36. Ross SB, Clark CW, Morton CA, Rosemurgy AS. Access for laparoendoscopic single site surgery. Diagn Ther Endosc. 2010;2010:943091.

Part II
NOTES (Natural Orifice Translumenal Endoscopic Surgery)

Chapter 13
NOTES: Laboratory Work

Candace F. Granberg and Matthew T. Gettman

Keywords NOTES • Laboratory • Transvaginal • Transvesical • Transgastric
Transcolonic • Hybrid

Transvaginal NOTES

The transvaginal approach to NOTES is particularly attractive, as many intraabdominal organs can be accessed in a linear fashion without the need for camera retroflexion. For the exposure necessary for transvaginal port placement, a combination of self-retaining vaginal retractors, Deaver retractors, and a weighted vaginal speculum may be used. An intravesical Foley catheter should be placed at the start of the procedure, and a rectal pack is optional. Multiple different ports and trocars have been used through the colpotomy with the transvaginal approach, as described below.

In the first experimental application of natural orifice surgery, Gettman et al. described a completely transvaginal nephrectomy in a porcine model [1]. Under the guidance of both rigid and flexible laparoscopes and cystoscopes, the procedure was performed transvaginally through modified plastic fascial dilators (Amplatz dilating set; Microvasive, Natick, MA) used as working ports (Fig. 13.1). Roticulating laparoscopic instruments with handles placed 180° apart were utilized for dissection. For hilar vascular control, an Endo-GIA™ stapler (U.S. Surgical, Dublin, Ireland) was used transvaginally under transvaginal cystoscopic guidance. The dissected kidney was placed in an EndoCatch™ (Covidien, Dublin, Ireland) device and

C.F. Granberg, M.D. (✉) • M.T. Gettman, M.D.
Department of Urology, Mayo Clinic,
200 First Street, SW, Rochester, MN 55905, USA
e-mail: granberg.candace@mayo.edu, candacegranberg@gmail.com;
gettman.matthew@mayo.edu

A. Rane et al. (eds.), *Scar-Less Surgery*,
DOI 10.1007/978-1-84800-360-6_13, © Springer-Verlag London 2013

Fig. 13.1 Transvaginal
NOTES access in the porcine
model

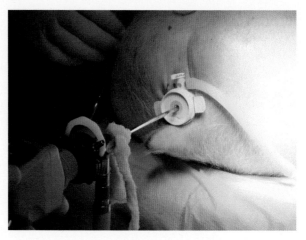

removed transvaginally, and the colpotomy was left open to heal by secondary intention. The limitations of this approach included anatomical constraints of the porcine GU sinus, as well as difficulty with existing laparoscopic instrumentation that made the procedure cumbersome.

Single-port multi-lumen platforms subsequently evolved in an effort to overcome the technical difficulties encountered with existing instrumentation. Clayman et al. utilized a TransPort™ Multi-Lumen Operating Platform (USGI Medical, San Clemente, CA) to perform transvaginal nephrectomy in a porcine model [2]. Through the four working channels of the TransPort, tissue-acquisition devices (g-Prox® and g-Lix™; USGI Medical, San Clemente, CA) were used in combination with other endoscopic instruments for dissection. An additional 12-mm transabdominal port was placed to maintain a pneumoperitoneum, confirm placement during transvaginal access, place a fan retractor, and apply a vascular GIA (Ethicon Endo-Surgery) for division of the renal artery and vein. Although the TransPort allowed for multiple instruments to be utilized through multiple channels within a single port, drawbacks with this experiment included difficulty with triangulation and an inability to secure the renal hilum through the existing channels in this platform due to size limitations.

Thus, multichannel single-port platforms with larger-caliber channels were developed. Aron et al. [3] used the QuadPort® (Advanced Surgical Concepts, Bray, Ireland) via a 3-cm colpotomy to perform transvaginal nephrectomy in a human cadaver. The port's inner ring was deployed through the posterior fornix into the peritoneum and the outer ring cinched over the vulva to serve as a self-retaining unit, although gas leaks were encountered in some cases. All straight and articulating instruments as well as a 10-mm camera were introduced and utilized to complete the procedure through the one 15-mm, two 10-mm, and one 5-mm channels. However, dissection of the upper pole proved challenging due to difficult angles and the distance from the introitus. Moreover, the port was not ideal for vaginal placement, particularly in the presence of an intact uterus, which may alter the working space as well as inhibit instrument movement.

Fig. 13.2 Intraperitoneal view of MAGS camera, with external manipulation of magnet (inset) (Courtesy of Dr. Jeffrey Cadeddu, UT-Southwestern, Dallas, TX)

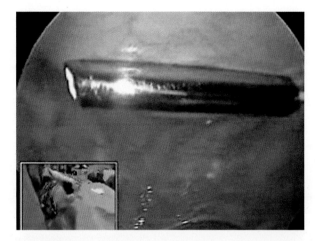

Fig. 13.3 Intraperitoneal view of MAGS cauterizer, with external manipulation of magnet (inset) (Courtesy of Dr. Jeffrey Cadeddu, UT-Southwestern, Dallas, TX)

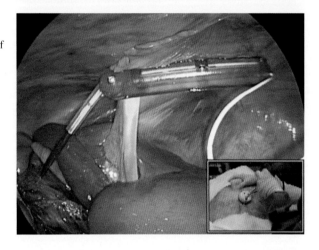

A major drawback to traditional single-port, multi-lumen platforms is having the camera adjacent to and in line with the instrument channels, at times leading to "sword-fighting" during procedures. Initially developed for laparoscopic procedures [4] and previously reported for use in single-port transabdominal nephrectomy [5] and transvaginal cholecystectomy [6], Raman et al. applied magnetic anchoring and guidance system (MAGS) technology to NOTES to perform a pure transvaginal NOTES nephrectomy in a porcine model [7]. The MAGS camera (Fig. 13.2) and cauterizer (Fig. 13.3) were deployed through a transvaginal port and manipulated within the abdomen with an external magnet. Instruments used through the trans-vaginal port included a prototype 70-cm articulating laparoscopic grasper (RealHand®; Novare Surgical Systems, Cupertino, CA) for dissection and an extra-long articulating endovascular stapler for hilar vascular control. The use of MAGS technology in this case helped to overcome limitations previously encountered dur-ing pure transvaginal procedures, including an improvement in triangulation and a decreased clashing of instruments. However, a major drawback to this technique was that electrical and hydraulic tethers to supply the MAGS equipment must be strung through the transvaginal port, causing leakage of insufflation, allowing for a maximum pneumoperitoneum of only 7–10 mmHg during the procedure. Moreover, the increased abdominal wall thickness, resulting in increased magnet-to-target distance, leads to an exponential decay in coupling strength of the magnets. This was confirmed with force-distance tests, delineating a drop-off threshold of 3.64 ± 0.8 cm [8]. Thus, the population in whom this technology could be currently utilized is restricted.

Since the inception of transvaginal NOTES nephrectomy, multiple other transvaginal procedures have been performed in porcine models, including cholecystectomy [9, 10], partial gastrectomy [11] and abdominal wall herniorrhaphy [12, 13], as well as retroperitoneal transvaginal procedures such as distal pancreatectomy [14], RPLND [15], nephrectomy [16], and adrenalectomy [17]. An important limitation of the porcine GU sinus as a transvaginal NOTES model is the smaller vaginal diameter (approximately 2 cm). Additionally, experimental porcine studies exclude potential anatomic variations that may occur in humans, such as previous pelvic or vaginal surgery, variation in uterine size and position, and increased distance from introitus to target organs, which need to be taken into account prior to the clinical application of techniques.

In less than a decade, significant advancements have been made in instrumentation and platforms available for transvaginal NOTES. This has resulted in the translation of procedural techniques from the laboratory to clinical applications, as evidenced by reports of transvaginal hybrid and pure NOTES nephrectomy in humans [18–22], among other procedures. However, technological advances must continue to evolve to develop site-specific NOTES devices that can overcome existing limitations and bring transvaginal NOTES to its full clinical potential. Initial work by engineers and researchers must continue in the laboratory setting prior to clinical application.

Transgastric NOTES

A transgastric approach introduces the risk of intraperitoneal contamination and infection due to exposure to gastric and bowel contents. In addition, maintaining the spatial orientation is difficult, and all instruments pass through working channels on the endoscope, with the light source and camera in line. With this approach, some maneuvers require working off-axis, further increasing the difficulty of complex procedures. Nevertheless, the transgastric route has garnered significant interest as a NOTES portal for a variety of surgical procedures.

Kalloo et al. was the first to describe the application of transgastric NOTES in an animal model in 2004 [23]. In 50-kg pigs, access to the peritoneal cavity was obtained perorally through an endoscope by needle-knife (Olympus, Center Valley, PA) puncture followed by either an extension of the incision with a sphincterotome or balloon dilation over a guidewire. Transgastric peritoneoscopy and liver biopsy were subsequently performed without complication in either acute or long-term survival animals, and the gastrotomy was closed with clips (EndoClips™; Olympus Optical Co., Tokyo, Japan).

Although the safety and feasibility of the transgastric approach were demonstrated in this initial study, subsequent attempts at organ resection via this portal exposed its limitations. Wagh et al. reported an inability to visualize the gallbladder in four of nine pigs and a difficulty identifying retroperitoneal structures; however, they did successfully perform oophorectomy and partial hysterectomy in some animals [24]. They also noted that the scope stability is limited when attempting to access upper abdominal organs in retroflexion. In another experiment, Merrifield et al. encountered a 40 % complication rate (two of five pigs) following transgastric partial hysterectomy, as one pig suffered peritonitis secondary to incomplete closure of the gastric incision and another was found to have a gastric abscess at the incision site [25]. Thus, full-thickness, watertight closure of the gastric incision site is crucial, and the development of improved closure techniques ensued. Currently, a plethora of NOTES gastrotomy closure devices exist, ranging from clips and staplers to threaded tags/anchors and endoscopic suturing tools, and further research and development are ongoing.

The development of a platform specific to flexible endoscopic procedures was investigated by Swanstrom et al. [26]. Following prototype testing in inanimate models, dogs and pigs were subsequently used in nonsurvival experiments, including transgastric liver biopsy, bowel retraction and manipulation, and cholecystectomy. Their novel instrumentation utilized the ShapeLock® technology (USGI Medical, San Clemente, CA), which allows a scope to be advanced, positioned, and then locked into place for stability. With larger working channels, a prototype 4-mm Pentax flexible scope, and independently movable arms, they were able to successfully perform the procedures with improved optics and triangulation. However, of concern was that despite gastrotomy closure in five animals, only one was found to have a watertight closure on explant testing.

Indeed, an efficient, reliable, and reproducible gastric closure technique is absolutely requisite to the acceptance of this NOTES approach. Moreover, the size of specimens extracted from a gastrotomy site is limited. Accordingly, these issues must be addressed in further ex vivo and animal models prior to routine application in humans.

Transcolonic NOTES

To overcome the limitations of the scope in retroflexion in the transgastric approach, attempts at transcolonic NOTES have been reported. Fong et al. described transcolonic peritoneoscopy in pigs, noting the feasibility of upper abdominal exploration [27]. At necroscopy there was evidence of incision-related adhesions as well as histopathologic evidence of microabscesses, mucosal ulcerations, and serositis at the closure site. The authors postulate these findings were secondary to colonic seepage into the peritoneal cavity as a sufficient seal could not be maintained around the endoscope, and it occurred despite a vigorous perioperative colon prep consisting of multiple tap water enemas, intracolonic cefazolin suspension for 10 min, 10 % povidone-iodine rectal lavage, and external gluteal anal scrub.

In the first report of transcolonic organ resection, Pai et al. performed cholecystectomy in survival porcine models [28]. After a similar surgical prep, they utilized a hot biopsy forceps, snare tip, hook knife, prototype endoscopic scissors (Microvasive), and insulated-tip needle-knife to carry out dissection, and the gallbladder was ultimately removed through the colonic incision. Again, at necroscopy there was evidence of adhesions, and one of five animals was prematurely euthanized due to concerns of peritonitis and found to have incomplete closure of the colonic incisions. In contrast, Dubcenco et al. reported no evidence of infection, perforation, or adhesions at necroscopy 2 weeks following combined transcolonic and transabdominal small bowel resection in pigs [29].

Advantages of the transcolonic versus transgastric approach include better access to organs within the upper quadrants, with improved scope stability and the ability to extract larger specimens via the colotomy. Although these feasibility studies in animal models are encouraging for the future implementation of transcolonic NOTES, a reliable and efficient closure of the colonic incision with the absence of long-term gross and histopathologic concerns for adverse events such as infection, adhesions, fistula, etc. must be developed.

Transvesical NOTES

In 2005 and 2006, Gettman utilized ex vivo and in vivo porcine models to evaluate the bladder as a portal for NOTES. To evaluate NOTES access techniques, ex vivo studies were first performed. As a bladder model, the stomach was harvested from euthanized pigs and placed in an analysis chamber, with an inflated latex balloon used to simulate the bowel and 30 Fr silicone tubing used to simulate the urethra (Fig. 13.4). Access techniques included two blunt-tip prototypes and the use of an injection needle with subsequent guidewire placement and balloon dilation. Data collected for evaluation included the force of entry, the size of the access defect, the occurrence of injury to simulated bowel, and a subjective assessment of the ease of entry. Regarding the force of entry, the preferred technique in this experiment was balloon dilation of the cystotomy tract, as the blunt-tip prototypes required increased force. However, the size of the defect created by the dilation technique was larger than that of the blunt-tip prototypes. There were no observed injuries to the simulated bowel with either technique.

In the in vivo model, two pigs were placed under general anesthesia, and access was obtained using a blunt-tip prototype in one and the needle/balloon dilation technique in the other. A pneumoperitoneum was achieved and maintained via insufflation through the irrigation port of the ureteroscope. Diagnostic peritoneoscopy was performed with a rigid ureteroscope (13.5 Fr; Richard Wolf, Knittlingen, Germany). Liver biopsies were performed utilizing endoscopic grasping forceps

Fig. 13.4 Custom device for ex vivo assessment of transvesical NOTES access using a porcine stomach simulating bladder and 30 Fr silicone tubing simulating urethra

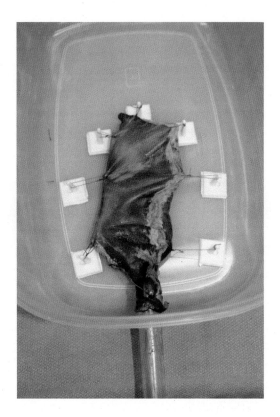

through the working channel of the ureteroscope, with cauterization of biopsy sites using an electrocautery probe. One access-related bowel injury occurred with the needle/balloon dilation technique; however, this did not preclude proceeding with and completing the procedure successfully. Studies were then carried out in human fresh-frozen cadavers, demonstrating the feasibility of transvesical peritoneoscopy (Fig. 13.5), appendectomy, and division of the falciform ligament.

Lima et al. [30] subsequently evaluated the utility of transvesical access in three acute and five survival porcine models. Through a cystoscope, an open-ended ureteral catheter was used to puncture the ventral bladder wall. A guidewire was advanced and a 5.5 Fr overtube was placed transvesically, and peritoneoscopy was performed using a 9.8 Fr ureteroscope. Liver biopsy and division of the falciform ligament were then successfully performed. Postoperatively, the survival animals were left with a catheter for 4 days, after which necroscopy revealed completely healed cystotomy sites. Moreover, there was no evidence of intraperitoneal complications.

Lima et al. later demonstrated the feasibility of transvesical thorascopy in a porcine model [31]. Through a transvesical port, a ureteroscope was introduced into the peritoneum and advanced into the thoracic cavity. Insufflation was achieved through the ureteroscope, and inspection of the pleural cavity and lung surface was carried out in addition to lung biopsies. Foley catheter was removed on postoperative day 4,

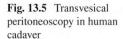

Fig. 13.5 Transvesical peritoneoscopy in human cadaver

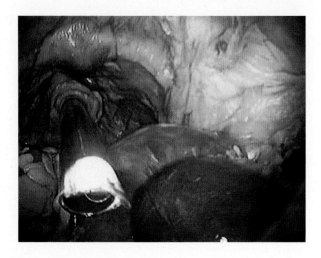

and necroscopy on postoperative day 15 revealed complete healing of the vesical and diaphragmatic incisions as well as the lung biopsy sites.

Although these initial laboratory studies substantiate the feasibility of a transvesical approach for simple NOTES procedures, technical challenges exist that warrant additional study. A major limitation to this access portal is the urethral diameter and the variable urethral length; thus, smaller instruments that allow for orientation in space as well as triangulation need to be developed. Moreover, a reliable method of bladder closure must be established to limit the time needed for postoperative indwelling catheter.

Hybrid NOTES

Employing more than one natural orifice to perform NOTES is termed "hybrid" NOTES, and many have reported on a variety of procedures performed using this approach in the laboratory setting [32–35]. Others have utilized a single natural orifice in combination with a standard transabdominal port(s) [36–39]. Both methods were developed to overcome limitations of single-orifice NOTES, such as a difficulty maintaining spatial orientation, a lack of triangulation, and an inability to extract specimens, and has proven beneficial for more complex procedures.

Recognizing the utility of more than NOTES portal, Box et al. [40] expounded on the hybrid NOTES approach by incorporating robotics to perform nephrectomy in a porcine model. Robotic ports were telescoped through transvaginal and transcolonic laparoscopic ports, and dissection was carried out robotically, with the hilum taken with an endovascular stapler placed transvaginally. Significant "swordfighting" was encountered due to the proximity of ports in this case. Haber et al. [41] hoped to decrease robotic arm collisions by moving one robotic arm to a transumbilical port while the other remained transvaginal to perform dismembered pyeloplasty, partial nephrectomy, and radical nephrectomy in porcine models. This arrangement did not eliminate all collisions, but the use of the robot was found to be beneficial for 3D vision and intracorporeal suturing.

NOTES Training

As with any new surgical technology, a new skill set must be learned and proficiency demonstrated prior to integration into routine practice. Although existing laparoscopic and robotic skills may be readily applied to NOTES procedures, access and exit techniques vary by portal. Moreover, NOTES portals lack a fascial layer that provides stability to traditional transabdominal laparoscopic ports, which creates an element of instability not typically experienced by those trained in minimally invasive surgery. Thus, ex vivo NOTES training systems have been developed. Gillen et al. [42] first reported on the ELITE (endoscopic-laparoscopic interdisciplinary training entity) female human-like simulator, assessing surgeon and endoscopist performance at retrieving anchor points within the abdomen as well as cholecystectomy via a trans-sigmoidal approach. They noted that experience (expert vs. novice) was positively correlated with procedural time; however, all participants demonstrated an improvement in procedural times during the experiment. Importantly, simulated trans-sigmoidal cholecystectomy was proven feasible. Similarly, others have described training exercises in ex vivo and animal models to define learning curves, assess instrument performance, and identify potential complications and limitations [43, 44]. Such training is critical to achieving success when implementing the technically demanding skills necessary for NOTES.

Conclusion

As patients and surgeons alike continue to strive toward progressively more minimally invasive procedures, NOTES has evolved to become acknowledged as the new frontier: surgery without visible scars. Significant strides have been made in operating platforms and instrumentation. Ex vivo, animal, and cadaveric laboratory studies have played an essential role in testing prior to human application as well as training and simulation models for prospective surgeons and endoscopists.

References

1. Gettman MT, Lotan Y, Napper CA, et al. Transvaginal laparoscopic nephrectomy: development and feasibility in the porcine model. Urology. 2002;59:446–50.
2. Clayman RV, Box GN, Abraham JBA, et al. Transvaginal single-port NOTES nephrectomy: initial laboratory experience. J Endourol. 2007;21:640–4.

3. Aron M, Berger AK, Stein RJ, et al. Transvaginal nephrectomy with a multichannel laparoscopic port: a cadaver study. BJU Int. 2009;103:1537–41.
4. Park S, Bergs RA, Eberhart R, et al. Trocar-less instrumentation for laparoscopy: magnetic positioning of intra-abdomial camera and retractor. Ann Surg. 2007;245:379–84.
5. Zeltser IS, Bergs R, Fernandez R, et al. Single trocar laparoscopic nephrectomy using magnetic anchoring and guidance system in the porcine model. J Urol. 2007;178:288–91.
6. Scott DJ, Tang SJ, Fernandez R, et al. Completely transvaginal NOTES cholecystectomy using magnetically anchored instruments. Surg Endosc. 2007;21:2308–16.
7. Raman JD, Bergs RA, Fernandez R, et al. Complete transvaginal NOTES nephrectomy using magnetically anchored instrumentation. J Endourol. 2009;23:367–71.
8. Best SL, Bergs R, Gedeon M, et al. Maximizing coupling strength of magnetically anchored surgical instruments: how thick can we go? Surg Endosc. 2011;25:153–9.
9. Bessler M, Stevens PD, Milone L, et al. Transvaginal laparoscopic cholecystectomy: laparoscopically assisted. Surg Endosc. 2008;22:1715–6.
10. Asakuma M, Perretta S, Allemann P, et al. Challenges and lessons learned from NOTES cholecystectomy initial experience: a stepwise approach from the laboratory to clinical application. J Hepatobiliary Pancreat Surg. 2009;16:249–54.
11. Nakajima K, Takahashi T, Souma Y, et al. Transvaginal endoscopic partial gastrectomy in porcine models: the role of an extra endoscope for gastric control. Surg Endosc. 2008;22: 2733–6.
12. Lomanto D, Dhir U, So JBY, et al. Total transvaginal endoscopic abdominal wall hernia repair: a NOTES survival study. Hernia. 2009;13:415–9.
13. Powell B, Whang SH, Bachman SL, et al. Transvaginal repair of a large chronic porcine ventral hernia with synthetic mesh using NOTES. JSLS. 2010;14:234–9.
14. Allemann P, Perretta S, Asakuma M, et al. NOTES retroperitoneal transvaginal distal pancreatectomy. Surg Endosc. 2009;23:882–3.
15. Nassif J, Zacharopoulou C, Marescaux J, et al. Transvaginal extraperitoneal lymphadenectomy by natural orifices transluminal endoscopic surgery (NOTES) technique in porcine model: feasibility and survival study. Gynecol Oncol. 2009;112:405–8.
16. Perretta S, Allemann P, Asakuma M, et al. Feasibility of right and left transvaginal retroperitoneal nephrectomy: from the porcine to cadaver model. J Endourol. 2009;23:1887–92.
17. Allemann P, Perretta S, Marescaux J. Surgical access to the adrenal gland: the quest for a "no visible scar" approach. Surg Oncol. 2009;18:131–7.
18. Branco AW, Branco Filho AJ, Kondo W, et al. Hybrid transvaginal nephrectomy. Eur Urol. 2008;53:1290–4.
19. Castillo OA, Vidal-Mora I, Campos R, et al. Laparoscopic simple nephrectomy with transvaginal notes assistance and the use of standard laparoscopic instruments. Actas Urol Esp. 2009;33:767–70.
20. Kaouk JH, White WM, Goel RK, et al. NOTES transvaginal nephrectomy: first human experience. Urology. 2009;74:5–8.
21. Alcaraz A, Peri L, Molina A, et al. Feasibility of transvaginal NOTES-assisted laparoscopic nephrectomy. Eur Urol. 2010;57:233–7.
22. Sotelo R, de Andrade R, Fernandez G, et al. NOTES hybrid transvaginal radical nephrectomy for tumor: stepwise progression toward a first successful clinical case. Eur Urol. 2010;57: 138–44.
23. Kalloo AN, Singh VK, Jagannath SB, et al. Flexible transgastric peritoneoscopy: a novel approach to diagnostic and therapeutic interventions in the peritoneal cavity. Gastrointest Endosc. 2004;60:114–7.
24. Wagh MS, Merrifield BF, Thompson CC. Endoscopic transgastric abdominal exploration and organ resection: limited experience in a porcine model. Clin Gastroenterol Hepatol. 2005;3: 892–6.
25. Merrifield BF, Wagh MS, Thompson CC. Peroral transgastric organ resection: a feasibility study in pigs. Gastrointest Endosc. 2006;63:693–7.

26. Swanstrom LL, Kozarek R, Parischa PJ, et al. Development of a new access device for transgastric surgery. J Gastrointest Surg. 2005;9:1129–37.
27. Fong DG, Pai RD, Thompson CC. Transcolonic endoscopic abdominal exploration: a NOTES survival study in a porcine model. Gastrointest Endosc. 2007;65:312–8.
28. Pai RD, Fong DG, Bundga ME, et al. Transcolonic endoscopic cholecystectomy: a NOTES survival study in a porcine model (with video). Gastrointest Endosc. 2006;64:428–34.
29. Dubcenco E, Grantcharov T, Eng FC, et al. "No scar" small bowel resection in a survival porcine model using transcolonic NOTES and transabdominal approach. Surg Endosc. 2011;25:930–4.
30. Lima E, Rolanda C, Pego JM, et al. Transvesical endoscopic peritoneoscopy: a novel 5 mm port for intra-abdominal scarless surgery. J Urol. 2006;176:802–5.
31. Lima E, Henriques-Coelho T, Rolanda C, et al. Transvesical thoracoscopy: a natural orifice translumenal endoscopic approach for thoracic surgery. Surg Endosc. 2007;21:854–8.
32. Lima E, Rolanda C, Pego JM, et al. Third-generation nephrectomy by natural orifice transluminal endoscopic surgery. J Urol. 2007;178:2648–54.
33. Isariyawongse JP, McGee MF, Rosen MJ, et al. Pure natural orifice transluminal endoscopic surgery (NOTES) using standard laparoscopic instruments in the porcine model. J Endourol. 2008;22:1087–91.
34. Mintz Y, Horgan S, Savu MK, et al. Hybrid natural orifice translumenal surgery (NOTES) sleeve gastrectomy: a feasibility study using an animal model. Surg Endosc. 2008;22:1798–802.
35. Auyang ED, Vaziri K, Volckmann E, et al. NOTES: cadaveric rendezvous hybrid small bowel resection. Surg Endosc. 2008;22:2277–8.
36. Mintz Y, Horgan S, Cullen J, et al. NOTES: the hybrid technique. J Laparoendosc Adv Surg Tech A. 2007;17:402–6.
37. Baldwin DD, Tenggardaja C, Bowman R, et al. Hybrid transureteral natural orifice translumenal endoscopic nephrectomy: a feasibility study in the porcine model. J Endourol. 2010;24:1–6.
38. Hagen ME, Wagner OJ, Swain P, et al. Hybrid natural orifice transluminal endoscopic surgery (NOTES) for Roux-en-Y gastric bypass: an experimental surgical study in human cadavers. Endoscopy. 2008;40:918–24.
39. Metzelder M, Vieten G, Gosemann JH, et al. Endoloop closure of the urinary bladder is safe and efficient in female piglets undergoing transurethral NOTES nephrectomy. Eur J Pediatr Surg. 2009;19:362–5.
40. Box GN, Lee HJ, Santos RJS, et al. Rapid communication: robot-assisted NOTES nephrectomy: initial report. J Endourol. 2008;22:503–6.
41. Haber GP, Crouzet S, Kamoi K, et al. Robotic NOTES (natural orifice translumenal endoscopic surgery) in reconstructive urology: initial laboratory experience. Urology. 2008;71:996–1000.
42. Gillen S, Wilhelm D, Meining A, et al. The "ELITE" model: construct validation of a new training system for natural orifice transluminal endoscopic surgery (NOTES). Endoscopy. 2009;41:395–9.
43. Becerra Garcia FC, Misra MC, Bhattacharjee HK, et al. Experimental trial of transvaginal cholecystectomy: an *ex vivo* analysis of the learning process for novel single-port technique. Surg Endosc. 2009;23:2242–449.
44. Fuchs KH, Breithaupt W, Kuhl HJ, et al. Experience with a training program for transgastric procedures in NOTES. Surg Endosc. 2010;24:601–9.

Chapter 14
NOTES: Appendectomy

D. Nageshwar Reddy, G. Venkat Rao, and Magnus Jayaraj Mansard

Keywords NOTES appendectomy • Transvaginal appendectomy • Transgastric appendectomy • Natural orifice translumenal endoscopic surgery • Endoscopic appendectomy

Introduction

Appendicitis is the most common surgical emergency, affecting between 7 % and 12 % of humans [1, 2]. Appendectomy is the treatment of choice. The first known surgical removal of the appendix occurred in 1,735 when Claudius Amyand explored the scrotal hernia of a boy with a fecal fistula [3]. With the risk for the development of appendicitis during one's lifetime being about 1 in 8, appendectomy is one of the most common surgeries performed around the world [4].

Open appendectomy is considered to be the gold standard in the treatment of appendicitis [5]. For years, appendectomies were performed by a right lower quadrant oblique or transverse incision. In 1983, Semm introduced laparoscopic surgery that proved to be useful for both the diagnosis and treatment of a variety of intraabdominal conditions [6]. With demonstrable advantages of lesser wound infection, lesser pain, better cosmesis, and improved diagnostics, the laparoscopic appendectomy has come to challenge the open technique as the standard treatment. The approach to this operation has been very standardized, and it now has a track record for reliable outcomes even in complicated cases [7, 8].

NOTES (natural orifice translumenal endoscopic surgery) seeks to improve upon the advantages of laparoscopic surgery by totally avoiding an external incision. The

---

D.N. Reddy, M.D., DM, DSc, FAMS, FRCP • G.V. Rao, M.S., FRCS, MAMS
M.J. Mansard, M.S., DNB (✉)
Department of Surgical Gastroenterology, Asian Institute of Gastroenterology,
6-3-661 Somajiguuda, Hyderabad 500082, Andhra Pradesh, India
e-mail: aigindiainfo@yahoo.co.in; drraogv@sify.com; jeymagnus@gmail.com

A. Rane et al. (eds.), *Scar-Less Surgery*,
DOI 10.1007/978-1-84800-360-6_14, © Springer-Verlag London 2013

goal is to perform abdominal surgery safely through the body's natural orifices, some even outside the operating room setting, and to avoid complications associated with abdominal incisions, such as wound infection, pain, herniation, and adhesions. The work of Kalloo et al. in the transgastric abdominal approach using endoscopy in animal experiments reported in 2004 sparked the current heavy interest in NOTES [9]. NOTES has been attempted worldwide and has improved tremendously in a short time. Work on porcine models has been progressing for many years and has now culminated in successful endoscopic surgery in human subjects [10]. Rao et al. (the senior authors of the chapter) presented the first clinical case, their work on the first transgastric appendectomy, at the World Congress of Gastroenterology in 2005 [11]. Since then, appendectomy has become the second-most common surgery, reported in peer-reviewed journals, performed through the NOTES approach [12]. World experience in human NOTES appendectomy, restricted to ethically approved studies, is growing, particularly in the field of transvaginal and transgastric access (Table 14.1).

NOTES Nomenclature

While ideally, a "pure NOTES" procedure entails no incision on the abdominal wall, the safety of this method has not been established enough to be used routinely in human subjects. Most of the NOTES appendectomy procedures performed are "hybrid NOTES," which involves inserting one or two trocars in the abdominal area and using laparoscopic equipment. These transabdominal instruments are used for assistance in retraction and visualization, while the main dissection is done with flexible endoscopes. Also, when the operation is performed by laparoscopy with a low natural orifice instrumentation contribution (retraction or visualization), it has been termed "NOTES-assisted laparoscopy" [12].

Table 14.1 NOTES appendectomies performed in humans to date

Authors	Route	Number of successful operations/ number of attempted operations	Year of publication
Palanivelu et al. [13]	Transvaginal	3/6	2008
Rao et al. [14]	Transgastric	8/10	2008
Bernhardt et al. [15]	Transvaginal	1	2008
Tabutsadze and Kipshidze [16]	Transvaginal	2	2009
Horgan et al. [17]	Transvaginal	1	2009
	Transgastric	1	
Zorron et al. [12]	Transvaginal	37	2010
	Transgastric	14	
Park and Bergstrom [18]	Transgastric	1/3	2010
Noguera et al. [19]	Transvaginal	2	2010
Shin et al. [20]	Transvaginal	1	2010

Preprocedure Preparation

Before embarking on the performance of any NOTES procedure, a well-trained multi-disciplinary team is required with advanced laparoscopic and endoscopic skills. It is important to invest time in gathering extensive experience on animal models [21]. This is not only for the surgeon/gastroenterologist who is to perform the procedure, but also for the operating room staff, scrub nurses, and anesthetists [18]. IRB approval and a detailed informed consent from the patient are other crucial requisites [22]. Close consultation with a gynecologist is essential if the transvaginal approach is chosen.

Patient Selection

The proper patient selection is required for the successful completion of appendectomy through the NOTES approach. Advanced and emergency procedures should be avoided in the early phase of technological development. The patient should not have "complicated" appendicitis. Preferably, a patient with pain of less than 48 h' duration and no history of recurrent pain in the past is chosen. A nonobese, nonpregnant patient not in the extreme age groups with no major medical comorbidity/bleeding disorder is favored. There should preferably be no previous history of abdominal surgery. For the transvaginal approach, a history of pelvic inflammatory disease, of severe endometriosis, of hysterectomy, of ectopic pregnancy, or of vaginal trauma; vaginal infection; pregnancy, and virgin patients constitute contraindications. Before surgery, a bimanual pelvic examination is essential. Because of the unresolved concern of the effect of the transvaginal route on fertility, women who had completed their family were chosen by some groups for this approach [12].

Sterilization of Equipment

Normally, endoscopes used for conventional purposes undergo bacteriostatic sterilization. However, for intraperitoneal use, bactericidal sterilization is required. Sterilization with ethylene oxide as per the guidelines of the Minimal Access Therapy Decontamination Working Group is recommended for a NOTES appendectomy procedure [20].

Patient Preparation and Anesthesia

For the transvaginal approach, disinfection of the vagina is achieved by topical iodopovidone or chlorhexidine solution, and a urinary catheter is installed after anesthesia [14]. For the transgastric approach, disinfection of the gastric lumen is achieved by intraoperative gavage with clorohexidine solution. Some centers have used no special cleaning besides aspiration [18].

Prophylactic antibiotic use is recommended by all centers. Usually, a single dose of an intravenous bolus of either 2 g of cefalexin or a combination of 400 mg of metronidazol and 400 mg of ciprofloxacin is given at the induction of anesthesia. The procedure is carried out under general anesthesia with a transnasal endotracheal intubation in a Lloyd–Davies/lithotomy position.

Creation of Pneumoperitoneum

The pneumoperitoneum can be created by insufflation through the transabdominal port, usually in the vicinity of the umbilicus, or through the endoscope. Translumenal endoscopic insufflation was obtained usually by attaching a laparoflator to a working channel of the endoscope or by tying an insufflation tube to the endoscope. Creating the pneumoperitoneum through endoscopic insufflation has been found to be more difficult to measure and maintain [23]. A wider variation in pressure has been observed than with laparoscopic insufflation. Hence, most of the groups have used the laparoscopic insufflation system, which ensures that any excess insufflation is noted and quickly addressed. CO_2 was the gas of choice to insufflate NOTES surgery, and pressures of 5–15 mmHg have been used.

Approach

Transrectal, transesophagic, and transurethral accesses have been described in animal experiments [24, 25]. But they are not suitable yet for clinical studies, due to a lack of sufficient experimental data and technical development for its safe use in trials. Silberhumer et al. described the design and development of devices that enable the inversion of the appendix through colonoscopy [26]. Such an inverted appendix has been excised akin to a colonoscopic polypectomy. All the other NOTES appendectomy described to date in humans have used the transvaginal and transgastric approaches.

Transvaginal Approach

The transvaginal access has become the preferred route for NOTES appendectomy in most clinical series. The use of the vaginal route for endoscopic procedures is not new. Ventroscopy was described as early as in 1901, followed by reports of culdoscopy and colpolaparoscopy [27]. Bueno described in 1949 the first successful performance of incidental vaginal appendectomy at the time of vaginal hysterectomy, and Reiner, in 1980, presented his experience with 100 consecutive appendectomies done incidentally at the time of vaginal surgery [28]. Culdolaparoscopy regained popularity at the end of the twentieth century when ports inserted transvaginally were used in the assistance of laparoscopic gynecologic procedures for the introduction of operative instruments and the extraction of specimens.

The peritoneum can be accessed transvaginally via two methods [12]. In the more common method, the laparoscopic port is inserted first in the periumbilical region. A pneumoperitoneum is created. The pelvis is visualized through a laparoscopic camera/needloscope to rule out adhesions. Under laparoscopic guidance, the posterior cul-de-sac is punctured in the avascular area between the two uterosacral ligaments with one or more trocars. Alternately, the incision in the center of the cul-de-sac is done via the mini-laparoscopy at a point stretched by an atraumatic plastic rod placed transvaginally. The trocar(s) is subsequently placed through this incision. A flexible endoscope introduced through this trocar(s) is used for the appendectomy.

In the second method, opening of the posterior vaginal sac is done with conventional instruments. A Sims speculum is inserted in the vagina, and two lateral retractors are used to retract the vaginal walls. The posterior fornix is stretched with a Pozzi clamp grasping the posterior lip of the cervix. A uterine manipulator can be utilized to assist in the procedure. The vaginal mucosa in the posterior cul-de-sac is opened at the cervicovaginal junction by a semilunar 2.5-cm incision. With a sharp dissection performed with scissors, the posterior cul-de-sac peritoneum is identified and opened.

Transgastric Approach

Transgastric appendectomy begins with the insertion of a two-channel gastroscope into the stomach, which is distended with carbon dioxide. Esophageal overtubes have been used by a few groups to prevent esophageal trauma caused by repeated passages of the endoscope. A needle-knife is used to incise the gastric wall, choosing a spot in the anterior wall midway between the vascular arcades along the curvatures. The needle-knife is withdrawn, and a guidewire is threaded through the incision. This hole is then dilated using a balloon dilator, threaded over the guidewire (Fig. 14.1). The scope is then advanced into the peritoneal cavity along with the dilator balloon through the gastrotomy [14]. The alternate way of gastrotomy with a sphincterotome is less favored as it leaves behind a larger incision in the stomach wall than the balloon-dilated puncture, which collapses as the uncut muscle contracts after withdrawal of the scope. The "needle-knife/guidewire/balloon" technique used to introduce the endoscope into the peritoneal cavity is easy, quick, and reliable [18].

Fig. 14.1 Balloon dilation of
anterior gastrotomy

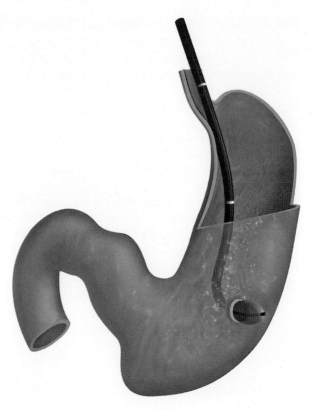

Procedure

The regular dual-channel gastroscope is used. Alternately, the colonoscope is used
[20]. The procedure is carried out with standard endoscopic accessories, such as a
grasper, hot biopsy forceps, needle-knife, snare, and endoloop passed through the
accessory channel of the endoscope. Rigid instruments passed through the laparoscopic port have been used by different groups for various activities, including visualization, retraction, dissection, ligation, and gastrotomy closure. Two monitors are
usually utilized, one for the laparoscopic view and another for the endoscopic
view.

After passing the endoscope into the peritoneal cavity, it is directed toward the
anterior abdominal wall for orientation. Visualization of the abdominal cavity is
simplified by tilting the patient into different positions, just as in traditional laparoscopy. However, tilting the table will result in not only the organs but also the scope
falling to that side by gravity [18]. Platforms or flexible overtubes that can be made
rigid in different positions might be helpful [29, 30].

The tip of the scope is then positioned in the right lower abdomen and the appendix is located. Even when the transvaginal route is used, this has been accomplished
by most workers without the need for retroflexion. Endoscopic graspers are used to

Fig. 14.2 Division of the mesoappendix with hot biopsy forceps

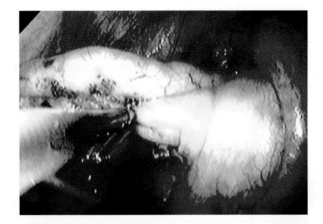

Fig. 14.3 Division of the appendix after application of loop at the base

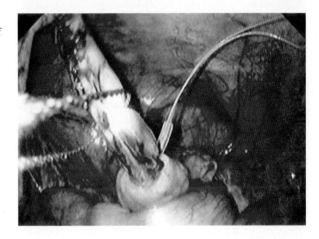

separate the appendix from adjacent tissues. The appendix is then luxated outward and moved into an optimal position. A rat-toothed biopsy is used to grasp and lift the appendix and stretch the mesoappendix. A hot biopsy forceps with monopolar cautery is used to dissect the mesoappendix from the appendix (Fig. 14.2). Cauterized tissue is cut with the needle-knife. Endoclips can be used to secure the appendicular artery pedicle. Once the appendix is entirely skeletonized, an endoloop is applied to the base, and the appendix is divided with an endosnare (Fig. 14.3). Because of concerns of the reliability of endoloops for this purpose, some groups have utilized laparoscopic loop ligatures to ligate the appendix base [20]. The endoscopic linear cutter has also been used to divide the base of the appendix along with the mesoappendix. The transected appendix is then extracted through the natural orifice along with the endoscope (Fig. 14.4). The use of an endoscopic bag in the extraction of the specimen has been advocated to restrict contamination. Irrigation and suction of the peritoneal cavity is then performed. A thorough exploration of the abdominal cavity is performed to look for injuries before withdrawal of the ports.

Fig. 14.4 Transoral extraction of the appendix

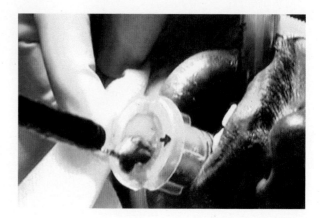

Closure

The vaginal incision closure is straightforward and is done externally under direct vision using conventional instruments and a single layer of absorbable sutures. However, there are serious concerns related to the closure of the gastric puncture, as anything other than a 0 % leak rate cannot be acceptable in practice. Because of these concerns, many centers have adopted a policy of routine laparoscopic closure of the gastric puncture [12]. Others have used T-tags, endoclips, g-Prox sutures, and other newly designed endoscopic closure devices with and without laparoscopic reinforcements [12, 17, 18, 31].

Operative Time

Operative time, as expected, is longer for NOTES appendectomy, at usually more than 100 min, than conventional appendectomies. The time was longer when the procedure was performed by the "pure NOTES" technique than the "hybrid" technique. Also, if the entry and closure time were excluded, the operation was performed faster through the transgastric approach than through the transvaginal approach [32]. This has been ascribed to the more direct approach of the scope to the appendix by the transgastric approach when compared to the transperineal approach. A learning curve could be demonstrated whereby the operating time decreased as experience increased [32]. However, when the closure time was included, the transvaginal approach was faster than the transgastric approach [12].

Postoperative Care

Patients are allowed a liquid diet 12–24 h after surgery. On the first postoperative day, solid meals are started. Antibiotics have been continued for 2–3 days by most [14]. Though the patient has been fit for discharge earlier, most of the patients have been kept in the hospital for 3 days as a precautionary measure.

If the transvaginal route has been used, the vaginal dressing is changed on the first postoperative day. Similar to the wound care after obstetrical gynecological surgery, antibiotic suppositories are inserted for 1 week. Abstinence from sexual intercourse is advised for 1 month. Regular follow-up in the first month is advised.

Transgastric Versus Transvaginal Approach

The transgastric approach was the first approach used in NOTES surgery both in the animal model and in humans [9, 14]. Also, it gives a more direct approach to the appendix [32]. However, more complications have been noted with the transgastric approach than with the transvaginal approach. Additionally, the issue of lack of reliable instruments to achieve a safe closure deters many workers from preferring this route.

The transvaginal route, though it can be applied to only 50 % of the population, has become the approach of choice. The closure is simple and the orientation problem is easily overcome with experience. Unlike the transgastric approach, where a long length of the scope is used up in transversing the esophagus and stomach and very little of the scope is available outside to work with, the transvaginal route is shorter, giving more freedom for manipulation of the scope [13]. Also, it allows larger instruments to be introduced, and larger specimens to be extracted, than the transgastric route. Despite these advantages, the sensitive and private nature of this approach makes it controversial. Fertility concerns and the risk of dyspareunia are other apprehensions that need to be addressed.

Complications

Reported complications have been few and of minor consequence. In the series reported by Rao et al., one patient who underwent a pure NOTES appendectomy sustained a needle-knife injury to the anterior abdominal wall during transgastric access. Another patient from the same series experienced postoperative ileus [14]. In the series from Palanivelu et al., two patients complained of postoperative vaginal discomfort on the second postoperative day, probably due to the colpotomy, which was relieved by oral analgesia. Hemorrhage from the appendicular artery was seen in one patient, which was controlled endoscopically [13]. In the series from Park et al., a T-tag used to close the gastrotomy had anchored the stomach wall to the left lateral thoracic wall and had penetrated the pleural cavity, resulting in a pneumothorax [18].

In the IMTN NOTES Study, four patients (three transvaginal and one transgastric) had bleeding of the appendicular vessel intraoperatively, which was managed with endoscopic or laparoscopic hemostasis. One other patient had abdominal wall injury during transgastric access that was managed conservatively. Postoperatively, one patient who underwent transgastric appendectomy had prolonged ileus, which was managed conservatively [12].

There was no reported wound complication, pelvic pain, or urinary difficulty and no mortality. None of the groups using the transvaginal approach reported postoperative dyspareunia in any of their subjects.

Benefits and Hurdles

Studies comparing laparoscopic with open surgeries have demonstrated lower pain scores and fewer analgesic needs for laparoscopic surgery. Laparoscopic surgery has also shown to have a lower stress response and less impaired immune functions when compared with open surgery [33]. NOTES surgery is likely to further these advantages by achieving a "scarless" status. Lesser or no pain, no wound-related complications, including wound infection and hernia, a shorter convalescence, and better cosmesis are the suggested advantages of a NOTES procedure.

Postoperative pain is less compared with patients undergoing laparoscopic appendectomy [13]. The NOTES IMTN Study has shown the lack of need for postoperative analgesia in a significant proportion of patients after NOTES procedures [12]. Also, a trend toward a lower end tidal CO_2 has been shown in the same study. Unpublished reports suggest that NOTES appendectomy has been performed with lesser insufflation pressures, 5–6 mmHg CO_2, than required for conventional laparoscopy, possibly because of less need for exposure and insufflation.

The physical restraints of operating exclusively through an endoscope with limited dexterity and rudimentary instrumentation compared with laparoscopy and traditional minimally invasive techniques remain the main hurdle to the universal acceptance of NOTES procedures. A limited operating field, lack of triangulation, disorientation, difficult navigation, and accessories with a high elasticity and low hardness incapable of exerting an adequate force are some of the impediments that need to be addressed before we see universal acceptance of this technique [10].

Conclusion

NOTES appendectomy is feasible with the available instruments, taking possibly longer operative times than laparoscopy until new endoscopic technology arises. Transvaginal and transgastric appendectomies can be performed safely with limited complications when performed by skilled operators with extensive training in veterinary NOTES surgery. Using a laparoscope for assistance in the initial experience appears to be a useful adjunct in improving safety. The initial studies have focused on feasibility and safety. The ultimate aim should be of conducting blinded, randomized controlled trials using comparisons with the current gold standard of open/laparoscopic appendectomy.

References

1. Nguyen DB, Silen W, Hodin RA. Appendectomy in the pre- and postlaparoscopic eras. J Gastrointest Surg. 1999;3(1):67–73.
2. Addiss DG, et al. The epidemiology of appendicitis and appendectomy in the United States. Am J Epidemiol. 1990;132(5):910–25.
3. Milanchi S, Allins AD. Amyand's Hernia: history, imaging, and management. Hernia. 2008;12(3):321–2.
4. Martin RF, Rossi RL. The acute abdomen. An overview and algorithms. Surg Clin North Am. 1997;77(6):1227–43.
5. Kapischke M, et al. Open versus laparoscopic appendectomy: a critical review. Surg Endosc. 2006;20(7):1060–8.
6. Semm K. Endoscopic appendectomy. Endoscopy. 1983;15(2):59–64.
7. Konstantinidis KM, et al. A decade of laparoscopic appendectomy: presentation of 1,026 patients with suspected appendicitis treated in a single surgical department. J Laparoendosc Adv Surg Tech A. 2008;18(2):248–58.
8. Markides G, Subar D, Riyad K. Laparoscopic versus open appendectomy in adults with complicated appendicitis: systematic review and meta-analysis. World J Surg. 2010; 34(9):2026–40.
9. Kalloo AN, et al. Flexible transgastric peritoneoscopy: a novel approach to diagnostic and therapeutic interventions in the peritoneal cavity. Gastrointest Endosc. 2004;60(1):114–7.
10. Mansard MJ, Reddy DN, Rao GV. NOTES: a review. Trop Gastroenterol. 2009;30(1):5–10.
11. ASGE/SAGES Working Group on natural orifice translumenal endoscopic surgery white paper, October 2005. Gastrointest Endosc. 2006;63(2):199–203.
12. Zorron R, et al. International multicenter trial on clinical natural orifice surgery – NOTES IMTN study: preliminary results of 362 patients. Surg Innov. 2010;17(2):142–58.
13. Palanivelu C, et al. Transvaginal endoscopic appendectomy in humans: a unique approach to NOTES – world's first report. Surg Endosc. 2008;22(5):1343–7.
14. Rao GV, Reddy DN, Banerjee R. NOTES: human experience. Gastrointest Endosc Clin N Am. 2008;18(2):361–70; x.
15. Bernhardt J, et al. NOTES – case report of a unidirectional flexible appendectomy. Int J Colorectal Dis. 2008;23(5):547–50.
16. Tabutsadze T, Kipshidze N. New trend in endoscopic surgery: transvaginal appendectomy NOTES (natural orifice transluminal endoscopic surgery). Georgian Med News. 2009;168:7–10.
17. Horgan S, et al. Natural orifice surgery: initial clinical experience. Surg Endosc. 2009;23(7):1512–8.
18. Park PO, Bergstrom M. Transgastric peritoneoscopy and appendectomy: thoughts on our first experience in humans. Endoscopy. 2010;42(1):81–4.
19. Noguera JF, et al. Emergency transvaginal hybrid natural orifice transluminal endoscopic surgery. Endoscopy. 2010;43:442–4.
20. Shin EJ, et al. Transvaginal endoscopic appendectomy. J Korean Soc Coloproctol. 2010;26(6):429–32.
21. Zacharakis E, et al. Natural orifices translumenal endoscopic surgery (NOTES) – who should perform it? Surgery. 2008;144(1):1–2.
22. Ponsky JL, Rosen MJ, Poulose BK. NOTES: of caution. Surg Endosc. 2008;22(7):1561–2.
23. Nakajima K, et al. Current limitations in endoscopic CO_2 insufflation for NOTES: flow and pressure study. Gastrointest Endosc. 2010;72(5):1036–42.
24. Pai RD, et al. Transcolonic endoscopic cholecystectomy: a NOTES survival study in a porcine model (with video). Gastrointest Endosc. 2006;64(3):428–34.
25. Lima E, Rolanda C, Correia-Pinto J. Transvesical endoscopic peritoneoscopy: intra-abdominal scarless surgery for urologic applications. Curr Urol Rep. 2008;9(1):50–4.

26. Silberhumer GR, et al. Design and instrumentation of new devices for performing appendectomy at colonoscopy (with video). Gastrointest Endosc. 2008;68(1):139–45.
27. Tsin DA, et al. Minilaparoscopy-assisted natural orifice surgery. JSLS. 2007;11(1):24–9.
28. Zorron R, et al. NOTES transvaginal cholecystectomy: preliminary clinical application. Surg Endosc. 2008;22(2):542–7.
29. Bessler M, et al. Transvaginal laparoscopically assisted endoscopic cholecystectomy: a hybrid approach to natural orifice surgery. Gastrointest Endosc. 2007;66(6):1243–5.
30. Swanstrom LL, Whiteford M, Khajanchee Y. Developing essential tools to enable transgastric surgery. Surg Endosc. 2008;22(3):600–4.
31. Sclabas GM, Swain P, Swanstrom LL. Endoluminal methods for gastrotomy closure in natural orifice transenteric surgery (NOTES). Surg Innov. 2006;13(1):23–30.
32. Jayaraman S, Schlachta CM. Transgastric and transperineal natural orifice translumenal endoscopic surgery (NOTES) in an appendectomy test bed. Surg Innov. 2009;16(3):223–7.
33. Buunen M, et al. Stress response to laparoscopic surgery: a review. Surg Endosc. 2004;18(7):1022–8.

Chapter 15
NOTES: Cholecystectomy (European Experience)

Silvana Perretta and Jacques Marescaux

Keywords Training • NOTES • Transluminal surgery • Simulation • Web-based education

Introduction

Recent decades have seen remarkable progress in medicine as minimally invasive procedures have replaced radical surgical resections. Natural orifice translumenal endoscopic surgery (NOTES) is an evolving minimally invasive technique that has the potential to break the physical barrier between incisions and surgery. The present-day concept of NOTES was articulated by Kalloo et al. in 2004, who challenged surgeons and endoscopists to focus research on finding the best translumenal endoscopic access to the peritoneal cavity, with the utmost attention to safety, including the reliable closure of the entry point [1]. The justifications for this technique are as follows: the reduction or absence of postoperative pain; the ease of access to some organs; the absence of trauma to the abdominal wall; ideal cosmetic results; and the psychological advantages of eliminating the trauma caused by transabdominal surgery. Both transvaginal and transgastric cholecystectomies have been translated from research into clinical applications, attracting an explosion of interest [2, 3]. Since the first report from Marescaux et al. [3] and Bessler et al. [2] in 2007, over 500 NOTES cholecystectomies have been reported in Europe, mostly using a hybrid approach between NOTES and laparoscopy. With the goal of tracking the evolution of new techniques, a global European NOTES activity registry, the Euro-NOTES

S. Perretta, M.D. • J. Marescaux, M.D. (Hon), FRCS, FACS (Hon), JSES (✉)
Department of Digestive and Endocrine Surgery,
University Hospital of Strasbourg,
1 Place de l'Hopital, Strasbourg 67091, France
e-mail: silvana.perretta@ircad.fr; jacques.marescaux@ircad.fr

A. Rane et al. (eds.), *Scar-Less Surgery*,
DOI 10.1007/978-1-84800-360-6_15, © Springer-Verlag London 2013

Registry (www.euronotes.world.it), was created among ten centers. An independent nationwide German registry was also established as an outcome database to allow the monitoring and safe introduction of NOTES [4]. Both registries invite surgeons who performed NOTES procedures to voluntarily contribute. Despite the fact that NOTES has just recently been introduced, the technique has already gained considerable clinical application in Europe, and it appears to be well accepted by patients [5]. According to the registries, cholecystectomies account for 89 % of all NOTES procedures in Europe. NOTES cholecystectomies have been described in Europe using the transvaginal approach with rigid in-line instruments, and through both the transvaginal and transgastric approaches with a flexible platform.

NOTES: Cholecystectomy (European Experience)

Transvaginal abdominal access has a longer track record of safety in the field of gynecology, and so, not surprisingly, it has been the leading access for NOTES. Transvaginal access for abdominal surgery is not new, with the first transvaginal appendectomy at the time of vaginal hysterectomy reported by Bueno in 1949 [6]. This first case report was followed soon after by the successful report of 12 and 8 cases from Pelosi and McGowan, respectively [7, 8]. The procedures were described as simple, quick, and safe. Posterior colpotomy as a route for specimen retrieval was described as early as 1896 when Howard Kelly [9] reported ten cases of ectopic pregnancies managed surgically through the vaginal route. NOTES has revisited the established concept of posterior colpotomy as a port to the abdomen. The experience by gynecologists performing transvaginal procedures has demonstrated safety in terms of pelvic infection. Data from transvaginal hysterectomies report an infection rate of 3.9 %, and fertiloscopy is associated with an extremely low infection rate (0.1 %) [10]. The transvaginal route was the access chosen for the first human NOTES cholecystectomies due to the benefits of (1) an established method of access and closure of the entry point, (2) a direct line of vision toward the gallbladder, and (3) the ability to introduce rigid laparoscopic instruments that could assist in different steps of the procedure. The most obvious limitation of this route is, of course, that it is applicable to only half of the population. Additionally, a major long-term concern is postoperative sexual function. Validated sexual function questionnaires exist, as sexual function can be difficult to characterize and track.

In contrast to the transvaginal route, only 12 transgastric cholecystectomies have been reported to date [11]. The use of a transgastric route to perform surgical procedures is not particularly new either. The first transgastric procedure dates back to percutaneous endoscopic gastrostomy (PEG) feeding tube placement reported in 1980 [12]. PEG is today a common, well-standardized transgastric procedure, with a low complication rate. In 1998, the Apollo group led by Kalloo brought new fuel and an innovative prospective to this approach. Many experts believe that the transgastric route will be the one to dominate NOTES in the future; today significant challenges remain for this approach before it becomes widespread. Unlike the transvaginal route supported by many years of experience, the transgastric route raises contentious issues of controlling contamination and safe closure of the stomach. J. Hazey investigated the bacterial load and contamination patients experience during laparoscopic Roux-en-Y gastric bypass while having their gastrotomy for gastrojejunostomy [13]. Of the 50 patients enrolled, only 5 patients demonstrated cross-contamination of bacterial loads from the stomach to the abdomen. None of these cross-contaminants resulted in significant infection. Thus, these findings support the hypothesis that while transgastric instrumentation does contaminate the abdominal cavity, the pathogens introduced are unlikely to cause a clinically significant infection.

The majority of NOTES cholecystectomies in Europe have been performed by a rigid hybrid technique either by a modified TEM instrumentation or using laparoscopic rigid instrumentation as described by Zornig in 2007 [14]. His technique became popular compared to the use of flexible endoscopes, as it relies on known laparoscopic skills and instrumentation over less familiar endoscopic techniques and less effective tools. In short, transvaginal access is performed under direct vision of a 5-mm optic at the umbilicus. A 5-mm mandarin is introduced in the posterior vaginal fornix and subsequently replaced by an extra-long dissector. A 10-mm trocar is inserted alongside the dissector to introduce an extra-long 10-mm 45° scope (Olympus, Hamburg, Germany). The optic at the umbilicus is then replaced by another dissector. In his initial series of 68 patients with uncomplicated cholelithiasis, Zornig described an acceptance rate of 23 % with an intention to treat feasibility of 98 %. The mean operative time was 53 min, with the need for an additional trocar in three cases, and no intraoperative complications [14]. One major complication of an abscess in the pouch of Douglas requiring laparoscopic drainage was reported 3 weeks after surgery. Recently, the same group reported a matched-pair analysis [15] comparing the transvaginal hybrid approach to the conventional laparoscopic technique in a series of 100 patients. In this study, the two techniques appeared similar in terms of reoperations, wound infection, postoperative pain, hospital stay, and sick leave. The operative time was significantly longer for the transvaginal approach (52 vs. 35 min, $p < 0.001$). Indications were mainly symptomatic gallstones, although cholecystitis was found pathologically in a small subset of patients. Obesity (BMI $\geq$ 25) and older age ($\geq$65 years) were associated with longer operative times and a higher likelihood of conversion. Sexual function was reported to be unchanged although it was not assessed with a validated questionnaire [4].

The popularity of this "rigid" transluminal technique was recently highlighted by the recent report from the German Society of General and Visceral Surgery (Deutsche Gesellschaft für Allgemein- und Viszeralchirurgie). More than 488 NOTES cholecystectomies have been performed in the country, almost all using the technique described by Zornig [14]. According to the German registry, the mean number of abdominal trocars used was 1.2±0.5 (1-4 trocars) with an overall reported conversion rate to laparoscopy of 4.9 %. Of all conversions, 44 % were related to technical problems concerning either transvaginal access or intraoperative findings. In the rigid approach, complications occurred in 3 % and included bladder injury, uterine perforation, rectal injury requiring a Hartmann procedure, postoperative vaginal bleeding, abscess, and vaginal infection. The institutional case volume was associated with shorter operative times and fewer additional trocars.

Another European group recently published on rigid hybrid transvaginal cholecystectomy in a series of 102 consecutive patients [5]. The authors included all patients older than 18 years who were candidates for laparoscopic cholecystectomy without restriction on BMI or clinical presentation. They treated symptomatic cholelithiasis (74) and cholecystitis (28) with an overall operative time of 62 ± 21.9 min. An additional assisting trocar was required in 19 patients, 11 of whom had cholecystitis. Two major complications (one stroke and one trocar herniation) and 13 minor complications were reported (12.7 %). Among the gynecological complications, infection and dehiscence of the colpotomy closure were reported. Postoperative sexual function was assessed using the gastrointestinal quality-of-life questionnaire (GIQLI) and one additional question related to dyspareunia. Using these measures, the authors reported an improvement in sexual life after surgery that they attributed to the amelioration of the overall quality of life occurring after cholecystectomy.

With appropriate training, experience, and patient selection, the use of a hybrid transvaginal rigid instrument technique seems feasible and applicable to routine clinical use. Nevertheless, it is important to note that new and unexpected complications unique to these techniques even distant from the targeted organ are possible, including rectal and uterine injury.

The performance of cholecystectomy using a flexible platform with endoscopic instruments is more technically challenging and has therefore remained less popular. Difficulty derives from the endoscopic skills required and the limited capabilities of flexible instruments. All the cholecystectomy techniques reported in the literature with a "flexible" technique highlighted the limitations related to the inadequacy of the current instrumentation, with the resulting lack of exposure, fine dissection, and safe cystic duct ligation. One or several transabdominal laparoscopic trocars, transcutaneous suspension sutures, internal retractors, or transvaginal laparoscopic graspers are currently used to reach satisfactory exposure and visualization of Calot's triangle and to allow the use of standard laparoscopic instruments, such as a clip applier and energy-driven dissection tools.

Another limiting factor is related to instrument sterility and the absence of a definitive consensus on a standardization of "surgical" endoscope processing. Whereas there is general agreement that a high-level disinfection is mandatory for endoscopes used for NOTES, the need for sterilization with ethylene oxide is unclear.

As a consequence, in Europe, the use of flexible endoscopes for transvaginal and transgastric NOTES procedures in humans is still very limited and is performed only in highly specialized centers.

At our institution, we choose to approach cholecystectomy using a flexible endoscopic operating platform for both the transgastric and transvaginal approaches. While technically challenging, it conforms more to the core principles of NOTES, as it enables interventions throughout the abdomen, it can be performed without abdominal trocars, and when applied transgastrically, it is applicable to all patients.

The transgastric and transvaginal routes were evaluated for ease of access to the peritoneal cavity, quality of exposure of the gallbladder, and manipulation of the endoscopic instruments before proceeding to clinical application. Between 2005 and 2007, over 400 procedures were performed in animal and ex vivo models.

After a few changes of the technique in the early learning curve, we have now developed a standardized hybrid approach for flexible endoscopic transvaginal cholecystectomy including both steps and instruments. With the patient placed in a modified Lloyd–Davies position, the operation begins with the introduction of a 5-mm trocar necessary for insufflation and monitoring of the pneumoperitoneum, and to introduce a 5-mm laparoscopic clip applier. The patient position is then changed to a steep Trendelenburg tilt to better expose the pelvis. Transvaginal access is obtained under laparoscopic control. The vagina is scrubbed with betadine and the posterior lip of the cervix is grasped with a Pozzi forceps and traction maintained in the direction of the symphysis pubis. A horizontal 2-cm cold blade posterior incision, 1 cm below the uterine os, is performed between the uterosacral ligaments. Two stay sutures are placed at the distal edges of the colpotomy to prevent tearing of tissue and to facilitate closure. A double-channel endoscope (Karl Storz Endoskope, Tuttlingen, Germany) together with a 60-cm-long laparoscopic grasper is introduced transvaginally under vision. In order to improve the exposure, an internally anchored, hands-free retracting device, EndoGrab™ (Virtual Port Caesarea, Israel), is now regularly used. Cholecystectomy is accomplished using alternatively flexible instruments introduced via the endoscope and 5-mm laparoscopic instruments via the umbilical port. The cystic duct and artery are clipped using a laparoscopic clip applier. The colpotomy is closed by separate 3/0 Vicryl stitches. Gynecological assessment is performed 1 and 3 months postoperatively and includes both a physical exam performed by a gynecologist and a quality-of-life questionnaire (GIQLI). Postoperative sexual function is evaluated using a dedicated questionnaire (Sexual Function Questionnaire 31).

A similar technique was used by Pugliese et al. on a series of 18 transvaginal cholecystectomies [16]. The authors reported no intraoperative complications and no conversions, an overall mean duration of procedures of 75 min (range 40–190), and one biliary leak treated with drainage. At a mean follow-up of 12 months (range 1–22), none of the patients complained of dyspareunia or other colpotomy-related complications.

For the transgastric cholecystectomy, in a similar fashion to the transvaginal approach, we use a hybrid format by means of a 5-mm umbilical trocar. Placement of this trocar is recommended when performing transgastric NOTES with contemporary instrumentation, to ensure an adequate exposure of the cystic duct and artery, to allow the use of a 5-mm laparoscopic clip applier, and to monitor the gastrotomy creation and closure. Endoscopic access to the peritoneum is obtained by a modified PEG technique. A needle-knife is used to create a 5-mm gastrotomy on the anterior gastric wall, which is then balloon-dilated to allow the passage of the endoscope.

With this starting one-trocar setup used initially to retract the gallbladder, the dissection can be carried out exclusively using flexible instruments inserted via the two working channels of the endoscope. These instruments are obviously not designed or adapted to perform such tasks and, as a result, the dissection becomes very time-consuming. The operating time can be dramatically improved with the use of standard endoscopic instruments such as the hook inserted through the umbilical port. Prevention of injury during cholecystectomy relies on the accurate dissection of the cystic duct and artery, and avoidance of major biliary and vascular structures. Specific anatomical distortions due to NOTES technique, along with the lack of exposure provided by present methods of retraction and retroflexion, tend to distort the Calot's triangle by flattening it rather than opening it out. Transparietal assistance, using suspension of the falciform ligament, internal retraction systems, or the introduction of an additional micro-laparoscopic grasper at the umbilicus or in the right hypochondrium, is added liberally in order to obtain the safest possible exposure of the operative field.

As the cholecystectomy is completed, the gallbladder is removed through the gastrotomy using a polypectomy snare. Preventive drainage of the gallbladder is carried out to reduce the bulk of the specimen to avoid rupture of the gallbladder during retrieval and consequently biliary spillage. Particular attention should be paid to gallstones size. Stones larger than 2 cm should be retrieved via the abdominal trocar incision, to avoid esophageal impaction or laceration at retrieval. The gastrotomy is then closed with extracorporeal interrupted 3/0 Vicryl stitches by means of a 2-mm laparoscope and a 3-mm needle holder that were inserted side by side into the 5-mm umbilical port. Gastroscopy is carried out to inspect the closure and to confirm an airtight seal by the attainment of a satisfactory pneumogastrium.

From September 2007 to March 2009, a total of 30 patients with a mean age of 48.5 years (range: 28–65), a mean BMI of 23.3 (range: 21–31 kg/m^2), underwent NOTES cholecystectomy at our institution under IRB approval [3, 11]. Eleven transgastric (6 men and 5 women) and 19 transvaginal cholecystectomies were performed. All operations were performed using standard dual-channel endoscopes with at least one 5-mm laparoscopic port for assistance. Transgastric procedures resulted in longer total operative times [132 min (range: 90-180 minutes) vs. 104 min (range: 20–270 min)], peritoneal access times, and access closure times. The postoperative day 1 pain score (EVA 2/10 vs. 0.5/10) was slightly higher in the transgastric group. None of the TV cholecytstectomy patients complained of pelvic pain. Transgastric and transvaginal peritoneal accesses were achieved without complications or injury to adjacent organs. In the transgastric group, dissection of the gallbladder was completely performed with flexible endoscopic instruments in two patients, while a combination with a laparoscopic hook dissector was used in the remaining patients. A 5-mm laparoscopic clip applier was systematically used to secure the cystic pedicle. In two patients, there was a need to switch to a laparoscopic view to assess the biliary anatomy. No vascular or biliary injury to the adjacent organs occurred during the procedure. The routine use of additional retraction via a transvaginal grasper and an internal retraction system (EndoGrab™) clearly simplified the procedure and improved the critical view of the triangle of Calot, with a consequent dramatic reduction in the mean cholecystectomy time to 25 min (range: 20–30). There were no intraoperative complications. In one patient, a postoperative hematoma due to oozing from the cystic artery occurred, requiring a longer hospital stay. The artery had been clipped using endoscopic clips. As a result, we are now routinely securing the artery and duct with standard laparoscopic clips.

No infectious complications, gastric leaks, or biliary leaks were noted at 30-day follow-up. The mean postoperative hospital stay was 2 days (range: 2–3) for the transgastric group and 2.8 days (range: 1–11) for the transvaginal cholecystectomy patients.

All 19 women who underwent transvaginal cholecystectomy healed successfully with no complications, were able to resume sexual activity without pain following the recommended recovery period of 4 weeks, and reported no change in sexual desire and function at a mean follow-up of 13.2 ± 4.8 months. None of the patients reported infection or abnormal vaginal discharge. Postoperative gynecologic assessment showed a soft, well-healed cervix and vaginal vault in all patients.

Conclusions

NOTES techniques are becoming increasingly attractive for the surgeon and the gastroenterologist. In Europe, NOTES cholecystectomy is growing with strong patient acceptance. According to the European registries, complications occurred in 3 % of all patients and "conversions" to laparoscopy in 4.7 %, which is comparable to current rates in minimally invasive surgery. Nevertheless, unexpected complications unique to the NOTES technique are being reported. Expected advantages of NOTES relative to infection, hernia, postoperative pain, hospital stay, and time off work are still only theoretical and have yet to be proven in randomized controlled trials. Of the two key challenges to transluminal techniques, contamination has not proven to be a significant problem, while luminal closure remains a concern for transgastric approaches. Long-term sexual function is a concern for the transvaginal approach. In most centers, collaboration with the gynecologist is reported at least initially, to assess the absence of gynecological contraindications, address specific patients' questions, and perform the colpotomy. So far reports indicate that postoperative sexual function is unchanged.

Transvaginal cholecystectomy with rigid instruments has been standardized and may become routine in the near future, although limited to specific procedures in 50 % of the population.

Currently, flexible endoscopic NOTES is only being performed at highly skilled centers under strict IRB supervision. The majority of centers consider NOTES suitable for uncomplicated symptomatic cholelithiasis and are hesitant to apply this emerging technique to complex cases. Prevention of injury at cholecystectomy remains an unbreakable rule relying on accurate exposure and visualization of the Calot's critical view of safety. Hybrid techniques are mandatory at this stage for monitoring and assistance with both flexible and rigid NOTES techniques.

The use of a flexible technique allows NOTES to be performed more in keeping with the original intent of flexible transluminal surgery, but is less adopted due to technical challenges and longer operative time. Technical improvements by means of a surgical endoscopic platform would greatly enable the advancement of pure NOTES into the operating room.

The success of the Euronotes Society meetings and demand for training in new techniques demonstrates surgeons' enthusiasm for NOTES. Cholecystectomy today might not be the killer application of NOTES but undoubtedly represents a steady step forward to usher in new clinical applications and push surgical innovation. As NOTES continues its translation into clinical use, training and technology development is critical to achieve widespread applicability.

References

1. Kalloo AN, et al. Flexible transgastric peritoneoscopy: a novel approach to diagnostic and therapeutic interventions in the peritoneal cavity. Gastrointest Endosc. 2004;60(1):114–7.
2. Bessler M, et al. Transvaginal laparoscopically assisted endoscopic cholecystectomy: a hybrid approach to natural orifice surgery. Gastrointest Endosc. 2007;66:1243–5.
3. Marescaux J, et al. Surgery without scars: report of transluminal cholecystectomy in a human being. Arch Surg. 2007;142(9):823–6; discussion 826–7.
4. Lehmann KS, et al. The German registry for natural orifice translumenal endoscopic surgery: report of the first 551 patients. Ann Surg. 2010;252(2):263–70.
5. Linke GR, et al. Transvaginal rigid-hybrid NOTES cholecystectomy: evaluation in routine clinical practice. Endoscopy. 2010;42(7):571–5.
6. Bueno B. Primer caso de apendicectomía por vía vaginal. Tokoginecol Pract. 1949;8:152–4 [in Italian].
7. Pelosi III MA, Pelosi MA. Vaginal appendectomy at laparoscopic-assisted vaginal hysterectomy: a surgical option. J Laparoendosc Surg. 1996;6(6):399–403.
8. McGowan L. Incidental appendectomy during vaginal surgery. Am J Obstet Gynecol. 1966;95(4):588.
9. Kelly HA. Treatment of ectopic pregnancy by vaginal puncture. Bull Johns Hopkins Hosp. 1986;7:208.
10. Gordts S, et al. Risk and outcome of bowel injury during transvaginal pelvic endoscopy. Fertil Steril. 2001;76(6):1238–41.
11. Dallemagne B, et al. Transgastric hybrid cholecystectomy. Br J Surg. 2009;96(10):1162–6.
12. Gauderer MW, Ponsky JL, Izant Jr RJ. Gastrostomy without laparotomy: a percutaneous endoscopic technique. J Pediatr Surg. 1980;15(6):872–5.
13. Hazey JW. Transgastric instrumentation and bacterial contamination of the peritoneal cavity. Surg Endosc. 2007;22(3):605–11.
14. Zornig C, et al. Transvaginal NOTES hybrid cholecystectomy: feasibility results in 68 cases with mid-term follow-up. Endoscopy. 2009;41(5):391–4.
15. Zornig C, et al. NOTES cholecystectomy: matched-pair analysis comparing the transvaginal hybrid and conventional laparoscopic techniques in a series of 216 patients. Surg Endosc. 2011;25(6):1822–6.
16. Pugliese R, et al. Hybrid NOTES transvaginal cholecystectomy: operative and long-term results after 18 cases. Langenbecks Arch Surg. 2010;395(3):241–5.

Chapter 16
NOTES: Cholecystectomy (U.S. Experience)

Saniea F. Majid, Bryan J. Sandler, and Santiago Horgan

Keywords Natural orifice • Cholecystectomy • Human • Scarless • Endoscopic Endoluminal surgery

> Someday in the future, people will look back at a regular surgical incision
> as something archaic and barbaric.
> —Paul A. Wetter, M.D.

Introduction

Medicine has taken an enormous step from the performance of life-saving open procedures to minimally invasive surgery that assures not only survival, but also a relatively good quality of life. The general acceptance of laparoscopic surgery has

S.F. Majid, M.D. (✉)
Center for the Future of Surgery/Minimally Invasive Surgery,
University of California at San Diego,
200 W. Arbor Dr, #8401, San Diego, CA 92103, USA
e-mail: sanieam@gmail.com

B.J. Sandler, M.D., FACS
Center for the Future of Surgery, UC San Diego Health System,
Medical Education and Telemedicine Building, 9500 Gilman Drive, MC 0740,
La Jolla, CA 92093, USA
e-mail: bsandler@ucsd.edu

S. Horgan, M.D., FACS
Center for the Future of Surgery, UC San Diego Health System,
Medical Education and Telemedicine Building, 9500 Gilman Drive, MC 0740,
La Jolla, CA 92093, USA

Department of Minimally Invasive Surgery, University of California at San Diego,
San Diego, CA 92103, USA
e-mail: shorgan@ucsd.edu

A. Rane et al. (eds.), *Scar-Less Surgery*,
DOI 10.1007/978-1-84800-360-6_16, © Springer-Verlag London 2013

made many procedures less invasive, safer, and cosmetically more acceptable. The idea of scarless surgery has now become a great challenge for the whole medical environment.

But this is nothing new. A desire to evaluate the inside of a patient's abdomen or chest with limited injury existed as far back as Hippocrates (460–375 BC). In the 1960s, Kurt Semm, a German gynecologist, invented the automatic insufflator. He performed an appendectomy during a gynecological procedure and opened a large door for a new surgery, and was almost removed from the Germany Physician Society because of it. In 1970, after Dr. Semm became the chairman of Obstetrics and Gynecology at the University of Kiel, his co-workers demanded that he undergo a brain scan because, they said, "Only a person with brain damage would perform laparoscopic surgery" [1–4].

Natural orifice translumenal endoscopic surgery (NOTES) is a novel surgical technique that may improve patient outcomes in minimally invasive surgery. The clearest benefit is cosmetic because surgeons use the body's natural orifices for access rather than transfascial incisions. Leaders in gastroenterology and surgery anticipate that NOTES will reduce the incidence of hernia and may improve pain and recovery [5].

In much the same way as laparoscopy 20 years ago, NOTES defies conventional surgical practices and has been the subject of some appropriate skepticism. In 2004, Kalloo et al. [6] described NOTES in an animal model as a potential next step in the evolution of therapeutic endoscopy. Although several variations of natural orifice operations predate the work of Kalloo et al. [6, 7], it was their first experiments that sparked the current heavy interest in NOTES.

In response to the clinical potential of NOTES, leaders from the pertinent surgery society [Society of American Gastrointestinal and Endoscopic Surgeons (SAGES)] and the American Society for Gastrointestinal Endoscopy (ASGE) generated a white paper that encouraged further NOTES research and outlined key research areas that needed to be addressed [8, 9]. This outline, generously funded, has led to a body of preclinical work over the past few years. Notably, leaders agreed that all NOTES cases be collated in a central database to ensure the accurate reporting of outcomes and to provide early evidence of important trends regarding the safety of NOTES.

A large body of preclinical evidence now exists, demonstrating that several types of NOTES operations can be performed in both acute and survival animal models through a variety of approaches, including access via the stomach, rectum, vagina, esophagus, and bladder. The NOTES procedure has moved quickly from a concept to preclinical studies to human clinical trials based on this preclinical work [10–14].

At the University of California, San Diego (UCSD)'s Center for the Future of Surgery, we invested nearly 2 years in preclinical research using both animate and anatomic material models to maximize patient safety and prepare the way for a clinical trial. Evidence from this intensive work was central to the successful application to the IRB. We described a dual-view hybrid NOTES technique previously, which we believe maximizes safety [15]. The vagina was selected initially as the safest access point for NOTES. Close consultation with the university's Reproductive Medicine and Gastroenterology departments was central to our planning of human NOTES operations. In the rest of the chapter, we will be focusing on our approach to NOTES cholecystectomies and the lessons we have learned during this period.

Two separate protocols for performing NOTES operations for the purpose of performing a cholecystectomy were approved by the IRB at UCSD. The transvaginal and transgastric approaches were separated into different protocols. The exclusion criteria for these approaches are:

1. Patients with a body mass index (BMI) greater than 35
2. Patients younger than 18 or older than 65
3. Patients with a history of severe endometriosis, pelvic inflammatory disease, or ectopic pregnancy
4. Patients with known common duct stones or presumed gallbladder mass
5. Patients with prior open abdominal operations
6. Pregnant women
7. Patients with severe medical comorbidities
8. Patients with a history of vaginal trauma
9. Patients with clotting or bleeding disorders and patients receiving anticoagulant or antiplatelet medications

Technique for Transvaginal Cholecystectomy

Patient Positioning and Preparation

General anesthesia is confirmed, sequential compression devices are applied, appropriate antibiotic prophylaxis is administered, and a nasogastric tube is placed. The patient is positioned in the dorsal lithotomy position. The abdomen and vagina are prepped in standard sterile fashion. A Foley catheter is placed on the operative field in sterile fashion.

Transvaginal Access and Establishment of Pneumoperitoneum

A 5-mm Visiport™ (Covidien, Dublin, Ireland) is placed at the umbilicus using an open Hassan technique. The abdomen is insufflated to 15 mmHg, and a diagnostic laparoscopy is performed. The diagnostic laparoscopy serves the purpose of assessing the presence or absence of adhesions both in the pelvis for a safe transvaginal access as well as in the right upper quadrant around the gallbladder. If too much inflammation or adhesions are found during inspection, we recommend converting to conventional laparoscopy.

Once the transvaginal approach is deemed feasible, the cervix is sequentially dilated and a uterine sound placed to measure the cervical length. A uterine retractor is used to lift the uterus and a 15-mm dilating, exchangeable head, dual-channel trocar (Applied Medical, Rancho Santa Margarita, CA) is placed in the posterior cul-de-sac. All this is performed under direct laparoscopic view. A sterile endoscope is placed into the abdomen. The dual-lumen trocar allows for placement of the scope as well as a 5-mm rigid or flexible instrument alongside the flexible endoscope. A key risk to the placement of a vaginal trocar is the possibility of unrecognized injury to nearby structures, particularly the rectum, sigmoid colon, bladder, and ureters. Currently, laparoscopic vision is the best way to visualize the pelvis directly to ensure that no injury occurs during transvaginal access.

Endoscopic insufflation may be used to maintain a pneumoperitoneum, but this approach is more difficult to manage and measure than a standard laparoscopic port approach, which is specifically designed for intraabdominal insufflation. A wider variation in pressure is observed than with laparoscopic insufflation [16]. The transumbilical laparoscopic port and insufflation system ensures that any excess insufflation is noted and quickly addressed. This port also allows the passage of a single laparoscopic instrument into the abdomen for use. Until better instruments are developed, having one port available for use with well-developed minimally invasive instruments is important for safe natural orifice surgery at this stage.

Gallbladder Retraction

Adequate retraction undoubtedly serves as an obstacle when performing these surgical procedures. Aside from its inevitable prolongation of operative time, inadequate retraction can potentially convert a technically straightforward case into a complex ordeal. Minimally invasive surgeons all over the world have been attempting to create novel methods of accomplishing adequate retraction without leaving any visible evidence of it. We will review some of the retraction methods here and go over the salient features of each.

Endoscopic Graspers

Natural orifice surgery requires more capability than current endoscopes offer. Retraction of the gallbladder is difficult with the currently available, flimsy endoscopic graspers that do not maintain a secure purchase on the gallbladder wall. Furthermore, dedicating one channel of an endoscope to retraction limits vision and prohibits use of that channel by a tissue manipulation instrument through a second channel.

Fig. 16.1 Long articulating
grasper (Developed by UCSD
and Novare Endosurgical,
now available from Intuitive
Surgical)

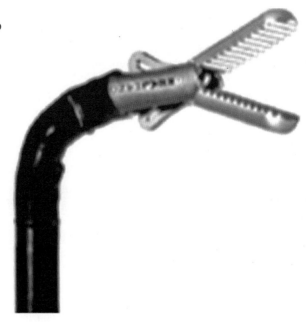

Articulating Graspers

A long articulating grasper (Fig. 16.1) placed adjacent to the endoscope through a second channel via a common port (developed by UCSD and Novare Endosurgical, now available from Intuitive Surgical, Sunnyvale, CA) allows for strong and flexible retraction independent of and offset from the endoscopic platform. This instrument, a 75-cm-long device, features a cable system that allows for flexibility at the tip and extra degrees of freedom, similar to the wrist of the da Vinci® robotic surgical system (Intuitive Surgical, Sunnyvale, CA). This device provides enough rigidity for strength of retraction, but with some flexibility to optimize exposure, and the strength of its grip on the gallbladder wall vastly exceeds that of an endoscopic grasper.

Transabdominal Stay Sutures

The sutures are placed through the fundus and infundibulum of the gallbladder using a straight Keith needle and then externalized in a transabdominal fashion to allow continuous extracorporeal manipulation, leaving only a negligible mark where the needle passed through the skin [17]. One limitation of the transabdominal stay-suture method of retraction is restricted retraction capability. In order to avoid entering the thoracic cavity and potential pneumothorax, the straight needle and stay sutures must be inserted inferior to the rib cage, resulting in anterior rather than complete anterior–superior retraction of the gallbladder fundus as performed in standard laparoscopy. Another drawback of this method is the potential for intraperitoneal bile leakage and possible rupture of the gallbladder as the needle must pierce the gallbladder wall. In addition, because these stay sutures serve as a fixed anchoring system, repositioning during surgery is not possible without the repeated passage of a second needle and suture [18].

Transabdominal Endoloop®

The Endoloop® (Ethicon Endo-Surgery, Cincinnati, OH) is introduced transabdominally into the peritoneal cavity through a 5-mm trocar and attached to the gallbladder fundus, which is then retracted anteriorly toward the abdominal wall [18]. Although similar conceptually to transabdominal stay sutures, an Endoloop provides two distinct advantages. First, because the Endoloop is used to grasp the gallbladder as opposed to piercing it, the potential for leakage and complete tearing of the gallbladder is minimized. Nevertheless, like stay sutures, because it must be introduced inferior to the rib cage, Endoloops cannot achieve complete superiorly directed retraction. In addition, fastening of the Endoloops may prove challenging in cases of scarred and distended gallbladders. The need for a 5-mm transabdominal trocar for the insertion and usage limits the usefulness of this device in the transvaginal approach.

R-Scope

The R-Scope (Olympus XGIF-2TQ240R, Olympus Corp., Tokyo, Japan) is a therapeutic endoscope equipped with two movable channels designed to enable both lifting and dissection of lesions. One channel is fitted with vertically moving grasping forceps to provide countertraction while the second uses a horizontally swinging electrocautery knife to dissect [19]. Using these two channels enables simultaneous retraction and dissection. Although initially used for endoscopic submucosal dissection of gastric lesions, Sumiyama et al. [20] report successful transgastric access to the gallbladder and cholecystectomy in four porcine models.

Magnetic Anchoring and Guidance System

Magnetic anchoring and guidance system (MAGS), developed by the group of Cadeddu and Scott in 2001 at UT Southwestern, employs intraabdominal magnetically anchored instruments to perform trocar-sparing laparoscopic surgery (Fig. 16.2). MAGS uses two internal neodymium–iron–boron magnetic platforms introduced into the abdomen through a 12-mm trocar. The internal platforms are magnetically anchored to external anchors on the patient's skin and are capable of manipulating and stabilizing these platforms [21, 22]. In Cadeddu's retraction

Fig. 16.2 MAGS retraction

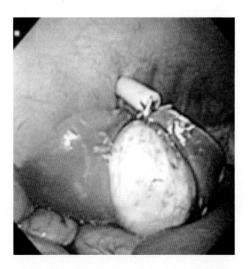

system, two internal magnetic platforms are coupled to either a latex sling or a three-fingered paddle, which allows nontraumatic elevation and retraction of organs like the liver and spleen. Ryou and Thompson [23] describe a modified MAGS retraction system whereby magnet-conjugated clips placed along the inferior edge of the liver are used to accomplish operative retraction. As yet, MAGS retraction has been used successfully in porcine models to perform transcolonic cholecystec-tomy and mesh implantation. In addition, MAGS instruments, cautery devices, and cameras have been used in single-port laparoscopic nephrectomies, freeing up the single port to be used for direct retraction [24].

We have described the use of MAGS safely and effectively in four patients who underwent transvaginal cholecystectomies [25].

Internal Retractors

The EndoGrab™ (Virtual Ports, Misgav, Israel) (Fig. 16.3) is an internally anchored retracting device that can be introduced into the abdomen at the outset of the opera-tion through a 5-mm port. Once deployed, one of the two grasping ends is attached to the gallbladder while the other is anchored to the abdominal wall. The main advantage of this device is that it not only leaves no visible marks but also can be anchored superiorly just below the diaphragm, thereby allowing retraction equiva-lent to that achieved with a designated retracting instrument. This device can be adjusted repeatedly throughout the operation to allow for optimal retraction and is removed at the end of surgery.

Each retraction method has its disadvantages, and not all of them can achieve the same degree of retraction, a point that becomes significant when less-than-ideal sur-gical anatomy is encountered. The ability of the EndoGrab to accomplish complete anterior and superior retraction of the gallbladder fundus is a distinct advantage over

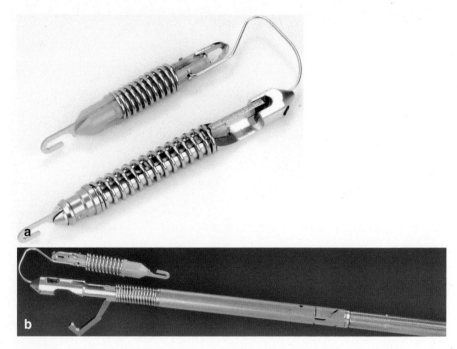

Fig. 16.3 (**a**) EndoGrab; (**b**) loaded EndoGrab (Courtesy of Virtual Ports, Misgav, Israel)

other methods. Because it is internally deployed, it can be attached high on the anterior abdominal wall just below the diaphragm without concern of entering the thoracic cavity. After being initially tested in porcine models, five successful transvaginal NOTES cholecystectomies were performed using this retraction device without complication [18]. A 70-cm introducer will be available for positioning the EndoGrab transvaginally, thereby obviating the need for transumbilical placement of the EndoGrab. These internal retractors are also currently being employed for colon retraction during colectomy and gastric retraction during sleeve gastrectomy.

Gallbladder Dissection and Ligating the Cystic Duct and Artery

Dissection of the gallbladder from the liver bed is difficult using the endoscopic needle hook or the L-shape hook device (Olympus America, Center Valley, PA). Although it is possible to dissect the gallbladder from the liver bed using this hook, its small size makes dissection cumbersome and lengthy. The use of a laparoscopic hook from the umbilical port, at least for the difficult portions of the dissection, allows for a safer and quicker procedure compared with the endoscopic counterparts.

Laparoscopic clips are absolutely necessary for patient safety. Endoscopic clips are not entirely occlusive and are not designed to secure the cystic duct. The development of new endoscopic instruments may improve upon current instrumentation, but until then, we believe the safest course is to use a single laparoscopic access umbilical port.

Extraction of Specimen

The gallbladder is removed easily from the trocar, either with or without an endobag.

Closure of the Vaginotomy

The abdomen is inspected and once good, hemostasis is confirmed. Using a vaginal speculum, the incision is easily visualized, and a single stitch with a 2-0 Vicryl can be placed to close the incision without difficulty. Because a dilating (nonbladed) trocar is used to stretch the incision, the incision quickly collapses to a smaller diameter after removal of the trocar. The 5-mm trocar is removed and the skin closed with a 4-0 monocryl suture. The patient is extubated and taken to the recovery room.

Postoperative Care

All patients are kept in the hospital overnight. The clinical protocol follow-up evaluation includes daily phone calls from the surgeon to check the temperature and pain levels postoperatively and clinic visits at 1 week and 1 month. No additional laboratory or radiographic testing is performed.

Results

NOTES cholecystectomy can be performed safely as shown by many clinical series from all over the world. A recent review of the published clinical NOTES cases by Auyang et al. [26] selected a total of 432 NOTES cases, with a majority (84 %) transvaginal procedures, followed by transgastric (13 %), transesophageal (4 %), and transrectal (0.5 %). Of all reported NOTES cases, 90 % were performed in hybrid fashion with transabdominal laparoscopic assistance. Cholecystectomy was the predominant procedure, accounting for 84 % of cases. The largest overall single-center experience consisted of 128 hybrid transvaginal cholecystectomies by Federlein et al. [27] in Germany, reported in 2010.

Compared with other natural orifice access routes, the transvaginal approach to NOTES imparts the least amount of risk to the patient. However, this approach is controversial given its sensitive and private nature. Numerous vaginal and transvaginal gynecologic procedures are performed daily across the United States. Furthermore, data have shown this approach to be safe and effective. It contrasts heavily with the transgastric approach, in which intentional perforation of the gastric wall is a novel concept.

One of the largest published series of 100 laparoscopic and combined culdoscopic procedures (hybrid NOTES) using multiple transabdominal instruments resulted only in a single uncomplicated postoperative fever [28]. Additionally, series comparing laparoscopically assisted vaginal hysterectomy with laparoscopic hysterectomy have found similar complication rates despite the use of the vaginal conduit [29, 30]. Published studies have demonstrated a higher incidence of certain complications (bladder injury, blood loss greater than 1 l, and vaginal hematoma) using a vaginal approach [31]. It also should be noted that the incision in a NOTES transvaginal procedure and the blood loss with this procedure are less than seen with vaginal hysterectomy. It could be surmised that the addition of laparoscopic vision used in a NOTES approach should reduce the likelihood of bladder injury or excess bleeding.

In recent years, vaginal hysterectomy has gained momentum in many countries as the operation of choice for benign uterine disease requiring an operation [32]. The route of hysterectomy appears to have little effect on postoperative sexual function [33]. Overall pain scores are improved by a vaginal approach compared with abdominal hysterectomy [34, 35]. This probably is due to the avoidance of an incision in the abdominal wall musculature. This benefit also extends to NOTES.

Clearly, it is critical to discuss all the potential known and unknown risks of a transvaginal NOTES procedure in obtaining informed consent. The risk of infertility after transvaginal NOTES procedures is unknown, but avoidance of bleeding and inflammation to the pelvis should minimize this potential risk. Although the mere suggestion that this procedure could lead to infertility may discourage many proponents of NOTES, the experience of reproductive medicine suggests that the risk is likely to be very small. The transvaginal approach is sometimes used for the delivery of therapy to women with refractory infertility [32, 36, 37], and transvaginal procurement of oocytes has been in practice for more than 20 years [38].

A survey conducted at our institution found that approximately 68 % of women ($N = 100$) would be willing to undergo a transvaginal procedure for gallbladder disease if the complication rate were similar. This is consistent with surveys regarding patient attitudes toward NOTES at other institutions [39].

Patients do not require the oral narcotic medications typically given after these procedures. This may be due in part to sparing of the muscle fibers of the abdominal wall. Placement of the transumbilical trocar also spares these fibers and makes use of an existing scar. Still, it is impossible to compare pain outcomes without a further prospective study comparing natural orifice surgery with laparoscopic surgery.

Table 16.1 Data from the first 11 NOTES cases performed by Horgan and colleagues

Patient	Operation	Age (years)	Time (min)	Abdominal trocars	Hospital stay	Complications
1	Transvaginal cholecystectomy	19	150	2	1 night	None
2	Transvaginal cholecystectomy	22	96	2	1 night	None
3	Transvaginal cholecystectomy	26	70	1	1 night	None
4	Transvaginal cholecystectomy	39	92	1	1 night	None
5	Transvaginal cholecystectomy	49	93	1	1 night	None
6	Transvaginal cholecystectomy	42	114	1	1 night	None
7	Transvaginal cholecystectomy	35	165	1	1 night	None
8	Transvaginal cholecystectomy	33	140	1	1 night	None
9	Transvaginal cholecystectomy	47	110	1	1 night	None
10	Transvaginal appendectomy	42	150	One plus two 2-mm ports	1 night	None
11	Transvaginal appendectomy	24	78	1	1 night	None

Source: With kind permission of Springer Science+Business Media. Reprinted with permission from Horgan et al. [40]

At the follow-up visit, no complications were reported by any of the patients. The patients were advised to observe pelvic rest for 4 weeks postoperatively. All sexually active patients reported a return to normal sexual activity. A summary of our previously published results of the first 11 human NOTES cases performed at UCSD is in Table 16.1.

Larger studies are needed to determine the true safety and efficacy of the transvaginal approach. A national database is the best means for collecting data on the natural orifice experience.

Technique Using the Incisionless Operating Platform

This section describes our technique using the incisionless operating platform (IOP) (USGI Medical, San Clemente, CA) (Fig. 16.4).

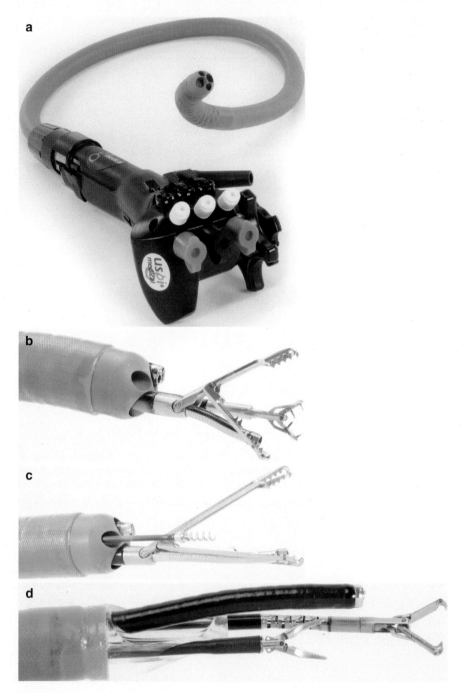

Fig. 16.4 (**a**) Transport multilumen operating platform: Incisionless Operating Platform (*IOP*); (**b–d**) close-up (All images courtesy of USGI Medical, San Clemente, CA)

Transvaginal Cholecystectomy

Patient positioning and the initial steps to accessing the cul-de-sac are the same as described above. The Transport™ device is then advanced into the abdomen and positioned facing the right upper quadrant. An endoscopic grasper is placed through the Transport to grasp the dome of the gallbladder and then retracted in a cephalad direction. This is performed under laparoscopic and endoscopic views. Endoscopic loop cautery is used for the careful dissection of the peritoneal layer from the gallbladder. The ultrasonic dissector is then used from the 5-mm trocar to remove the peritoneum further and delineate the anatomy.

An articulating Maryland dissector is introduced through the 5-mm port to create the cystohepatic window. Another endoscopic grasper is used to grasp the infundibulum of the gallbladder for lateral retraction to provide a clear critical view. Once this is accomplished, a 5-mm clip applier (Ethicon) is used from the umbilical port to clip the cystic duct. Endoscopic shears are used through the Transport to transect the cystic duct. An endoscopic snare is used with electrocautery to dissect the gallbladder from the liver bed. Hemostasis is ensured. The gallbladder is grasped using an endoscopic snare and removed from the abdomen via the vaginotomy. The abdomen is desufflated, and the vaginotomy is closed primarily using 2-0 Vicryl suture. The skin is closed, and the patient is awakened from anesthesia.

Transgastric Cholecystectomy

General anesthesia is induced, and a Foley catheter is placed. The patient's abdomen is prepped and draped in standard sterile fashion. A 3-mm Visiport (Ethicon) is placed in the umbilicus using a Hassan technique. The abdomen is insufflated to 15 mmHg, and diagnostic laparoscopy is performed. The decision is then made to proceed with transgastric cholecystectomy. Upper GI endoscopy is performed, and the Transport device is advanced into the stomach. Using an endoscopic needle-knife, a small gastrotomy is made in the anterior gastric wall and a guidewire is placed through the small gastrotomy. This is performed under direct laparoscopic vision, performed through the transumbilical trocar to avoid injury to the adjacent colon, liver, or spleen.

A standard wire-guided, endoscopic dilating balloon is advanced over the guidewire through the gastrotomy site, and the balloon is filled to dilate the gastrostomy site. Once this is achieved, the Transport device is advanced along with the wire and balloon into the peritoneal cavity. All this is performed under direct laparoscopic view.

The use of the USGI Transport system allows for using additional tools to accomplish the procedure along with an Olympus GIF-N180 endoscope that allows visualization of the target tissue, seen through the USGI Transport device.

A reliable and reproducible closure of the gastrotomy remains the largest challenge for the successful development of NOTES. Although many endoscopic suturing methods or devices are in use or development, most are cumbersome and require extensive training and lab time for their effective use.

Dilation of the gastrotomy appears to be preferable to cutting a long gastrotomy because after the endoscope or operating platform is removed, the dilated gastrotomy shrinks down in size as the uncut muscle contracts. Control of both the pnuemoperitoneum and gas volume inside the stomach is essential to the success of transgastric NOTES.

The Future of NOTES

The NOTES procedure must be safe and the operations easily replicated if the new technique is to become clinically relevant. The described operative approach addresses many of the technical challenges that hinder NOTES and provides solutions for a safe, rapid, and duplicable operation. Laparoscopic assistance allows for safe vision, minimizing the risk for unrecognized injury during access. The 5-mm port also provides control of insufflation, which may be difficult to maintain and measure using an endoscope alone.

The end effect is a procedure that is virtually scarless. A pure natural orifice approach may eliminate postoperative ventral hernias altogether.

Further data are needed to determine the true safety and efficacy of clinical NOTES. The creation of the NOSCAR (Natural Orifice Surgery Consortium for Assessment and Research) patient registry ensures an honest review of this emerging technology. This technique has created large interest among researchers and industry to create the next wave of developments in minimally invasive surgery, a rapidly evolving field.

References

1. Marescaux J. History of NOTES. Epublication: WeBSurg.com. 2007;7(11).
2. Valdivieso E, Saenz R, Claudio N. Natural orifice transluminal endoscopic surgery: putting together minimally invasive techniques for new era. Gastrointest Endosc. 2007;66:340–2.
3. Swain P. A justification for NOTES – natural orifice translumenal endosurgery. Gastrointest Endosc. 2007;65(3):514–6.
4. Gettman MT, Lotan Y, Nappèr CA, et al. Transvaginal laparoscopic nephrectomy: development and feasibility in the porcine model. Urology. 2002;59(3):446–50.
5. Wallace MB. Take NOTES (natural orifice transluminal endoscopic surgery). Gastroenterology. 2006;131:11–2.
6. Kalloo AN, Singh VK, Jagannath SB, et al. Flexible trans-gastric peritoneoscopy: a novel approach to diagnostic and therapeutic interventions in the peritoneal cavity. Gastrointest Endosc. 2004;60:114–7.
7. McGee MF, Rosen MJ, Marks J, et al. A primer on natural orifice trans-lumenal endoscopic surgery: building a new paradigm. Surg Innov. 2006;13:86–93.

8. ASGE Sages. ASGE/SAGES working group on natural orifice translumenal endoscopic surgery white paper, October 2005. Gastrointest Endosc. 2006;63:199–203.
9. Yusuf TE, Baron TH. Endoscopic transmural drainage of pancreatic pseudocysts: results of a national and an international survey of ASGE members. Gastrointest Endosc. 2006;63:223–7.
10. Hazey JW, Narula VK, Renton DB, et al. Natural-orifice transgastric endoscopic peritoneoscopy in humans: initial clinical trial. Surg Endosc. 2008;22(1):16–20.
11. Onders RP, McGee MF, Marks J, et al. Natural orifice transluminal endoscopic surgery (NOTES) as a diagnostic tool in the intensive care unit. Surg Endosc. 2007;21:681–3.
12. Zornig C, Mofid H, Emmermann A, et al. Scarless cholecystectomy with combined transvaginal and transumbilical approach in a series of 20 patients. Surg Endosc. 2008;22:1427–9.
13. Zorron R, Maggioni LC, Pombo L, et al. NOTES transvaginal cholecystectomy: preliminary clinical application. Surg Endosc. 2008;22:542–7.
14. Palanivelu C, Rajan PS, Rangarajan M, et al. Transvaginal endoscopic appendectomy in humans: a unique approach to NOTES: World's first report. Surg Endosc. 2008;23(3):668.
15. Mintz Y, Horgan S, Cullen J, et al. NOTES: the hybrid technique. J Laparoendosc Adv Surg Tech A. 2007;4:402–6.
16. Meireles O, Kantsevoy SV, Kalloo AN, et al. Comparison of intraabdominal pressures using the gastroscope and laparoscope for transgastric surgery. Surg Endosc. 2007;21:998–1001.
17. Navarra G, Rando L, La Malfa G, et al. Hybrid transvaginal cholecystectomy: a novel approach. Am J Surg. 2009;197(6):e69–72.
18. Schlager A, Horgan S, Talamini M, et al. Providing more through less: current methods of retraction in SIMIS and NOTES cholecystectomy. Surg Endosc. 2010;24:1542–6.
19. Yonezawa J, Kaise M, Sumiyama K, et al. A novel double-channel therapeutic endoscope ("R-scope") facilitates endoscopic submucosal dissection of superficial gastric neoplasms. Endoscopy. 2006;38(10):1011–5.
20. Sumiyama K, Gostout CJ, Rajan E, et al. Transgastric cholecystectomy: transgastric accessibility to the gallbladder improved with the SEMF method and a novel multibending therapeutic endoscope. Gastrointest Endosc. 2007;65(7):1028–34.
21. Park S, Bergs RA, Eberhart R, et al. Trocar-less instrumentation for laparoscopy: magnetic positioning of intra-abdominal camera and retractor. Ann Surg. 2007;245(3):379–84.
22. Scott DJ, Tang SJ, Fernandez R, et al. Completely transvaginal NOTES cholecystectomy using magnetically anchored instruments. Surg Endosc. 2007;21:2308–16.
23. Ryou M, Thompson CC. Magnetic retraction in natural-orifice transluminal endoscopic surgery (NOTES): addressing the problem of traction and countertraction. Endoscopy. 2009;41(2):143–8.
24. Zeltser IS, Cadeddu JA. A novel magnetic anchoring and guidance system to facilitate single trocar laparoscopic nephrectomy. Curr Urol Rep. 2008;9(1):62–4.
25. Horgan S, Mintz Y, Jacobsen GR, et al. Magnetic retraction for NOTES transvaginal cholecystectomy. Surg Endosc. 2010;24:2322.
26. Auyang ED, Santos BF, Enter DH, et al. Natural orifice translumenal endoscopic surgery (NOTESÒ): a technical review. Surg Endosc. 2011;25(10):3135–48.
27. Federlein M, Borchert D, Muller V, et al. Transvaginal video-assisted cholecystectomy in clinical practice. Surg Endosc. 2010;24:2444–52.
28. Tsin DA, Colombero LT, Lambeck J, Manolas P. Mini-laparoscopy-assisted natural orifice surgery. J Soc Laparendosc Surg. 2007;11:24–9.
29. Ghezzi F, Cromi A, Bergamini V, et al. Laparoscopic-assisted vaginal hysterectomy versus total laparoscopic hysterectomy for the management of endometrial cancer: a randomized clinical trial. J Minim Invasive Gynecol. 2006;13:114–20.
30. Muzii L, Basile S, Zupi E, et al. Laparoscopic-assisted vaginal hysterectomy versus minilaparotomy hysterectomy: a prospective, randomized, multicenter study. J Minim Invasive Gynecol. 2007;14:610–5.
31. Milad MP, Morrison K, Sokol A, et al. A comparison of laparoscopic supracervical hysterectomy vs. laparoscopically assisted vaginal hysterectomy. Surg Endosc. 2001;15:286–8.

32. McCracken G, Lefebvre GG. Vaginal hysterectomy: dispelling the myths. J Obstet Gynaecol Can. 2007;29:424–8.

33. Roussis NP, Waltrous L, Kerr A, et al. Sexual response in the patient after hysterectomy: total abdominal versus supracervical versus vaginal procedure. Am J Obstet Gynecol. 2004;190: 1427–8.

34. Morelli M, Caruso M, Noia R, et al. Total laparoscopic hysterectomy versus vaginal hysterectomy: a prospective randomized trial. Minerva Ginecol. 2007;59:99–105.

35. Abdelmonem A, Wilson H, Pasic R. Observational comparison of abdominal, vaginal, and laparoscopic hysterectomy as performed at a university teaching hospital. J Reprod Med. 2006;51:945–54.

36. Casa A, Sesti F, Marziali M, et al. Transvaginal hydrolaparoscopic ovarian drilling using bipolar electrosurgery to treat anovulatory women with polycystic ovary syndrome. J Am Assoc Gynecol Laparosc. 2003;10:219–22.

37. Fernandez H, Alby JD, Gervaise A, et al. Operative transvaginal hydrolaparoscopy for treatment of polycystic ovary syndrome: a new minimally invasive surgery. Fertil Steril. 2001;75: 607–11.

38. Schulman JD, Dorfmann AD, Jones SL, et al. Outpatient in vitro fertilization using transvaginal ultrasound-guided oocyte retrieval. Obstet Gynecol. 1987;69:665–8.

39. Varadarajulu S, Tamhane A, Drelichman ER. Patient perception of natural orifice transluminal endoscopic surgery as a technique for cholecystectomy. Gastrointest Endosc. 2008;67: 854–60.

40. Horgan J, Cullen JP, Talamini MA, et al. Natural orifice surgery: initial clinical experience. Surg Endosc. 2009;23:1512–8.

Chapter 17
NOTES Gastrojejunostomy

Per-Ola Park and Maria Bergström

Keywords NOTES • Anastomosis • Gastroentero-anastomosis • Gastrojejunostomy Endoscopic suturing • Compression anastomosis • Gastric outlet obstruction

Introduction

Anastomosis is a common surgical procedure in which two hollow organs are joined together to maintain an opening between them. Gastroentero-anastomoses have been performed since the days of J. E. Péan, L. Rydigier, and C. A. T. Billroth in the late 1800s [1]. The major indications for gastroentero-anastomoses have been gastric outlet obstruction due to cancer in the distal stomach, the duodenum, the head of the pancreas, or peptic ulcer disease (acute or chronic). Lately, different types of bariatric surgery, mainly gastric bypass, have been added to the indications for anastomosing the stomach to the small intestine.

The treatment of gastric outlet obstruction has traditionally been different types of surgery, open or laparoscopic. Gastric resections with either gastroduodenal anastomosis (Bilroth I) or gastrojejunal anastomosis (Bilroth II or Roux-en-Y) or just bypass surgery with gastrojejunal anastomosis without resection or pyloroplasty have been performed. The traditional way to attach the intestine to the stomach or another part of the intestine is to stitch it in place. Today the use of staplers to form anastomoses has become standard. Surgery is, however, associated with mortality and a high incidence of morbidity as the treated patients often are in bad condition [2, 3]. As an alternative to surgery in gastric outlet obstruction, endoscopic treatment has been introduced. In benign disease, balloon dilation has been tried with success [4] but is associated with a high rate of recurrence [5].

P.-O. Park, M.D., Ph.D. • M. Bergström, M.D., Ph.D. (✉)
Department of Surgery and Urology, South Älvsborg Hospital,
Bramhultsvagen 53, Boras 50182, Sweden
e-mail: per-ola.park@telia.com; emc.bergstrom@telia.com

A. Rane et al. (eds.), *Scar-Less Surgery*,
DOI 10.1007/978-1-84800-360-6_17, © Springer-Verlag London 2013

The introduction of self-expandable metal stents (SEMS) in the 1990s changed the routine treatment of gastric outlet obstruction from surgery to endoscopy. Duodenal stenting has been shown to be a reliable and safe method to restore the gastric outlet in malignant obstructions [6]. Studies comparing SEMS placement with surgical bypass anastomoses showed just as good clinical outcome with stents but these patients had a shorter hospital stay and lower overall costs [2, 7]. However, in a recent study, the patency of stents was shorter and the authors suggested stent treatment when life expectancy was shorter than 2 months and surgical bypass when life expectancy was longer [8].

In recent decades there has been an interest in performing "nonsurgical" gastroentero-anastomoses, either to overcome gastric outlet obstruction or as a part of gastric bypass in bariatric surgery. With the introduction of NOTES, this interest has grown. At the moment there are two different approaches to achieve gastroentero-anastomoses using endoscopic or NOTES techniques: tissue compression or suturing/stapling.

Compression Anastomoses

The concept of creating an anastomosis by means of steady compression between two ring-shaped discs without a need for sutures originates from Denan in 1821 [9]. In 1892 J. B. Murphy popularized anastomoses in laparotomies by introducing a compression button method allowing circular gastrointestinal anastomoses to be formed by the ischemic compression of tissue between two buttons held together by a spring [10]. A century later, P. Swain described a technique to achieve a compression anastomosis with flexible endoscopy in an experimental model [11]. An enterotomy was performed through a small laparotomy and a gastroscope was introduced into the intestine. With a PEG-like technique, a needle and thread were introduced from the endoscope into the stomach and grabbed by a snare from a second endoscope in the stomach. The parts of the compression device were brought together over the thread, one from the stomach side and one from the intestinal side, and locked together with a compression spring. The ischemia of the tissue between the two buttons caused by the compression induces a tissue reaction with a release of inflammatory mediators, activation of fibrinogen, and recruitment of inflammatory cells that stimulates tissue repair mechanisms. The compression device will in most cases erode through the ischemic tissue and leave the gastroentero-anastomosis. In a survival experiment by Swain, eight anastomoses were performed in six greyhounds. The compression complex passed the stools within 2–4 days. At endoscopy on postoperative day 7, five anastomoses could be passed by a standard 9-mm gastroscope.

In 1995, Cope reported the creation of compression gastroentero-anastomoses by means of oral introduction of magnets [12]. A guidewire through the mouth was placed into the proximal part of the jejunum with the assistance of fluoroscopy, and a magnet attached to the guidewire was passed into the jejunum and positioned close to the stomach wall. With a second guidewire passed into the stomach, another magnet was passed in the stomach and manipulated until it contacted the transmural jejunal magnet. Anastomoses of 16–24 Fr width were achieved within 7–13 days. Cope later refined the technique and prolonged the patency of the gastroenteric fistula for up to 6 months by placing a stent through the fistula [13].

In 2010, van Hooft et al. presented an endoscopically achieved enteric compression anastomosis in patients with malignant disease. Eight to 14 days later, a stent was placed in the formed gastroenteric fistula [14]. However, in this study, the necessity of a stent led to serious morbidity and even mortality, and the study was terminated after the inclusion of 18 patients.

A limitation of compression anastomoses is that one of the magnet components has to pass the obstruction, which in many cases is impossible. To overcome this problem, Anette Fritscher-Ravens et al. described a technique using endoscopic ultrasound to access the bowel distal to the stricture to perform a compression anastomosis [15]. An anastomotic device was formed by using two 7 Fr catheter segments, which were pushed over a guidewire into the less accessible target, the lumen. When released, by withdrawing the guidewire, the catheters formed a cross shape and created an anastomosis when compressed against a plate from the accessible side.

One major disadvantage of all compression anastomoses is that it takes several days to form a stoma. Other disadvantages include the limited stoma size [13] and the problem that compression anastomoses formed by the described techniques can only be performed to adjacent viscera if laparoscopy or laparotomy is not utilized [11].

NOTES Gastroentero-anastomoses

By definition, the described endoscopically achieved compression anastomoses are not performed using NOTES technique as the endoscope never leaves the gut lumen. In the beginning of the NOTES era, interest was focused on bariatric and bypass procedures. A NOTES bypass procedure includes access to the abdominal cavity, finding the correct part of the small bowel and bringing it up to stomach the wall. Finally, a gastroentero-anastomosis needs to be formed.

The most commonly reported technique to date for NOTES access of the abdominal cavity is the use of a needle-knife to puncture the gastric wall, followed by the introduction of a guidewire into the abdominal cavity. A sphincterotome or balloon dilator is used over the guidewire to widen the perforation and gain endoscopic access to the peritoneal cavity [16–18]. The location of the gastrotomy will become the gastric side of the anastomosis. Therefore, it is important to choose the place of entry depending on the reason for the anastomosis. The abdominal entry site for a gastrojejunal-anastomosis due to gastric outlet obstruction should be in the antrum area. If the anastomosis is a part of a gastric bypass procedure for weight reduction, the entry should be situated close to the cardia [19].

At the moment, there is no method to identify a specific part of the small intestine with NOTES technique. With the Olympus R-scope or different platforms,

Fig. 17.1 Bard EndoCinch™
T-tags (Bard, Murray Hill,
NJ) together with a Cook
EchoTip® needle (Cook,
Bloomington, IN) and Bard
EndoCinch™ locks (Bard,
Murray Hill, NJ) were
initially used for endoscopic
suturing

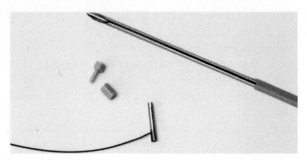

there is a theoretical possibility to run the bowel up and down to find the exact place for a gastroentero-anastomosis, but with the endoscopic graspers available, it is cumbersome even in a pig, with its thin omentum. However, it is possible to select upper, mid, and lower jejunum or ileum by using clues provided by transillumination and anatomic position in relation to other structures (e.g., bladder, right and left ovaries) [20].

The creation of NOTES gastroentero-anastomoses could be either sutured [20, 21] or stapled. However, a pure NOTES stapled anastomosis has not been reported, only stapled gastro-cystostomies [22]. Chiu et al. recently described a stapled gastrojejunostomy using a hybrid technique with a staple introduced through a laparoscopic port placed percutaneously into the stomach [23].

Different techniques have been tried to achieve a method for suturing or stitch placement using a flexible endoscope, for example, the EndoCinch™ (Bard, Murray Hill, NJ) [24], the Eagle Claw (Olympus and the Apollo Group, Japan) [25], NDO [26], and T-tags [27].

Suturing with T-Tags

Our group has developed a method for stitching through a standard gastroscope using T-tags [28]. Initially, we used Bard EndoCinch T-tags together with a Cook EchoTip® (Cook, Bloomington, IN) needle and Bard EndoCinch locks (Fig. 17.1). No extra device needs to be mounted outside the endoscope and no overtube is needed. Stitches can be placed anywhere you can reach with your endoscope. The T-tags are attached to a prolene thread, anchoring the thread in the tissue. One T-tag is placed on either side of a defect or one in each organ that is to be joined together, and the two threads can then be cinched together through a plastic lock (Fig. 17.2). A series of T-tag pairs can be used to perform a suture line [27] (Fig. 17.3). We have used this method in several animal models and also in human cases, for suturing ulcer perforation, bleeding ulcer, and an anastomotic leak [29], and also for closure after transgastric NOTES procedures [18]. The T-tag system has been refined by Ethicon Endosurgery, creating the TAS (Tissue Apposition System), and by Olympus, creating the BraceBar™ [30].

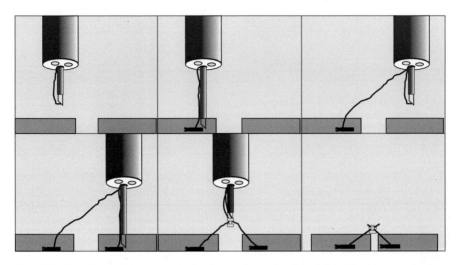

Fig. 17.2 One T-tag with the attached polypropylene thread is delivered with a needle into the tissue on one side of the defect. Another T-tag and thread are positioned on the other side of the defect. The threads are tied together by passing a thread through a cylinder to approximate the tissue edges. A pin is forced into the cylinder and locks the two threads

Fig. 17.3 A series of T-tag pairs can be used to perform a suture line

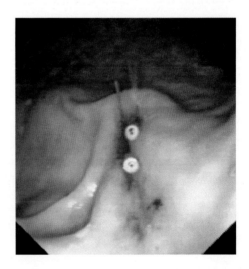

NOTES Sutured Gastroentero-anastomoses

The T-tag stitching technique was developed as a part of a project to perform endoscopic gastric bypass. As the gastroenterostomy is a crucial part of this procedure, we first aimed at creating patent and reliable anastomoses. Our aim was to create a NOTES gastrojejunostomy with an instant opening using only the gastroscope.

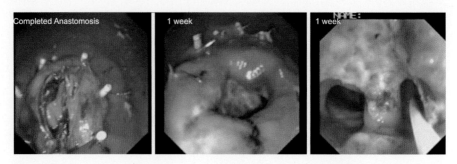

Fig. 17.4 Six to eight pairs of T-tags are placed around the bowel loop attaching it to the stomach. Eventually, the bowel is cut open and the gastrojejunostomy is ready and patent. At 1 week, an endoscope can pass into the afferent end efferent loop of the gastroentero-anastomosis

Technique

The abdominal cavity is entered through a NOTES access. For the purpose of anastomoses, the access is created by cutting the stomach wall with a sphincterotome instead of balloon dilation to reduce the risk of contraction of the stoma. After the abdominal cavity is entered, a piece of small bowel is caught on a snare and brought up into the stomach along with the double-channel gastroscope. Keeping the snare in place, the first four pairs of T-tags are placed around the bowel loop, attaching it to the stomach. The snare then needs to come off and another two to four pairs are placed to complete a suture line around the trapped loop of small bowel. Eventually, the bowel is cut open and the gastrojejunostomy is ready and patent (Fig. 17.4).

In a series of six nonsurvival pigs, we were able to create a gastrojejunostomy that was patent and seemed robust at postmortem. These anastomoses were all placed on the front side of the stomach at the mid-antrum. In a following series of six survival animals, a gastrojejunostomy was performed with the same technique. The small bowel was anastomosed to the stomach using T-tags and the pylorus was left open. The pigs were allowed immediate intake of ordinary feed. They were survived for 1 week. At the follow-up endoscopy, it was possible to identify the openings of the gastrojejunostomy and to enter both of them with a standard (9-mm) gastroscope. The pigs were sacrificed, and no signs of infection or leakage were present postmortem.

Other methods for suturing have also been used for creating anastomoses in a similar way. Kantsevoy et al. used the Eagle Claw suturing device to create sutured gastrojejunostomies in pigs. The Eagle Claw is a suturing device that is mounted on the outside of the endoscope and needs an overtube to protect the esophagus during introduction. In their study, they present two survival animals with gastrojejunostomies performed with pure NOTES technique, sutured in place using the Eagle Claw. Both animals survived for 2 weeks and had patent robust anastomoses at postmortem and no sign of leakage in the abdominal cavity [21].

NOTES Compression Anastomoses

Compression anastomoses with NOTES techniques, entering the endoscope into the abdominal cavity, have been performed in the same way as described above, but with two balloons compressing the tissue instead of magnets [31]. A device with two separate balloons is brought down through the working channel of the endoscope. The distal balloon is introduced into a piece of small bowel and inflated. The bowel is then brought up to the stomach's serosal side and the proximal balloon is inflated inside the stomach, creating both compression and fixation. However, no instant open stoma is created. The small fistular tract between the joined organs is dilated after 1 week and the stoma is ready. We explored this method in a series of five nonsurvival and four survival pigs, placing the device through a gastroscope with a 6-mm working channel (Olympus GIF-XTQ160). In the survival pigs, the device had fallen out and a fistular tract was established at 5–10 days. After balloon dilation, a 9-mm gastroscope could be passed down into both the afferent and efferent limbs of small bowel [32].

With the new technique called "smart self-assembling magnets for endoscopy" (SAMSEN), Marvin Ryou et al. described a magnet compression anastomosis with immediate gastrojejunostomy [33]. Four magnets form a 2.25 cm square frame, but for delivery they are pinched in a linear shape. The magnets are made of neodymium-iron-boron rare earth magnets (KJ Magnetics, Jamison, PA) covered by acrylonitrile-butadienestyrene plastic. Through a gastrostomy, a gastroscope with an overtube was introduced into the abdominal cavity to grab a loop of small bowel. An enterotomy was performed and the SAMSEN magnet attached to two guidewires was introduced into the bowel to form the square frame around the enterotomy. The overtube was retracted into the stomach and a second SAMSEN magnet was introduced over the guidewires to form the compression anastomosis under fluoroscopic guidance. The gastroscope was then passed through the anastomosis into the small bowel to ensure the opening. These anastomoses have been tested in animal and human cadaver studies and in acute animal studies and showed no leakage. The SAMSEN gastroentero-anastomosis is an interesting and promising technique. However, further studies, including survival studies, have to be presented before conclusions can be drawn regarding the reliability and safety of this anastomotic technique.

Conclusions

There is an increasing interest in performing less invasive gastrojejunostomies, and different types of devices and techniques have been developed during the last decade. No pure NOTES techniques have been used in man. Only compression anastomoses performed with a radiological or endoscopic technique have reached beyond benchtop and animal experiments into clinical use. The limitation of the compression anastomoses with no instant formation of a gastrojejunostomy may have been solved with the SAMSEN technique even if this technique has to be simplified and proven safe in survival settings. However, there is a need to develop an endoscopic stapling device to perform a fast, immediate, and reliable anastomosis before the clinical use of NOTES gastrojejunostomies will become a standard technique.

References

1. Santoro E. The history of gastric cancer: legends and chronicles. Gastric Cancer. 2005;8: 71–4.
2. Johnsson E, Thune A, Liedman B. Palliation of malignant gastroduodenal obstruction with open surgical bypass or endoscopic stenting: clinical outcome and health economic evaluation. World J Surg. 2004;28:812–7.
3. Lillemoe KD, Cameron JL, Hardacre JM, et al. Is prophylactic gastrojejunostomy indicated for unresectable periampullary cancer? A prospective randomized trial. Ann Surg. 1999;230: 322–8; discussion 328–330.
4. Griffin SM, Chung SC, Leung JW, Li AK. Peptic pyloric stenosis treated by endoscopic balloon dilatation. Br J Surg. 1989;76:1147–8.
5. Boylan JJ, Gradzka MI. Long-term results of endoscopic balloon dilatation for gastric outlet obstruction. Dig Dis Sci. 1999;44:1883–6.
6. Tang T, Allison M, Dunkley I, et al. Enteral stenting in 21 patients with malignant gastroduodenal obstruction. J R Soc Med. 2003;96:494–6.
7. Graber I, Dumas R, Filoche B, et al. The efficacy and safety of duodenal stenting: a prospective multicenter study. Endoscopy. 2007;39:784–7.
8. Jeurnink SM, Steyerberg EW, van Hooft JE, et al. Surgical gastrojejunostomy or endoscopic stent placement for the palliation of malignant gastric outlet obstruction (SUSTENT study): a multicenter randomized trial. Gastrointest Endosc. 2010;71:490–9.
9. Hardy KJ. Non-suture anastomosis: the historical development. Aust N Z J Surg. 1990;60: 625–33.
10. Murphy JB. Cholecysto-intestinal, gastro-intestinal, entero-intestinal anastomosis, and approximation without sutures (original research). Med Rec NY. 1892;42:665–76.
11. Swain CP, Mills TN. Anastomosis at flexible endoscopy: an experimental study of compression button gastrojejunostomy. Gastrointest Endosc. 1991;37:628–31.
12. Cope C. Creation of compression gastroenterostomy by means of the oral, percutaneous, or surgical introduction of magnets: feasibility study in swine. J Vasc Interv Radiol. 1995;6: 539–45.
13. Cope C, Ginsberg GG. Long-term patency of experimental magnetic compression gastroenteric anastomoses achieved with covered stents. Gastrointest Endosc. 2001;53:780–4.
14. van Hooft JE, Vleggaar FP, Le Moine O, et al. Endoscopic magnetic gastroenteric anastomosis for palliation of malignant gastric outlet obstruction: a prospective multicenter study. Gastrointest Endosc. 2010;72:530–5.
15. Fritscher-Ravens A, Mosse CA, Mukherjee D, et al. Transluminal endosurgery: single lumen access anastomotic device for flexible endoscopy. Gastrointest Endosc. 2003;58:585–91.
16. Kalloo AN, Singh VK, Jagannath SB, et al. Flexible transgastric peritoneoscopy: a novel approach to diagnostic and therapeutic interventions in the peritoneal cavity. Gastrointest Endosc. 2004;60:114–7.
17. Park PO, Bergstrom M, Ikeda K, et al. Experimental studies of transgastric gallbladder surgery: cholecystectomy and cholecystogastric anastomosis (videos). Gastrointest Endosc. 2005;61:601–6.

18. Park PO, Bergstrom M. Transgastric peritoneoscopy and appendectomy: thoughts on our first experience in humans. Endoscopy. 2010;42:81–4.
19. Park PO, Bergstrom M, Ikeda K, Swain P. Towards obesity surgery at flexible endoscopy: gastric bypass with a small pouch formation in a porcine model. Gastrointest Endosc. 2005;61:AB235.
20. Bergstrom M, Ikeda K, Swain P, Park PO. Transgastric anastomosis by using flexible endoscopy in a porcine model (with video). Gastrointest Endosc. 2006;63:307–12.
21. Kantsevoy SV, Jagannath SB, Niiyama H, et al. Endoscopic gastrojejunostomy with survival in a porcine model. Gastrointest Endosc. 2005;62:287–92.
22. Romanelli JR, Desilets DJ, Earle DB. Pancreatic pseudocystgastrostomy with a peroral, flexible stapler: human natural orifice transluminal endoscopic surgery anastomoses in 2 patients (with videos). Gastrointest Endosc. 2008;68:981–7.
23. Chiu PW, Wai Ng EK, Teoh AY, et al. Transgastric endoluminal gastrojejunostomy: technical development from bench to animal study (with video). Gastrointest Endosc. 2011;71:390–3.
24. Swain P, Park PO, Mills T. Bard EndoCinch: the device, the technique, and pre-clinical studies. Gastrointest Endosc Clin N Am. 2003;13:75–88.
25. Hu B, Chung SC, Sun LC, et al. Eagle Claw II: a novel endosuture device that uses a curved needle for major arterial bleeding: a bench study. Gastrointest Endosc. 2005;62:266–70.
26. Chuttani R, Kozarek R, Critchlow J, et al. A novel endoscopic full-thickness plicator for treatment of GERD: an animal model study. Gastrointest Endosc. 2002;56:116–22.
27. Raju GS, Fritscher-Ravens A, Rothstein RI, et al. Endoscopic closure of colon perforation compared to surgery in a porcine model: a randomized controlled trial (with videos). Gastrointest Endosc. 2008;68:324–32.
28. Ikeda K, Mosse CA, Park PO, et al. Endoscopic full-thickness resection: circumferential cutting method. Gastrointest Endosc. 2006;64:82–9.
29. Bergstrom M, Swain P, Park PO. Early clinical experience with a new flexible endoscopic suturing method for natural orifice transluminal endoscopic surgery and intraluminal endosurgery (with videos). Gastrointest Endosc. 2008;67:528–33.
30. Calisto JL, Kawamura J, Trencheva K, et al. Fixation of intestinal tissue using a novel endoscopic device. Surg Innov. 2011;18:44–7.
31. Swain P. NOTES and anastomosis. Gastrointest Endosc Clin N Am. 2008;18:261–77; viii.
32. Bergstrom M, Swain CP, Lichtenborgen E, et al. Double balloon anastomsis: a new technique to achieve transgastric gastro-jejunostomy. Gastrointest Endosc. 2006;63:AB79.
33. Ryou M, Cantillon-Murphy P, Azagury D, et al. Smart self-assembling magnets for endoscopy (SAMSEN) for transoral endoscopic creation of immediate gastrojejunostomy (with video). Gastrointest Endosc. 2011;73:353–9.

Chapter 18
NOTES: Nephrectomy

Scott Leslie, Tania Gill, and Mihir M. Desai

Keywords NOTES • Scarless • Minimally invasive • Nephrectomy • Single-port
Transvaginal • Kidney

Introduction

Surgery is in a constant state of flux. In the last 20 years there has been a dramatic
shift from large, open incisions for surgical extirpation to ever-smaller incisions to
achieve the same surgical goals. Surgical removal of the kidney is a procedure that
dates back to 1869 and up until the 1990s necessitated a large, morbid incision, a
significant "surgical footprint" if you will. With technological advancement and
surgical ingenuity, this "surgical footprint" has diminished with time. First, with the
introduction of conventional laparoscopic nephrectomy [1], followed by LESS
nephrectomy [2], and finally with the advent of NOTES nephrectomy, this "surgical
footprint" has all but been abolished. Perhaps this is the final chapter in the evolution of scarless surgery?

The benefits of NOTES nephrectomy are more than simply cosmetic. Minimizing
pain, having a shorter convalescence, as well as eliminating abdominal wound complications such as infection and hernias are other potential advantages of NOTES.
However, despite the appealing nature of NOTES nephrectomy, it has yet to receive
universal acceptance among urologists. The principal hurdle for widespread adoption is the technical challenge NOTES nephrectomy presents. Although transvesical, transgastric, transureteric, and transcolonic NOTES nephrectomy have all been
described in animal models [3–5], only the transvaginal route has been performed
in humans. This technical necessity naturally eliminates 50 % of patients that would

S. Leslie, B.Sc., (Med), MB BS (Hons), FRACS (Urol) (✉) • T. Gill, BS • M.M. Desai, M.D.
Department of Urology, Keck Medical Center,
University of Southern California Institute of Urology,
1441 Eastlake Avenue, Suite 7416, Los Angeles, CA 90033, USA
e-mail: scottleslie@me.com; adityadesai2003@gmail.com

A. Rane et al. (eds.), *Scar-Less Surgery*,
DOI 10.1007/978-1-84800-360-6_18, © Springer-Verlag London 2013

otherwise be suitable for the procedure. In addition, approaching the kidney through vaginal access presents the surgeon with unique obstacles. These include an unfamiliar view of the relevant anatomy and inadequate instrumentation that lacks the appropriate triangulation. Despite the use of flexible laparoscopes and extra-long and articulated instruments in an attempt to overcome these hurdles, it is clear that at this time the technology is not at the stage to facilitate a global acceptance of NOTES nephrectomy.

In this chapter, we review the peer-reviewed literature of human cases of NOTES nephrectomy that has been published over the last 5 years (Table 18.1).

NOTES Nephrectomy Terminology

As the clinical application of NOTES is in its infancy, there is as yet no agreed-upon nomenclature defining what constitutes NOTES. The *precursor* to NOTES nephrectomy might be considered conventional laparoscopic nephrectomy with vaginal extraction of the kidney. In 1993, Breda et al. described the first case of laparoscopic nephrectomy with removal of the specimen via the vagina [6]. Gill subsequently reported the technical steps and outcomes of conventional laparoscopic nephrectomy with vaginal extraction in a series of ten cases [7]. In these examples, where the dissection is performed completely through transabdominal ports, but the specimen is removed via the natural orifice, it is referred to as *natural orifice specimen extraction* (NOSE) [8]. Similarly, in instances where the natural orifice is used for the insertion of an endoscope for visualization, and the dissection is otherwise completely performed using conventional laparoscopic ports, this is referred to as *natural orifice visualization* (NOV) [9, 10].

The term "hybrid" NOTES defines procedures in which one or more transabdominal ports *assist* the transvaginal dissection. In contrast, "pure" NOTES refers to procedures where the whole case is performed *entirely* via the natural orifice. The literature demonstrates that hybrid procedures constitute over 90 % of NOTES cases [11]. Indeed, in the case of nephrectomy, there is only one published case of a pure transvaginal NOTES nephrectomy [12]. The ability to safely access the peritoneum through the abdomen, as well as more effective retraction and dissection, are reasons that hybrid NOTES is favored over pure NOTES. Although additional abdominal ports are required for hybrid NOTES, it preserves the main advantage of pure NOTES, which is avoidance of a large abdominal incision to extract the specimen.

Indications and Patient Selection

NOTES nephrectomy has been performed for both benign and malignant conditions of the kidney.

Table 18.1 Published NOTES nephrectomy series

	Branco et al. [13]	Kaouk et al. [12]	Alcaraz et al. [17]	Sotelo et al. [18]	Kaouk et al. [12]	Porpiglia et al. [16]	Alcaraz et al. [15]
Patients	1	1	14	4	1	5	20
Pure vs. hybrid	Hybrid	Hybrid	Hybrid	Hybrid	Pure	Hybrid	Hybrid
TVD[a]	No	Yes	No	Yes	Yes	Yes	Yes
NOV[b]	Yes	Yes	Yes	Yes	Yes	No	No
Optics	Gastroscope Double-channel, flexible	EndoEYE	EndoEYE	EndoEYE	EndoEYE	3-mm laparoscope	Standard laparoscope
Specialized instruments	–	Graspers and scissors 45-cm Articulating J-hook 65-cm Articulating	–	–	Graspers and scissors 45-cm Articulating J-hook 65-cm Articulating	3-mm instruments	–
Abdominal port(s)	X2 standard ports (5 mm)	X1 standard port (5 mm)	X2 standard ports (5-mm, 12-mm)	TriPort	Nil	X3 mini-laparoscopic ports (3.5-mm)	X3 standard ports (10-, 10-, 5-mm)
Vaginal port	No port	TriPort and GelPort	Bariatric port	TriPort	GelPort and TriPort	Bariatric port	Bariatric port
Operative time (min)	170	307	133	222	420	120	117
EBL[c]	350	100	111	150	50	160	215
Complications and technical difficulties	–	Instrument clashing with the TriPort	Colon injury	Colon injury intraabdominal collection	Air leak with the GelPort	–	Postoperative bleed
Hospital LOS[d] (h)	12	23	96	24	19	62	98

(continued)

Table 18.1 (continued)

	Branco et al. [13]	Kaouk et al. [12]	Alcaraz et al. [17]	Sotelo et al. [18]	Kaouk et al. [12]	Porpiglia et al. [16]	Alcaraz et al. [15]
Pain VAS[e] (0–10)	–	1/10	–	3/10	0/10	–	–
Pathology	Benign	Benign	Malignant (10), benign (4)	Malignant (3), benign (1)	Benign	Malignant (2), benign (3)	Benign (donor kidneys)

[a]Transvaginal dissection
[b]Natural orifice visualization
[c]Estimated blood loss
[d]Length of stay
[e]Visual analog score

Benign Conditions

NOTES nephrectomy was first performed for atrophic, nonfunctioning kidneys [12–14]. Recently Alcaraz et al. demonstrated the feasability of NOTES in the setting of living-donor nephrectomy [15]. In this series, the outcomes of 20 patients who underwent transvaginal NOTES donor nephrectomy were compared to a contemporaneous matched group who underwent conventional laparoscopic living-donor nephrectomy. Although a longer warm ischemia time was associated with the NOTES group (5 vs. 2.6 min), this did not translate into any difference between the two groups in terms of graft function. They concluded that NOTES living-donor nephrectomy was feasible; however, further randomized controlled trials with a longer follow-up were required.

Malignant Conditions

Three groups have described NOTES nephrectomy for renal cell carcinoma [16–18]. Typically, these tumors are T1b, with the mean diameter being 5 cm. Given the superior renal functional outcomes of partial nephrectomy over radical nephrectomy, smaller tumors that are amenable to nephron-sparing surgery should be excluded from NOTES nephrectomy.

NOTES nephrectomy has been performed for both upper pole and lower pole tumors. However, dissecting around the upper pole is particularly challenging in cases of NOTES given that the upper pole is farthest away from the ports. In addition, the inability to effectively retract an overlapping liver or spleen makes upper pole dissection even more difficult. For this reason, lower pole tumors may be better suited to NOTES nephrectomy at this time.

Patient Factors

A history of prior abdominal surgery may complicate a NOTES nephrectomy procedure given the possibility of intraabdominal adhesions. This is particularly relevant for pure transvaginal NOTES, where access to the peritoneal cavity is via the posterior fornix of the vagina. An inability to recognize adherent bowel within the pelvis during peritoneal access could result in inadvertent small bowel enterotomy.

As the kidney is removed via the vagina in NOTES nephrectomy, it is important that the specimen can be safely extracted. Patients who have not had a previous vaginal delivery, or whose vagina is not distensible on digital examination, are not appropriate candidates for NOTES nephrectomy. Similarly, in obese patients, where there may be a significant amount of perinephric fat, safe transvaginal extraction may not be possible for such voluminous specimens.

Fig. 18.1 Supine lithotomy position.
Transvaginal and transumbilical TriPort
(Advanced Surgical Concepts, Dublin,
Ireland) (Reprinted with permission from
Elsevier from Sotelo et al. [18])

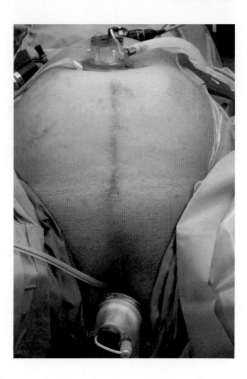

Patient Positioning

As there is no one standard technique for NOTES nephrectomy, there are many descriptions in the literature of how the patient should be positioned. Sotelo et al. described having the patient in the supine lithotomy position initially for placement of the umbilical and vaginal ports (Fig. 18.1). Once the ports are in position, the table is rotated such that the patient is in a 45° lateral decubitus position [18]. Similarly, in the case of pure NOTES nephrectomy described by Kaouk et al., the patient is initially in lithotomy for the placement of the vaginal port [12]. A wedge is placed on the side of the nephrectomy to accentuate the retroperitoneum, and the operating table is tilted as required to facilitate reflection of the colon away from the renal hilum. Porpiglia et al. described placing the patient in a lateral decubitus position from the outset, with the legs separated to allow vaginal access (Fig. 18.2) [16].

As these procedures are often of long duration, irrespective of the way the patient is positioned, it is important that pressure areas are padded and that appropriate DVT prophylaxis is maintained throughout the procedure and in the immediate postoperative period. A thorough vaginal and perineal scrub with iodine solution is imperative to minimize postoperative infection. The addition of metronidazole to the conventional cephazolin antibiotic regimen is important to cover for anaerobic organisms that may reside in this area.

Fig. 18.2 Lateral decubitus position (Reprinted with permission from Elsevier Porpiglia et al. [16])

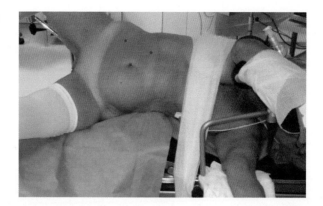

Translumenal Access to the Peritoneal Cavity

Translumenal access to the peritoneum through the natural orifice is achieved by one of two methods. In the case of pure NOTES, the peritoneal cavity is accessed through the vagina itself. This is achieved by using a vaginal retractor to help identify the cervix, followed by the creation of a colpotomy in the posterior vaginal cul-de-sac, directly entering the peritoneal cavity in the pouch of Douglas. Once there is access to the peritoneal cavity, a transvaginal port can be placed to allow insufflation and pneumoperitoneum.

In the case of hybrid NOTES, where one or more abdominal ports will be placed, it is preferable to *initially* access the peritoneum transabdominally. Using a 2-mm Veress needle or using an open Hassan technique may achieve this. Once a pneumoperitoneum has been created and the abdominal port(s) placed, the pelvis is inspected under direct vision for any adhesions or small bowel within the pouch of Douglas. Adhesions can be lysed and the posterior vaginal cul-de-sac can be cleared, to allow a transvaginal port to be placed under direct vision. This method of first accessing the peritoneum transabdominally is the preferred choice in the setting of prior pelvic surgery. In this way, injury to small bowel that may be stuck down in the pelvis can be avoided.

Ports

In the case of hybrid NOTES nephrectomy, various *abdominal* ports have been utilized. They include conventional laparoscopic ports, 3.5-mm *mini*-laparoscopic ports (Karl Storz Medical System, Tuttlingen, Germany) [16], and the TriPort® (Advanced Surgical Concepts, Dublin, Ireland) [18].

In the published literature, three types of *transvaginal* ports have been used for NOTES nephrectomy:

1. TriPort
2. GelPort® (Applied Medical, Rancho Santa Margarita, CA)
3. 12-mm bariatric port (Applied Medical, Rancho Santa Margarita, CA)

TriPort

Sotelo et al. described the simultaneous use of the TriPort (Fig. 18.1) in both the umbilicus and the vagina for NOTES nephrectomy [18]. The TriPort is a single-access port with three inlet channels (one 12-mm and two 5-mm). The port is secured in position by two plastic rings (one within the peritoneum and the other remaining outside); a sliding plastic sleeve connects both. Pulling up on the sleeve removes its slack, thereby tightly approximating the two rings against each other and creating an airtight seal for the pneumoperitoneum. Various standard 5-, 10-, and 12-mm laparoscopic instruments, as well as articulated instruments, can be inserted through this port.

GelPort

Kaouk et al. utilized this transvaginal port in their published NOTES nephrectomy cases [12, 14]. Similar to the TriPort, tightening the slack of the plastic sleeve that connects the inner and outer rings creates a seal. However, the GelPort is slightly larger than the TriPort and allows the use of two 10-mm trocars and a 5-mm trocar at the same time.

12-mm Bariatric Port

This was the preferred vaginal port of Alcaraz and Porpiglia [15–17] in their hybrid NOTES nephrectomy series. Bariatric ports are extra-long ports (15 cm in length) that are well suited for positioning in the vagina. Their added length permits them to extend from the introitus to where they enter the peritoneal cavity in the posterior vaginal fornix.

Optics and Instruments

In the case of hybrid NOTES, standard laparoscopes may be suitable if used via one of the abdominal ports. However, in the case of pure NOTES, or where the vaginal port is used to introduce the camera, then the standard laparoscope may be inadequate. With the laparoscope placed through the vagina, the caudal vision of the

Fig. 18.3 Deflectable-Tip EndoEYE™ Laparoscope (Olympus, Orangeburg, NY) (Reprinted with permission from Elsevier from Sotelo et al. [18])

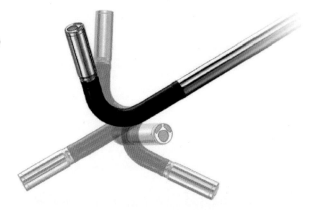

Fig. 18.4 Lack of instrument triangulation (Reprinted with permission from Elsevier from Sotelo et al. [18])

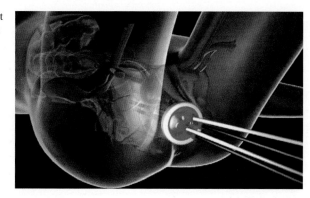

kidney is significantly different when compared to conventional laparoscopy. Visualization of the renal hilum and upper pole is particularly challenging given how far away these structures are from the vaginal port. Even with the use of a 30° camera, the visualization is often suboptimal. In order to help overcome this difficulty, a 5-mm laparoscope with a deflectable tip (EndoEYE™; Olympus, Orangeburg, NY) has been utilized (Fig. 18.3). Its ability to provide a perpendicular view to the kidney and hilar structures, even from the transvaginal vantage point, may help prevent clashing with other instruments that are using the same vaginal access.

One of the principles of conventional multiport laparoscopy is to space the ports far enough apart to allow for optimal triangulation. In so doing, clashing of instruments can be avoided and the tissues can be retracted adequately. In the case of pure NOTES, this triangulation is lacking, as each of the instruments is arising from the same reference point (Fig. 18.4). In order to minimize the resulting clashing, extra-long, articulating instruments have been developed. These include 45-cm articulating graspers and scissors (Novare Surgical Systems, Cupertino, CA), as used by Kaouk et al. However, these novel instruments lack tensile strength and

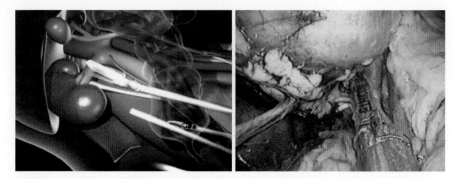

Fig. 18.5 Renal vein controlled by Endo GIA™ (Covidien, Dublin, Ireland) stapler (Reprinted with permission from Elsevier from Sotelo et al. [18])

maneuverability, often making dissection, tissue grasping, and retraction of intraabdominal structures challenging.

Dissection

Once the ports have been placed, the essential technical aspects of laparoscopic nephrectomy are duplicated. The colon is mobilized medially to allow access to the ureter and renal hilum. In the case of a hybrid procedure, retraction of the colon is best accomplished using a grasper placed through one of the abdominal ports. Once the renal artery and vein have been adequately skeletonized, they may be secured either with Hem-O-Lok® clips (Weck Closure Systems, Research Triangle Park, NC) or with an Endo GIA™ (Covidien, Dublin, Ireland) stapler (Fig. 18.5). As mentioned previously, one of the more difficult areas of dissection is the upper pole of the kidney. Its distance from the vaginal port makes it particularly challenging. Kaouk et al. used an articulating 65-cm J-hook to facilitate this upper pole dissection.

Specimen Extraction and Closure of Entry Site

Once the kidney has been completely dissected and is free from all surrounding attachments, it is extracted intact via the vagina. This is achieved by placing the kidney in an EndoCatch™ bag (Covidien, Norfolk, CT) that is introduced transvaginally under laparoscopic guidance.

Two methods have been described for closing the colpotomy incision. In the majority of series, the colpotomy is closed from within the vagina, typically using an absorbable 2-0 suture. Alcaraz makes the point of ensuring the vaginal closure includes the entire wall thickness to maximize hemostasis and reduce the risk of

Fig. 18.6 Internal picture showing the inner ring of the transvaginal TriPort (Advanced Surgical Concepts, Dublin, Ireland) sitting in the cul-de-sac (note the absence of the uterus) (Reprinted with permission from Elsevier from Sotelo et al. [18])

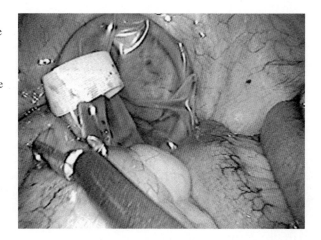

postoperative bleeding [15]. Sotelo et al. described closure of the colpotomy incision via laparoscopically placed sutures using the abdominal port. Of course, this is only possible in the case of hybrid NOTES nephrectomy [18].

Complications and Technical Difficulties

Table 18.1 outlines the complications and technical obstacles encountered in the early published series of NOTES nephrectomy. Although instrument clashing was ubiquitous in many of the NOTES nephrectomy series, it was particularly relevant for Kaouk et al. in their attempt to complete all of the dissection transvaginally. Despite their use of extra-long and articulated instruments, as discussed previously, significant clashing persisted, which in one case required exchanging the TriPort for the GelPort, thus allowing slightly better triangulation and dissection. However, in their case of pure NOTES nephrectomy, where they started with the GelPort, a persistent air leak necessitated changing from the GelPort to the TriPort. What is clear is that currently there is no ideal transvaginal port to facilitate pure NOTES nephrectomy. The unique anatomical characteristics of the vagina are prohibitive for the proper functioning of current ports that have been designed for the abdomen. Sotelo et al. argue that a prior hysterectomy, although predisposing to pelvic adhesions, may allow better functioning of the TriPort by allowing the inner ring to be more effectively deployed within the peritoneal cavity and thus optimizing an airtight seal (Fig. 18.6).

A complication described by Sotelo et al. is a case of an intraabdominal abscess occurring postoperatively that required percutaneous drainage and antibiotics [18]. This complication highlights the importance of a thorough perineal and vaginal iodine solution scrub and the use of broad-spectrum antibiotics at induction.

In the NOTES living-donor nephrectomy series of Alcaraz, there was one significant complication related to transvaginal access [15]. An acute postoperative hemorrhage occurred in one donor due to a uterine artery injury during transvaginal trocar insertion that was not identified at the time of the initial procedure. The patient required surgical intervention to control the bleeding, and the author concluded that placement of the vaginal trocar in the midline is important in order to avoid damage to the nearby uterine vessels.

Perhaps the most concerning complication of NOTES nephrectomy is colon injury, which has been described twice in the NOTES nephrectomy literature [17, 18]. In one case, a 2-cm injury to the rectum resulted from the attempted transvaginal insertion of the TriPort. Of note, the attempted insertion was performed *without* direct visualization from an abdominally placed laparoscope. The enterotomy was repaired with laparoscopically placed sutures, and the patient made an uneventful postoperative recovery. In the second case, the colon injury was not recognized intraoperatively, instead diagnosed on postoperative day 2 when the patient experienced abdominal pain and fevers. A CT scan confirmed the diagnosis and the patient required a diverting colostomy.

If we look further afield to nonurological transvaginal NOTES procedures (e.g., transvaginal NOTES cholecystectomy), we note other significant access-related complications, including bladder perforation, ureteric injury, and ureterovaginal fistula [11]. These serious complications serve to emphasize the care that must be taken when gaining peritoneal access through the natural orifice. It remains to be seen whether these complications are related to the early learning curve associated with transvaginal NOTES or if they reflect unacceptably high risks associated with transvaginal access that would otherwise be avoided with conventional laparoscopy.

One of the concerns of transvaginal access for NOTES procedures is the possibility of sexual dysfunction after surgery. However, the current literature on this topic, mainly in the gynecologic field, indicates that sexual dysfunction is a rare event after vaginal surgery [19]. Furthermore, in the Alcaraz series of NOTES donor nephrectomy, sexual function was measured preoperatively and 4 months after surgery. Sexual function was assessed using the Female Sexual Function Index (FSFI). No difference in FSFI was observed following surgery, and the women indicated there was no change in their sexual life [15].

Future Developments and Conclusions

NOTES procedures represent the pinnacle of *scarless* surgery. The published literature of NOTES nephrectomy demonstrates that not only is it technically feasible, but that the benefits of reducing postoperative pain, minimizing the hospital length of stay, and improving cosmesis are promising. However, NOTES nephrectomy is still in its infancy and the clinical data are limited to a small number of case series. The significant complications encountered in these studies and the difficulties of dissection (in particular with pure NOTES) are reminders that further advancements in technology and surgical ingenuity are required before NOTES nephrectomy is to become the gold standard.

In order to achieve this goal, a further refinement of ports, instrumentation, and robotics is required. As these new developments enter the clinical arena, additional studies will be required to uncover the future role of transvaginal NOTES (both pure and hybrid) in the management of urologic disease.

References

1. Clayman RV, et al. Laparoscopic nephrectomy: initial case report. J Urol. 1991;146(2): 278–82.
2. Raman JD, et al. Laboratory and clinical development of single keyhole umbilical nephrectomy. Urology. 2007;70(6):39–42.
3. Swain P. Nephrectomy and natural orifice translumenal endoscopy (NOTES): transvaginal, transgastric, transrectal, and transvesical approaches. J Endourol. 2008;22(4):811–8.
4. Bazzi WM, et al. Transrectal hybrid natural orifice transluminal endoscopic surgery (NOTES) nephrectomy in a porcine model. Urology. 2011;77(3):518–23.
5. Baldwin DD, et al. Hybrid transureteral natural orifice translumenal endoscopic nephrectomy: a feasibility study in the porcine model. J Endourol. 2011;25(2):245–50.
6. Breda G, et al. Laparoscopic nephrectomy with vaginal delivery of the intact kidney. Eur Urol. 1993;24(1):116–7.
7. Gill IS, et al. Vaginal extraction of the intact specimen following laparoscopic radical nephrectomy. J Urol. 2002;167(1):238–41.
8. Palanivelu C, et al. An innovative technique for colorectal specimen retrieval: a new era of "natural orifice specimen extraction" (N.O.S.E). Dis Colon Rectum. 2008;51(7):1120–4.
9. Zorron R, et al. International multicenter trial on clinical natural orifice surgery – NOTES IMTN study: preliminary results of 362 patients. Surg Innov. 2010;17(2):142–58.
10. Box G, et al. Nomenclature of natural orifice translumenal endoscopic surgery (NOTES) and laparoendoscopic single-site surgery (LESS) procedures in urology. J Endourol. 2008;22(11): 575–81.
11. Santos BF, et al. Preoperative ultrasound measurements predict the feasibility of gallbladder extraction during transgastric natural orifice translumenal endoscopic surgery cholecystectomy. Surg Endosc. 2011;25(4):1168–75.
12. Kaouk JH, et al. Pure natural orifice translumenal endoscopic surgery (NOTES) transvaginal nephrectomy. Eur Urol. 2010;57(4):723–6.
13. Branco AW, et al. Hybrid transvaginal nephrectomy. Eur Urol. 2008;53(6):1290–4.
14. Kaouk JH, et al. NOTES transvaginal nephrectomy: first human experience. Urology. 2009;74(1):5–8.
15. Alcaraz A, et al. Feasibility of transvaginal natural orifice transluminal endoscopic surgery-assisted living donor nephrectomy: is kidney vaginal delivery the approach of the future? Eur Urol. 2011;59(6):1019–25.
16. Porpiglia F, et al. Transvaginal natural orifice transluminal endoscopic surgery-assisted mini-laparoscopic nephrectomy: a step towards scarless surgery. Eur Urol. 2011;60(4):862–6.
17. Alcaraz A, et al. Feasibility of transvaginal NOTES-assisted laparoscopic nephrectomy. Eur Urol. 2010;57(2):233–7.
18. Sotelo R, et al. NOTES hybrid transvaginal radical nephrectomy for tumor: stepwise progression toward a first successful clinical case. Eur Urol. 2010;57(1):138–44.
19. Tunuguntla HS, Gousse AE. Female sexual dysfunction following vaginal surgery: a review. J Urol. 2006;175(2):439–46.

Chapter 19
NOTES: Challenges

Oussama M. Darwish, Matthew J. Maurice, and Lee E. Ponsky

Keywords NOTES • Natural orifice • Translumenal • Transgastric • Transvaginal Transurethral • Minimally invasive • Laparoscopy • Endoscopic

Introduction

In an era of evolving minimally invasive surgical techniques, natural orifice translumenal endoscopic surgery (NOTES) has emerged as an exciting, innovative, and yet challenging adjunct to laparoscopic surgery [1]. The desire to decrease postoperative morbidity, shorten hospitalizations and convalescence, improve cosmesis, and "push the envelope" continues to drive innovation in the field of minimally invasive surgery [2].

NOTES involves gaining access to the abdominal cavity through a viscera (e.g., stomach, rectum, vagina, urinary bladder) in order to perform intraabdominal surgery. Originally introduced by a consortium of gastroenterologists and general

O.M. Darwish, M.D. • M.J. Maurice, M.D.
Urology Institute, University Hospitals Case Medical Center, 11100 Euclid Avenue,
Cleveland, OH 44106, USA
e-mail: oussama_darwish@hotmail.com; matthew.maurice@uhhospitals.org

L.E. Ponsky, M.D., FACS (✉)
Urology Institute, Urologic Oncology and Minimally Invasive Therapies Center,
Case Western Reserve University School of Medicine, University Hospitals Case Medical Center,
Cleveland, OH 44106, USA

11100 Euclid Avenue, Cleveland, OH 44106, USA
e-mail: lee.ponsky@uhhospitals.org

A. Rane et al. (eds.), *Scar-Less Surgery*,
DOI 10.1007/978-1-84800-360-6_19, © Springer-Verlag London 2013

surgeons in 2005 [3] with the support of their respective professional organizations, NOTES has gained popularity in other surgical specialties, including urology [4].

Besides the improved cosmesis of surgery without a visible scar, NOTES may offer other potential advantages over traditional laparoscopic surgery, including pain reduction, decreased anesthesia requirements, fewer adhesions, and a decreased risk of surgical site infections and incisional hernias [5, 6]. NOTES also may offer technical advantages in the morbidly obese patient population. However, despite over half a decade of advancements in the field of NOTES, many contemporary challenges remain, including obtaining reliable intraabdominal access through the viscera, closing incisions in a field necessarily contaminated by the natural orifice's bacterial colonization, and adapting equipment and instruments designed for other purposes to NOTES.

Conceptually, NOTES has stimulated a revolution, sparking an interest in *scarless* surgery and challenging the traditional paradigm of the triangulation of instruments. While the full realization of NOTES in clinical practice is hindered by technical limitations, the enthusiasm behind the concept has spawned other endeavors, including the development of laparoendoscopic single-site (LESS) surgery. Now, LESS is becoming increasingly popular in its own right. Furthermore, two offshoot endeavors that straddle the concepts of NOTES and LESS, namely, *hybrid* NOTES and *hybrid* LESS, have arisen, involving a combination of natural orifice and transcutaneous approaches [4].

The aim of this chapter is to describe current applications of NOTES, particularly focusing on the challenges of translumenal approaches.

Procedure

As mentioned previously, NOTES has been performed through such natural orifices as the oral cavity, vagina, urethra, and rectum to gain intraperitoneal or retroperitoneal access. The terminology used to describe the NOTES procedure relies on the nomenclature of the organ used for entry.

The basic steps of any NOTES procedure include [7]:

1. Entering the natural orifice
2. Incision of the viscera
3. Dilation of the access tract
4. Port placement by means of a catheter or guide tube for reliable CO_2 insufflation
5. Advancement of the scope into the peritoneal cavity or retroperitoneal space, and
6. Closure of the viscerotomy

Transgastric

Kalloo et al. first described the transgastric approach to the peritoneum for intraabdominal surgery in the porcine model [8]. Soon thereafter, Reddy and Rao boldly demonstrated the success of a therapeutic transgastric NOTES appendectomy in a patient on video display at the 45th Annual Conference of the Society of Gastrointestinal Endoscopy of India in 2004 [9]. Marks et al. described a bedside transgastric PEG-tube *rescue* in a patient with a dislodged gastrotomy tube in 2007 [6]. A prospective study by Hazey et al. reported favorable results with transgastric diagnostic peritoneoscopy in ten patients, further supporting the feasibility of transgastric NOTES [10].

In the field of urology, multiple transgastric NOTES procedures have been performed and currently are under further investigation. Our group described a combined transgastric and transvaginal NOTES renal surgery in the porcine model [11]; Lima et al. described combined transgastric and transvesical nephrectomy [12]; and Boylu et al. described transgastric partial nephrectomy [13]. We also have evaluated transgastric and transvesical partial cystectomy [15].

Despite promising initial results with transgastric surgery, certain insurmountable barriers continue to stymie progress to this day. Indeed, under the best circumstances, transgastric NOTES is feasible. However, evidence demonstrating the reliable, safe delivery of this technique is lacking. Currently, the major limitations include the difficulty obtaining peritoneal access, the significant degree of endoscopic retroflexion required for upper abdominal procedures, and, most importantly, the problematic nature of endoscopic closure of the gastrotomy.

An effective and safe closure of the access gastrotomy remains the most significant barrier to human applications of transgastric surgery. A faulty gastrotomy closure and the resultant gastric leak are a potentially devastating complication, exposing the patient to otherwise unnecessary risks of peritonitis, reoperation, including possible laparotomy, sepsis, and even death. Many experimental devices have been tested to solve this technical dilemma with mixed results, including endoscopic clips [15, 16], various suture devices [16], the NDO tissue plicating device [17], and a flexible stapler [18].

Transvaginal

The transvaginal approach, historically extensively utilized in gynecologic procedures for specimen extraction, is a proven method of access to the peritoneum with a low complication rate. The main advantages of this approach are its accessibility and improved visualization. Specifically, it permits the use of rigid instruments and allows for direct in-line viewing of most abdominal structures without retroflexion. Of course, the obvious drawback of the transvaginal approach is its limited application in only female patients.

Gettman et al. reported the first transvaginal NOTES procedure, a nephrectomy, in a porcine model in 2002 [19]. The clinical application of transvaginal NOTES in humans became relevant in 2007 when Zorron et al. reported the first successful cholecystectomy [20], followed shortly thereafter by the first reported appendectomy using this approach from Palanivelu et al. in 2008 [21].

In 2007, Branco et al. described a hybrid transvaginal NOTES nephrectomy with two 5-mm abdominal trocars and a transvaginal scope [22]. In 2008, in an attempt to improve cosmesis, Sotelo et al. reported a hybrid transvaginal NOTES nephrectomy using only a single umbilical transabdominal access port [23]. In 2009, Allaf et al. described a hybrid transvaginal donor nephrectomy involving three abdominal incisions [24]. Transvaginal NOTES also has been applied to retroperitoneal nephrectomy in the porcine model [14]. This growing cumulative experience culminated in 2009, when Kaouk et al. performed the first pure NOTES urologic procedure, a transvaginal radical nephrectomy [25]. It was especially noteworthy because all the operative steps were performed transvaginally, including removal of the intact kidney.

Secure closure of the vagina after transvaginal surgery is readily attainable using standard surgical techniques that are well documented in the gynecological literature. The success with vaginal closure in gynecology is mirrored in the NOTES experience. In 2001, Gill et al. reported ten cases of the transvaginal extraction of kidneys after laparoscopic nephrectomy. They described excellent patient satisfaction on postoperative questionnaire, and the only adverse event was self-limited vaginal spotting in a single patient [26]. In an early clinical experience of transvaginal NOTES cholecystectomy, the authors reported minimal discomfort and morbidity in a small study of four patients [27].

Transvesical

Transvesical access, unique in its relative sterility and applicability to both genders, suffers from the physical limitations of the urethral orifice, which restrict instrument size and mobility. In the porcine model, Lima et al. were the first to perform transvesical peritoneoscopy and thoracoscopy using a ureteroscope [28, 29]. In 2007, Gettman and coworkers successfully translated transvesical peritoneoscopy to the clinical realm, using a flexible ureteroscope through a vesicotomy that had been balloon-dilated [27]. Later, in 2009, Humphreys et al. remarkably described a transurethral NOTES radical prostatectomy in a human cadaveric model [30].

The combination transgastric and transvesical approach aims to overcome the limitations of either approach alone. Lima et al. investigated the viability of this concept in a porcine model with a pure NOTES nephrectomy without specimen extraction [12].

Our group has performed transvesical peritoneoscopy using both the dual-channel rigid cystoscope and pediatric gastroscope in a porcine model [31]. We also have performed transurethral NOTES partial cystectomy with full-thickness bladder resection in the porcine model [15].

Closure of the transvesical access vesicostomy is an area of particular interest to urologists as it is relevant not only in NOTES but also in the management of traumatic and iatrogenic bladder injuries. While classic teaching dictates surgical closure for intraperitoneal bladder injuries, it may be possible to manage small vesicotomies with simple catheter drainage [32]. In the NOTES literature, Lima et al. reported no complications due to an unclosed vesicotomy made by a uretero-scope in a chronic transvesical study [28]. Despite their success, a reliable endo-scopic method of bladder closure would be ideal. And, in 2008, Lima et al. demonstrated just that with successful bladder closure using endoscopically applied sutures in a chronic porcine model [33]. Our group also has described successful bladder closure with standard endoscopic metal clips in a chronic porcine model [15]; however, the duration of clip attachment and the potential for stone formation are potential drawbacks of this technique.

Transcolonic

A colorectal access point for NOTES offers theoretical advantages afforded by a large natural orifice, including accommodating larger-diameter instruments and permitting the extraction of large specimens. Compared to transgastric NOTES, the transcolonic approach carries similar, if not greater, risks of infection and raises serious concerns over safe, effective closure. According to traditional colorectal teaching, certain small colonic defects may safely undergo primary repair, while larger defects with significant fecal contamination may require proximal diversion [34]. Certainly, the need for this type of operation is incongruous with the mini-mally invasive intent of transcolonic NOTES. These considerations make transco-lonic NOTES the most controversial access point of all. Nevertheless, this approach has been tested in multiple animal studies, including transcolonic cholecystectomy [35], ventral hernia repair, and distal pancreatectomy [36]. Of note, Box et al. described the first urologic application of this approach in 2008 with a hybrid NOTES nephrectomy in a porcine model. Using the assistance of a da Vinci® S surgical system (Intuitive Surgical, Sunnyvale, CA), they performed their nephrec-tomy using three trocars (transvaginal, transcolonic, and transabdominal) with transvaginal specimen extraction [37].

   As discussed, the safe and reliable closure of transcolonic access is paramount when taking into consideration the high underlying bacterial load of the colon, the risk of severe intraabdominal infections, and the disastrous consequences of a col-orectal leak.

Technical Challenges

In 2006, a consortium of gastroenterologists and general surgeons called NOSCAR™ (Natural Orifice Surgery Coalition for Assessment and Research) identified a num-ber of specific barriers to NOTES procedures. These challenges included coaxial limitations, peritoneal access, maintenance of spatial orientation, access closure, control of hemorrhage, development of suturing and anastomotic devices, and the need to develop new innovative platforms [3]. While the group mainly focused on access from the gastrointestinal tract, the issues they raised apply to vaginal and bladder access as well.

Coaxial Limitations

Coaxial positioning, operating working instruments in parallel, is a technical limitation of single-access-site surgery, including general endourology and NOTES. The resulting visual and mechanical impairments created by a lack of instrument triangulation create a significant challenge for the surgeon. Even dual-lumen scopes, which accommodate two working instruments, are extremely limited with regards to the working distance between instruments and the visualization via the scope. Strategies have been developed to address some of these coaxial limitations during NOTES procedures. One strategy is a combined-orifice approach to achieve traditional triangulation. Examples include the combined transgastric and transvaginal approach, the combined transgastric and transvesical approach, or the use of a *hybrid* approach. While improving technical ease, a combined approach may cause increased morbidity and requires a multidisciplinary operating team. Another strategy involves the development of novel platforms with dedicated NOTES scopes, magnetic instruments, and micro-robots.

Access

As emphasized earlier in the chapter, establishing translumenal access while maintaining sterility of the abdomen is a significant barrier to NOTES, particularly for access through the gastrointestinal tract. To date, given its significant advantages, the transvaginal approach is the most popular access site used clinically, typically via a posterior colpotomy. The benefits of transvaginal surgery include direct in-line visualization of most retroperitoneal structures without the need for retroflexion and maintenance of spatial orientation. Furthermore, rigid instruments can be inserted via this approach either directly or via a preloaded overtube. Overtubes allow the easy reinsertion and exchange of instruments; however, these devices are mostly experimental, such as the modified trocar our group has used, a plastic overtube connected to a standard laparoscopic trocar.

Gettman and Blute described the first human transvesical peritoneoscopy using a ureteroscope through a vesicostomy made by balloon dilation over a transvesical wire [32]. Our group's technique for bladder access in the porcine model involves three steps: incising the porcine bladder with wire electrocautery, passing a wire through the vesicotomy, and then performing balloon dilation over the wire to safely enlarge the incision. The greatest challenge we have encountered is maintaining bladder distention given the organ's natural tendency to collapse on itself when perforated. In our experience, the porcine bladder generally maintains its shape with dilation of the vesicotomy to 10 mm but not to 20 mm [38]. Lima et al. used a 5.5-mm port for transvesical procedures with a ureteroscope in a porcine model [28], avoiding difficulties with bladder collapse while permitting the periodic removal and insertion of the scope.

Conventional Scopes

Early work in NOTES has involved the use of existing traditional endoscopic equipment. Important properties to consider in scope selection include scope size, flexibility, maneuverability, number of channels, channel size, ability to insufflate gas through the scope, ability to adequately illuminate the abdominal cavity, and ease of cleaning the lens. For most natural orifices, flexible scopes have proven to be advantageous, and in the case of transgastric access, they are essential for the purposes of reaching the stomach and visualizing the upper abdominal cavity. The most common scopes described in the literature for transgastric or transvaginal access are the dual-channel standard gastric endoscopes or colonoscopes, or the single-channel pediatric gastroscopes. The standard gastric endoscopes have numerous advantages over other traditional scopes, including maneuverability in both the vertical and horizontal planes, the ability to remotely clean the lens by depressing a button, and good illumination of the abdominal cavity. Advantages of smaller flexible scopes include maneuverability within the abdominal cavity and the potential for retroflexion.

Scope size is an important consideration. With the exception of the recent use of combination port devices transvaginally, the scope is the sole conduit for instruments for most pure NOTES procedures. A tradeoff exists among the scope size, the number and size of channels, and the size of the visceral defect. We prefer to have at least a dual-channel scope that can accommodate standard endoscopic equipment for procedures involving the manipulation of tissues. However, scope selection is limited by the size of the access site. For example, urethral caliber limits access to scopes less than 30 Fr, which precludes the entry of even the smallest standard dual-channel adult gastric endoscope but does allow the passage of a single-channel pediatric gastroscope in our experience [39]. Very small scopes such as ureteroscopes introduced through the bladder may not even require closure of the defect [28].

While a flexible cystoscope was employed in Gettman et al.'s original description of a transvaginal nephrectomy, urologic scopes play a limited role in clinical NOTES [19]. Lima described the use of flexible ureteroscopes; however, their size accommodates only small instruments [32]. Our group described the use of a standard rigid cystoscope, which we found provides reasonable illumination and accommodates two standard gastrointestinal endoscopic instruments [31].

Additional challenges of traditional scopes include maintaining the spatial orientation and operating instruments through the scope. Flexible scopes, in particular, are prone to causing disorientation, especially in the retroflexed position, where the view may flip completely upside down. Instrument manipulation through the working channel of a flexible scope is further hindered by the scope's natural tendency to recoil during instrument advancement. As noted previously, traditional scopes also suffer from coaxial limitations.

Pneumoperitoneum

Surprisingly, establishing and maintaining a pneumoperitoneum has proven relatively easy with the full gamut of currently available scopes, including gastric endoscopes, rigid cystoscopes [39], and even ureteroscopes [32]. However, since instruments and the insufflant compete for space within the working channels, we have found that instruments may occlude the flow of gas and significantly affect insufflation pressures, particularly in the smaller single-channel scopes such as the pediatric gastroscope. One practical solution to this problem involves using a transabdominal needle port for insufflation in what might be considered *hybrid* NOTES. Furthermore, conventional scopes were never designed to regulate pressures; therefore, new platforms with the ability to regulate insufflation pressures are being explored.

Closure of Access

Secure closure of the access portal is one of the most important factors to consider when performing NOTES. For this reason, tissue approximation has become an intense focus of research and development in the NOTES community, spawning a variety of novel devices that serve as suturing substitutes. The ideal device would facilitate intracorporeal suturing. An early prototype described in the literature was the Eagle Claw™ (Olympus, Tokyo, Japan). This was followed by the OverStitch™ device (Apollo Endosurgery, Austin, TX), which attaches to the end of the gastroscope and allows both running and interrupted sutures. Various other manufacturers have produced suturing devices that facilitate suture placement, tissue approximation, and securing of the closure with a fastening device, essentially replacing the need for knot tying. Two such devices include the T-tag™ system and TAS™.

Endoscopic Instruments

Like traditional open and laparoscopic approaches, NOTES requires tools with which to carry out the basic surgical techniques—incision, dissection, retraction, specimen retrieval, and tissue approximation. In NOTES, these tools are limited by the small working channels of existing scopes. In fact, size is the greatest challenge to devising instruments capable of executing theses tasks. To date,

NOTES lacks a working complement of instruments specifically designed to address and meet the challenges of translumenal endoscopic surgery. Using currently available endoscopic instruments, tissue incision can be carried out with needle-knife electrocautery, snare-wire cautery, or flexible scissors. However, in comparison to open or laparoscopic instruments, these tools are substandard. We eagerly await the development of more robust and effective instruments in the future. Until then, we feel that NOTES is unlikely to advance significantly in the clinical realm.

Complications

Most complications after NOTES are largely theoretical. Like most invasive intraabdominal surgeries, NOTES carries risks of bleeding, infection, hernia formation, and damage to surrounding structures, including the bowel and vasculature. Given the infancy of the field and its steep learning curve, NOTES procedures may be more prone to these complications than the equivalent open or laparoscopic surgery. NOTES carries the unique risks inherent to gaining access via a perforated viscus, including peritonitis and intraabdominal sepsis. The transvaginal approach involves a risk of dyspareunia and peritoneal leakage from the vagina.

Conclusions

Incision-less minimally invasive surgery was once science fiction. NOTES is an exciting new approach to minimally invasive surgery, demonstrating that *scarless* surgery is at least conceptually possible. Although NOTES has remained relevant since its introduction in 2005, it is still in its infancy, troubled by many contemporary challenges that impede its full clinical realization.

Despite promising early reports, many technical barriers and safety considerations exist that hinder the widespread clinical use of NOTES. Innovative techniques and technical advances are necessary to overcome these challenges. Until we demonstrate that NOTES is safe, effective, and functionally operational, its future role in clinical practice is uncertain.

References

1. Gettman MT, Box G, Averch T, et al. Consensus statement on natural orifice transluminal endoscopic surgery and single-incision laparoscopic surgery: heralding a new era in urology? Eur Urol. 2008;53:1117–20.
2. Pemberton RJ, Tolley DA, van Velthoven RF. Prevention and management of complications in urological laparoscopic port site placement. Eur Urol. 2006;50:958–68.

3. Rattner D, Kalloo A, ASGE/SAGES working group. ASGE/SAGES working group on natural orifice translumenal endoscopic surgery. Surg Endosc. 2006;20:329.

4. Box G, Averch T, Cadeddu J, et al. Nomenclature of natural orifice translumenal endoscopic surgery (NOTES) and laparoendoscopic single-site surgery (LESS) procedures in urology. J Endourol. 2008;22(11):2575–81.

5. Isariyawongse JP, McGee MF, Rosen MJ, et al. Pure natural orifice transluminal endoscopic surgery (NOTES) nephrectomy using standard laparoscopic instruments in the porcine model. J Endourol. 2008;22(5):1087–91.

6. Marks JM, Ponsky JL, Pearl JP, McGee MF. PEG "Rescue": a practical NOTES technique. Surg Endosc. 2007;21(5):816–9.

7. White WM, Haber GP, Doerr MJ, Gettman M. Natural orifice translumenal endoscopic surgery. Urol Clin North Am. 2009;36:147–55. vii.

8. Kalloo AN, Singh VK, Jagannath SB, et al. Flexible transgastric peritoneoscopy: a novel approach to diagnostic and therapeutic interventions in the peritoneal cavity. Gastrointest Endosc. 2004;60:114–7.

9. Reddy N, Rao P. Per oral transgastric endoscopic appendectomy in humans. In: 45th annual conference of the society of gastrointestinal endoscopy of India. Jaipur; 2004. p. 28–9.

10. Hazey JW, Narula VK, Renton DB, et al. Natural-orifice transgastric endoscopic peritoneoscopy in humans: initial clinical trial. Surg Endosc. 2008;22(1):16–20.

11. Isariyawongse JP, McGee MF, Rosen MJ, et al. Pure natural orifice transluminal endoscopic surgery (NOTES) nephrectomy using standard laparoscopic instruments in the porcine model. J Endourol. 2008;17:22.

12. Lima E, Rolanda C, Pego JM, et al. Third-generation nephrectomy by natural orifice transluminal endoscopic surgery. J Urol. 2007;178(6):2648–54.

13. Boylu U, Oommen M, Joshi V, et al. Natural orifice translumenal endoscopic surgery (NOTES) partial nephrectomy in a porcine model. Surg Endosc. 2010;24(2):485–9.

14. Perretta S, Allemann P, Asakuma M, et al. Feasibility of right and left transvaginal retroperitoneal nephrectomy: from the porcine to the cadaver model. J Endourol. 2009;23(11):1887–92.

15. Sawyer MD Cherullo EE, Elmunzer BJ, Schomisch S, Ponsky LE. Pure natural orifice translumenal endoscopic surgery partial cystectomy: intravesical transurethral and extravesical transgastric techniques in a porcine model. Urology. 2009;74(5):1049–53.

16. Swanstrom LL, Whiteford M, Khajanchee Y. Developing essential tools to enable transgastric surgery. Surg Endosc. 2008;22(3):600–4.

17. McGee MF, Marks JM, Jin J, et al. Complete endoscopic closure of gastric defects using a full-thickness tissue plicating device. J Gastrointest Surg. 2008;12(1):38–45.

18. Meireles OR, Kantsevoy SV, Assumpcao LR, et al. Reliable gastric closure after natural orifice translumenal endoscopic surgery (NOTES) using a novel automated flexible stapling device. Surg Endosc. 2008;22(7):1609–13.

19. Gettman MT, Lotan Y, Napper CA, Cadeddu JA. Transvaginal laparoscopic nephrectomy: development and feasibility in the porcine model. Urology. 2002;59(3):446–50.

20. Zorron R, Filgueiras M, Maggioni LC, et al. NOTES. Transvaginal cholecystectomy: report of the first case. Surg Innov. 2007;14(4):279–83.

21. Palanivelu C, Rajan PS, Rangarajan M, et al. Transvaginal endoscopic appendectomy in humans: a unique approach to NOTES-world's first report. Surg Endosc. 2008;22(5):1343–7.

22. Branco AW, Filho AJ, Kondo W, et al. Hybrid transvaginal nephrectomy. Eur Urol. 2007; 53:1290–4.

23. Sotelo R, de Andrade R, Fernandez G, et al. NOTES hybrid transvaginal radical nephrectomy for tumor: stepwise progression toward a first successful clinical case. Eur Urol. 2010; 57(1):138–44.

24. Quasi-NOTES surgery used to remove donor kidney. Medical News, surgery. Available from: http://www.medpagetoday.com/Surgery/GeneralSurgery/12744. 22. Accessed 4 February 2009.

25. Kaouk JH, Haber GP, Goel RK, et al. Pure natural orifice translumenal endoscopic surgery (NOTES) transvaginal nephrectomy. Eur Urol. 2009;57:723–6.

26. Gill IS, Cherullo EE, Meraney AM, et al. Vaginal extraction of the intact specimen following laparoscopic radical nephrectomy. J Urol. 2002;167(1):238–41.
27. Zorron R, Maggioni LC, Pombo L, et al. NOTES transvaginal cholecystectomy: preliminary clinical application. Surg Endosc. 2008;22(2):542–7.
28. Lima E, Rolanda C, Pego JM, et al. Transvesical endoscopic peritoneoscopy: a novel 5 mm port for intra-abdominal scarless surgery. J Urol. 2006;176(2):802–5.
29. Lima E, Henriques-Coelho T, Rolanda C, et al. Transvesical thoracoscopy: a natural orifice translumenal endoscopic approach for thoracic surgery. Surg Endosc. 2007;21(6):854–8.
30. Humphreys MR, Krambeck AE, Andrews PE, et al. Natural orifice translumenal endoscopic surgical radical prostatectomy: proof of concept. J Endourol. 2009;23(4):669–75.
31. Sawyer MD, Cherullo EE, Ponsky LE. Transvesical NOTES peritoneoscopy: initial experience with standard rigid cystoscope in a chronic porcine model. J Endourol. 2008;22 Suppl 1:A188.
32. Gettman MT, Blute ML. Transvesical peritoneoscopy: initial clinical evaluation of the bladder as a portal for natural orifice translumenal endoscopic surgery. Mayo Clin Proc. 2007;82(7):843–5.
33. Lima E, Rolanda C, Osorio L, et al. Endoscopic closure of transmural bladder wall perforations. Eur Urol. 2008;53:1117–20.
34. Stone HH, Fabian TC. Management of perforating colon trauma: randomization between primary closure and exteriorization. Ann Surg. 1979;190(4):430–6.
35. Pai RD, Fong DG, Bundga ME, et al. Transcolonic endoscopic cholecystectomy: a NOTES survival study in a porcine model (with video). Gastrointest Endosc. 2006;64(3):428–34.
36. Shin EJ, Kalloo AN. Transcolonic NOTES: current experience and potential implications for urologic applications. J Endourol. 2009;23(5):743–6.
37. Box GN, Lee HJ, Santos RJ, et al. Rapid communication: robot-assisted NOTES nephrectomy: initial report. J Endourol. 2008;22(3):503–6.
38. Sawyer MD, Cherullo EE, Ponsky LE. Vesicotomy closure: a novel method using endoscopic clips in a porcine model (meeting abstract). J Endourol. 2008;22(11):2621.
39. Sawyer MD, Cherullo EE, Ponsky LE. Visualization into the peritoneum: a urologic perspective on transvesical access including novel use of a rigid cystoscope. In: 3rd international conference on NOTES. San Francisco; 10–12 July 2008.

Part III
LESS (Laparo-Endoscopic Single Site Surgery)

Chapter 20
LESS: Pyeloplasty

Sara L. Best and Jeffrey A. Cadeddu

Keywords Minimally invasive surgery • Pyeloplasty • Laparoendoscopic single-site
(LESS) surgery • Laparoscopy • Ureteropelvic junction obstruction

Introduction

Laparoscopy has emerged as the primary management modality for a variety of renal
abnormalities. Increasing one's proficiency with complex laparoscopic tasks such as
suturing has allowed many urologists to tackle even difficult reconstructive procedures
such as pyeloplasty in a minimally invasive fashion. As the benefits of laparoscopy have
been better understood and embraced by the urologic community at large, there has been
increasing interest in developing techniques to make surgery even less invasive.

One direction this interest has taken is in the development of laparoendoscopic
single-site (LESS) pyeloplasty. As in other LESS renal procedures, access points to
the abdomen are clustered at a single location, typically the umbilicus, rather than
strategically spread across the abdominal wall.

Pyeloplasty is a desirable target for LESS for several reasons. First, there is no
large specimen to be removed and therefore no extraction incision at the completion
of the operation. Keeping the incision small increases the chances that the maximum
benefits of LESS may be obtained, such as optimizing the ability to hide the incision
completely within the umbilicus and minimizing the size of painful muscle-splitting
incisions. Second, ureteropelvic junction (UPJ) obstructions are often discovered in

S.L. Best, M.D. (✉)
Department of Urology, University of Wisconsin School of Medical and Public Health,
1685 Highland Ave, MFCB-3229, Madison, WI 53705, USA
e-mail: best@urology.wisc.edu

J.A. Cadeddu, M.D.
Department of Urology,
University of Texas Southwestern Medical Center, Dallas, TX, USA

A. Rane et al. (eds.), *Scar-Less Surgery*,
DOI 10.1007/978-1-84800-360-6_20, © Springer-Verlag London 2013

younger patients who are more likely to have had few prior abdominal surgeries and to be thinner, conditions that tend to be favorable for a successful LESS operation. Last, younger patients may also be more interested in "scarless" surgery.

Despite its desirability, LESS pyeloplasty has several challenges associated with it, namely related to the complex task of suturing the anastomosis. The loss of triangulation that affects all LESS procedures particularly encumbers sewing. Strategies for dealing with these challenges will be discussed.

Preoperative Planning and Evaluation

As is the case for the surgical management of UPJ obstructions regardless of approach, imaging studies such as diuretic renography, computerized tomographic (CT) angiography, intravenous urogram, and/or retrograde pyelography may be useful in determining the site or source of obstruction as well as the renal function. Additionally, CT can demonstrate the amount of perinephric fat tissue, a large amount of which can amplify the challenges of LESS, especially early in one's experience.

Factors that may affect the decision to proceed with a LESS rather than traditional laparoscopic pyeloplasty are patient characteristics such as body habitus and prior abdominal surgical history. Substantial abdominal girth increases the distance between the operative site and the umbilicus, which can make the procedure more difficult. Additionally, the clustering of instruments and the resultant loss of triangulation can make adhesions from prior abdominal surgeries difficult to manage. Thus, thinner patients with few or no prior abdominal operations may be prime candidates for LESS, though certainly these challenges can be overcome with patience and experience.

A limited bowel preparation with a bottle of magnesium citrate is advisable as it may improve the ease of visualization. Confirmation of a sterile urine culture is also prudent.

Finally, consideration should be given to retrograde (cystoscopic) stent placement immediately prior to pyeloplasty on the day of surgery. While many surgeons place the ureteral stent in an antegrade fashion after transection of the UPJ during traditional laparoscopic pyeloplasty, the limited working angles created by LESS can make this difficult.

Patient Positioning

The positioning for LESS pyeloplasty essentially mirrors that of traditional laparoscopic pyeloplasty. The patient can be placed in full or modified flank position, depending on the surgeon's preference. A Foley catheter draining to gravity should be placed. Careful attention to padding is also important. Mild flexion of the table may be helpful in some cases though is not always necessary.

Fig. 20.1 Use of three separate 5-mm ports, clustered at umbilicus, for LESS pyeloplasty

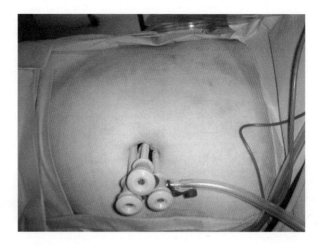

Access to the Abdominal Cavity

The incision location for LESS pyeloplasty is typically at the umbilicus, which provides a "straight-on" view of the UPJ as well as an opportunity to conceal the scar. A 2–3-cm incision is typically sufficient and can be made in a semilunar fashion, following the circle of the umbilicus itself. A variety of purpose-built LESS ports have been developed, and the surgeon should feel free to use whichever port he or she is most comfortable using. The insertion of these ports is typically performed in a Hasson fashion, under direct vision.

As an alternative to using a custom LESS port, three standard 5-mm trocars can be used instead. These can be inserted through a semilunar umbilical incision, similar to a custom LESS port, or they can each be inserted through separate skin incisions, clustered at the umbilicus (Fig. 20.1).

In right-sided procedures, the insertion of a 2- or 3-mm grasper in the subxyphoid region can provide helpful liver retraction. In order to diminish the cosmetic impact, this instrument can often be passed across the abdominal wall through a tiny skin incision without the actual port.

Procedure

The goal of LESS pyeloplasty is to reproduce the operation as it is performed during traditional laparoscopy. Therefore, the steps of the operation remain unchanged, though the loss of triangulation and potential clashing of instruments may require some special maneuvers. These difficulties can often be overcome using the standard principles of LESS, such as crossing the instruments just inside the fascial incision,

Fig. 20.2 The angle for the scissors to spatulate the ureter can be improved by drawing the transected ureter toward the port

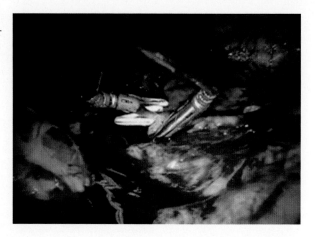

using a flexible endoscope, and using bent or articulating instruments. While the merits of each of the modifications are discussed elsewhere, it is important to point out that there is no "right way" to deal with these challenges and surgeons should use whichever combination of tools they are most comfortable using.

After port placement (and cystoscopic retrograde stent placement), the colon is first reflected medially. The proximal ureter is identified and mobilized, along with the renal pelvis. A careful effort is made to identify and preserve any cross-ing vessels. After mobilization, if a dismembered pyeloplasty is planned, the ureter is transected at the level of the UPJ, using caution not to cut the stent if it has already been placed. The proximal curl of the stent is dislodged from its position inside the renal pelvis so that the transected ureter is more mobile. In order to spatulate the ureter, due to the loss of triangulation, we find it helpful to draw the ureter toward the port, such that the cut end of the ureter is perpen-dicular to the scissors tips (Fig. 20.2). The spatulated ureter and renal pelvis are then brought anterior to any crossing vessels prior to anastomosis. The hiatus in the renal pelvis can also be widened and any redundant tissue excised at this time as well.

While some authors have reported accomplishing the LESS pyeloplasty anasto-mosis without assistant trocars [1], most report using a 3-mm instrument placed laterally to facilitate the complex task of sewing. It has been our practice to place a 3-mm port in the mid-axillary line, through which the surgical drain can also be drawn at the end of the procedure. Through this port, a 3-mm grasper can be placed and used along with a standard 5-mm laparoscopic needle driver, placed through the LESS port, to sew the anastomosis in a fashion that replicates standard laparoscopic pyeloplasty. We typically use 3-0 polyglactin running sutures, sewing the posterior wall first, then the anterior portion.

It is advisable to leave an intraabdominal closed bulb suction drain near the site of the anastomosis. We place a 10 Fr Jackson–Pratt drain through the site of our mid-axillary line trocar. If a lateral assistant trocar is not used, the drain can alterna-tively be brought out through the umbilical incision (Fig. 20.3).

Fig. 20.3 Immediate post-operative image of the LESS umbilical incision, with the surgical drain exiting

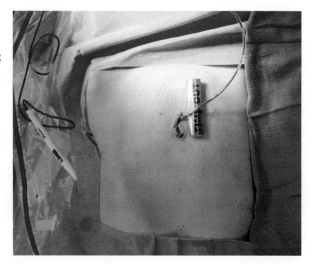

Upon completion of the procedure, the port(s) are removed. The fascia does not need to be closed if it was only traversed with separate 5-mm ports. If a purpose-built LESS port was used, the fascial incision can be closed under direct vision with an absorbable suture, making sure not to catch the drain with the needle if it is exiting through the incision. The skin itself can then be closed in whichever cosmetically pleasing way the surgeon prefers.

Postoperative Management

The care of a patient undergoing LESS pyeloplasty is essentially the same as that of traditional laparoscopy. Admission is typically about 48 h long so that postoperative drain output can be monitored. A Foley catheter is left place in order to maximally drain the urinary system, and this is usually removed after 24 h. Once this is removed, the drain output is carefully monitored for 8–12 h to make sure there is no urine leakage. The stent is left in place for 4–6 weeks. A diuretic renogram is typically obtained 6 weeks after the stent removal to make sure that the kidney drains well.

Robotic LESS Pyeloplasty

The triangulation challenges of LESS have led surgeons to explore a variety of possible tools to make LESS easier. The da Vinci® Surgical System (Intuitive Surgical, Sunnyvale, CA), with its articulating, wristed instruments, has been adapted for

Fig. 20.4 Port placement for a robotic LESS pyeloplasty, (**a**) before and (**b**) after docking of the robot. In this case, two 5-mm robotic cannulas were used, along with two 12-mm laparoscopic ports. The robot's camera arm is docked to the top port and the lens is inserted in a "30° up" configuration. The bottom 12-mm trocar is used by the bedside assistant

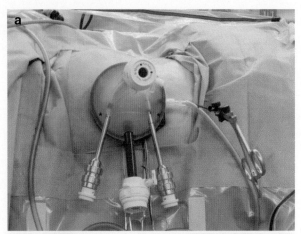

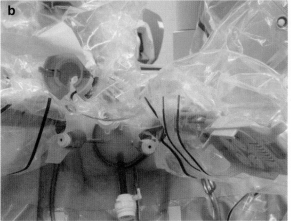

LESS by some authors. Just as in multiport surgery, robotics may be particularly helpful for reconstructive operations, such as pyeloplasty, where sewing is required.

A few cases of robotic LESS pyeloplasty have already been reported in the literature, and more are anticipated [2–4]. Our experience with robotic LESS pyeloplasty (unpublished data) suggests there are several modifications that can make this procedure easier to perform. We make a 2.5–3-cm curved umbilical incision and insert a GelPOINT® device (Applied Medical, Rancho Santa Margarita, CA) using the Hasson technique. Two pediatric 5-mm robotic ports, a 12-mm camera port, and a 10-mm assistant trocar are then preplaced through the gel in a diamond configuration (Fig. 20.4), with the camera port at the top and the assistant's trocar at the bottom. Pediatric instrumentation, as opposed to the standard 8-mm robotic instruments, occupies less of the limited incision space, reducing instrument conflict. The robot is then docked. We use an 8-mm robotic camera lens oriented in the 30° up configuration. This modification,

Fig. 20.5 The remote centers of the robotic ports ("*black lines*") are set at the level of the fascial incision and then the ports are arranged to "cross" each other. This increases the separation of the instrument tips, which decreases clashing and restores a degree of triangulation

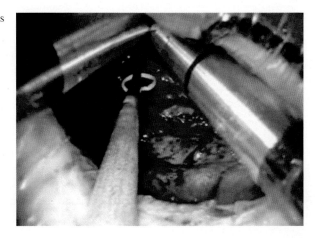

while different from what is typically used for robotic renal surgery, diminishes clashing between the camera and the robotic instruments as well as helps keep the assistant trocar from being blocked externally. A 5-mm hook cautery device and graspers are then inserted into the robotic cannula, whose "black lines," the remote centers, are set at the level of the fascial incision. We have found it very useful to insert the robotic instruments such that they cross each other just inside the fascial incision (Fig. 20.5). This crossing technique, also used by some surgeons in standard nonrobotic LESS, results in greater separation of the instruments, both in and outside the body, reducing clashing. In standard LESS, this technique can be challenging, since the instrument that comes in from the left side of the screen on the monitor is actually controlled by the surgeon's right hand, and vice versa. An advantage of the robotic platform is that the master controllers (right and left "hands") on the console can be swapped, avoiding this problem.

Once inserted and crossed, the tips of the instruments can be brought back toward each other using the wristed segment. One other difference we have noted, compared to traditional robotic renal surgery, is that all three of the robotic components (camera and two instruments) must be moved in unison in order to avoid clashing. In other words, if the surgeon wishes to move to a different part of the surgical field, he or she must alternately move the camera and working instruments together small distances in the same direction; otherwise, the camera would bump into them and be unable to move. In our experience, these modifications on traditional robotic surgery have a fairly short learning curve.

Once the robot is docked and the instruments positioned in this way, the rest of the steps of the procedure are unchanged. Due to the ease of sewing with robotic instrumentation, the use of the robotic platform negates the need for an additional instrument outside the LESS incision, used by many LESS surgeons to facilitate sewing the anastomosis.

Outcomes

Due to the relatively recent adoption of the LESS technique, the literature outlining outcomes of LESS pyeloplasty, particularly in the long term, is limited. Since the first LESS pyeloplasty was reported by Desai and colleagues in 2008 [5], a number of other series have been described using various port types as well as varying combinations of straight and articulating instruments [1, 2, 6–10]. Several authors have reported utilizing an additional small-caliber grasper, inserted through the lateral abdominal wall (outside the LESS port) to facilitate sewing.

There is a learning curve associated with any new technique, and LESS is no exception, particularly for a complex reconstructive operation such as pyeloplasty. This learning curve may result in an increased rate of complications early in one's experience. Indeed, an investigation into the complications associated with this learning curve by Best and colleagues found that 71 % of complications occurred in the first 10 cases of their 28 case series, with an overall complication rate of 25 % during their preliminary experience [11]. While most of the individual case series reported in the literature reported a low complication rate, a multiinstitutional study focusing on complication rates for a variety of LESS procedures found the incidence of complications to be 25.7 %, though most of these were minor and self-limited [7]. Importantly, the authors found a significant difference in complication rates between reconstructive and extirpative LESS procedures (27.1 vs. 7.8 %). While no prospective, randomized comparisons have been conducted to date, two institutions have performed matched comparisons between patients undergoing LESS or standard laparoscopic pyeloplasty. Stein et al. (16 LESS patients) [8] and Tracy et al. (14 LESS patients) [9] both found an equivalent length of stay, postoperative pain measures, and complication rates. They also found similar early success rates between conventional laparoscopic and LESS pyeloplasty. A longer follow-up will help determine if long-term success rates are indeed equivalent.

References

1. Rais-Bahrami S, Montag S, Atalla MA, et al. Laparoendoscopic single-site surgery of the kidney with no accessory trocars: an initial experience. J Endourol. 2009;23(8):1319–24.
2. Desai MM, Berger AK, Brandina R, et al. Laparoendoscopic single-site surgery: initial hundred patients. Urology. 2009;74(4):805–12.
3. Kaouk JH, Goel RK, Haber GP, et al. Robotic single-port transumbilical surgery in humans: initial report. BJU Int. 2009;103(3):366–9.
4. Stein RJ, White WM, Goel RK, et al. Robotic laparoendoscopic single-site surgery using GelPort as the access platform. Eur Urol. 2010;57(1):132–6.
5. Desai MM, Rao PP, Aron M, et al. Scarless single port transumbilical nephrectomy and pyeloplasty: first clinical report. BJU Int. 2008;101(1):83–8.
6. Desai MM, Stein R, Rao P, et al. Embryonic natural orifice transumbilical endoscopic surgery (E-NOTES) for advanced reconstruction: initial experience. Urology. 2009;73(1): 182–7.

7. Irwin BH, Cadeddu JA, Tracy CR, et al. Complications and conversions of upper tract urological laparoendoscopic single-site surgery (less): multicentre experience: results from the NOTES Working Group. BJU Int. 2011;107(8):1284–9.
8. Stein RJ, Berger AK, Brandina R, et al. Laparoendoscopic single-site pyeloplasty: a comparison with the standard laparoscopic technique. BJU Int. 2011;107(5):811–5.
9. Tracy CR, Raman JD, Bagrodia A, et al. Perioperative outcomes in patients undergoing conventional laparoscopic versus laparoendoscopic single-site pyeloplasty. Urology. 2009;74(5): 1029–34.
10. White WM, Haber GP, Goel RK, et al. Single-port urological surgery: single-center experience with the first 100 cases. Urology. 2009;74(4):801–4.
11. Best SL, Donnally C, Mir SA, et al. Complications during the initial experience with laparoendoscopic single site (LESS) pyeloplasty. BJU Int. 2011;108(8):1326–9.

Chapter 21
LESS: Extirpative Renal Surgery Including Donor

Dennis J. Lee and Mihir M. Desai

Keywords LESS • Nephrectomy • Robotic • Donor nephrectomy • Partial nephrectomy • Nephroureterectomy

Introduction

Since the first laparoscopic nephrectomy by Clayman et al. in 1991 [1], there has been a progressive development of minimally invasive urologic procedures. Upper and lower urinary tract procedures can be performed laparoscopically through the use of three to five laparoscopic ports. However, there are well-recognized complications related to port placement. These include risk of bleeding, infection, organ damage, and scar formation.

Ongoing refinement in surgical technique to reduce surgical morbidity and improve cosmesis has led to the development of laparoscopic surgery through a single incision site. Multiple monikers have been used to describe this approach, such as "single-port laparoscopic surgery" (SILS), "scarless surgery," and "one-port umbilical surgery" [2]. In 2010, the term "laparoendoscopic single-site surgery" and the LESS acronym were coined by consensus [3].

The initial reports of LESS nephrectomy were described by Rane and Raman [4, 5]. The usage of fewer port sites is believed to be associated with reduced morbidity, a lower incidence of port-site hernia, and improved cosmesis [6]. In addition, LESS has the potential to decrease postoperative pain, length of hospital stay (LOS), duration of recovery, and time to return to work in comparison with traditional laparoscopic surgery [7].

D.J. Lee, M.D. (✉) • M.M. Desai, M.D.
Department of Urology, University of Southern California Institute of Urology,
1441 Eastlake Avenue, Suite 7416, Los Angeles, CA 90089 USA
e-mail: dennisjl@use.edu; adityadesai2003@gmail.com

A. Rane et al. (eds.), *Scar-Less Surgery*,
DOI 10.1007/978-1-84800-360-6_21, © Springer-Verlag London 2013

267

The evolution of the LESS technique required the concomitant development of new laparoscopic access devices, instrumentation, and optics in order to accommodate the unique requirements of LESS.

Access during LESS can be obtained through multiple small-diameter trocars or through the use of multichannel ports [8]. Multichannel ports allow for the insertion of instruments and a camera through a single fascial incision. There are multiple ports made for LESS, such as TriPort®, previously known as R-Port (Olympus, Tokyo, Japan), and GelPOINT® (Applied Medical, Rancho Santa Margarita, CA). Due to the limited commercial availability of multichannel ports in some regions and the higher associated costs of multichannel ports, handmade ports have also been described in the literature. These handmade ports are made by placing an Alexis® wound retractor (Applied Medical, Rancho Santa Margarita, CA) into the incision and then placing trocars into the cut ends of a surgical glove. The trocars are then fixed into place using a silk tie or a rubber band [9].

Instrumentation also creates a distinct challenge in LESS. Conventional laparoscopic instruments can be used for LESS, but often result in suboptimal ergonomics for the surgeon. The parallel insertion of the instruments results in internal and external clashing and decreased maneuverability. These challenges have resulted in the development of articulating and prebent instruments. The modified instruments provide working space for the surgeon's hands, while keeping the instrument tips triangulated in the operative field. These changes result in better ergonomics and force application. In addition, needlescopic instruments have increased in popularity as an adjunct to LESS, as they can be introduced through a small puncture without a formal closure [8, 10].

Optics have also been optimized to accommodate the needs of LESS. Conventional laparoscopes result in external clashing because of their large camera head and light cable exiting at 90°. Newer scopes combine light and camera systems to keep the camera head and light cord out of the operative field. In addition, extra-long scopes allow the camera operator to work outside the operative space, providing the surgeon with more room to operate [8].

Robotic LESS urologic surgery has also been described in the literature using the da Vinci® Surgical System (Intuitive Surgical, Sunnyvale, CA). The robotic console provides a more ergonomic work setting for the surgeon and the EndoWrist® (Intuitive Surgical, Sunnyvale, CA) allows for more facile suturing. Access can be obtained via a GelPort. However, robotic LESS surgery still encounters problems inherent to the LESS approach: namely, limited range of motion, extracorporeal instrument clashing, and inability to use the fourth arm for tissue retraction [11]. Modifications to the existing platform have been tested in the experimental setting to overcome the parallel arrangement of instruments. The technique of "chopstick" surgery arranges ports so that instruments cross at the abdominal wall, thus separating the robotic arms. The left- and right-hand assignments are subsequently reassigned in the console to correct for the change in handedness [12]. New robotic equipment is also currently being developed for the application of LESS surgery. One such prototype is the VeSPA® surgical instrument (Intuitive Surgical, Sunnyvale, CA) designed for use with the da Vinci Si

Surgical System. The system involves semirigid instruments that are inserted through a multichannel port with curved cannulae. Initial studies have demonstrated feasibility in the porcine model [11].

LESS Nephrectomy

LESS nephrectomy is performed through the umbilicus or a single incision in the suprapubic crease. The operative steps follow that of conventional laparoscopic nephrectomy. Early reports mainly focused on the treatment of benign conditions, but more recent studies have expanded to include LESS for the management of renal tumors.

In their series of 100 LESS cases, Desai et al. reported the outcomes of 14 patients undergoing LESS simple nephrectomies (Table 21.1). The mean operative time (ORT) was 145 ± 69 min, the estimated blood loss (EBL) was 109 ± 81 ml, the hospital length of stay (LOS) was 2 ± 1 days, and the time to complete recovery was 32 ± 6 days. There were no conversions, and surgical outcomes were found to be comparable to conventional laparoscopy [10].

Raman et al. performed a retrospective case control study comparing LESS nephrectomy in 11 patients with conventional laparoscopic nephrectomy in 22 patients. The mean tumor size was 5.5 cm. The study found no difference in ORT, EBL, analgesic use, LOS, and complication rate. Patient benefit was found to be limited to a cosmetic advantage [13]. Raybourn et al. also found no difference when comparing ten LESS nephrectomies to ten laparoscopic simple nephrectomies [2].

Tugcu et al. subsequently performed a prospective randomized trial comparing LESS nephrectomy in 14 patients to standard laparoscopic nephrectomy in 13 patients for the treatment of benign disease. No difference was observed in ORT, EBL, transfusion rates, and LOS. However, the visual analog pain score (VAS) and use of postoperative analgesics were significantly lower in the LESS nephrectomy group in the days immediately following surgery (postoperative days 1–3). In addition, the time to return to normal activities was significantly shorter in the LESS nephrectomy group (10.7 vs. 13.5 days, $p = 0.001$). There were no intraoperative or postoperative complications in either group. LESS nephrectomy was found to be more expensive than conventional laparoscopy ($1,600–2,000 vs. $450–600) [14].

Stolzenburg et al. described their experience with LESS radical nephrectomy (RN) in 42 patients. The mean tumor size was 5.45 cm, ORT was 135 min (75–200), and EBL was 158 ml (50–1,100). All surgical margins were negative. An extra 3-mm needlescopic instrument was used in 19 patients. The authors found needlescopic instruments helpful for retraction of the liver in right-sided cases. Three cases were converted to conventional laparoscopy due to the need for retraction and hemostasis in two patients and extensive adhesions in one patient. Intraoperatively, a bowel injury was identified in one patient and repaired without need for colostomy [15].

Greco et al. reported their experience with LESS RN in 33 patients for renal tumor. The mean tumor size was 4.1 ± 1.4 cm, ORT was 143.7 ± 24.3 min, EBL was

Table 21.1 Summary of literature

Group (year)	Summary	Operative time (min) (range)	Complications	Comments
Nephrectomy				
Raman et al. (2009) [13]	Retrospective case control study: LESS NPX (N=11) vs. Lap NPX (N=22)	122 (90–210) vs. 125 (90–240), p=0.78	No complications	LESS NPX benefit limited to cosmesis
Tugcu et al. (2010) [14]	Prospective randomized trial – LESS NPX (N=14) vs. Lap NPX (N=13)	118±13 vs. 114±15, p=0.52	No major complications	Lower post-op analgesic requirements and shorter return to normal activities in LESS group
Stolzenberg et al. (2011)	LESS RN (N=42)	135 (75–200)	Three conversions to Lap, 1 bowel injury	
Robotic nephrectomy				
White et al. (2011) [22]	Matched comparison: R-LESS RN (N=10) vs. Lap RN (N=10)	167.5 (150–210) vs. 150 (150–173), p=0.28	No major complications	Lower narcotic usage and shorter LOS in R-LESS RN group
Retroperitoneal nephrectomy				
Chen et al. (2011) [23]	Retroperitoneal LESS NPX (N=16) for benign nonfunctional kidneys	85 (75–140)	No major complications	Use of one bent instrument and one straight instrument found to aid in triangulation
Partial nephrectomy				
Aron et al. (2009) [21]	LESS PN (N=5) with hilar clamping	270 (240–345)	Pseudoaneurysm requiring angio-embolization	LESS PN best suited for small, exophytic, anterior, lower pole tumors
Kaouk et al. (2009) [26]	Clampless LESS PN (N=5) and R-LESS PN (N=2)	160±25 and 170±57	One conversion to Lap	
Han et al. (2011) [28]	R-LESS PN (N=14) using homemade port	205 (140–365)	Two conversions to open surgery	
Nephroureterectomy				
Lee et al. (2011) [30]	LESS NephU (N=10) using homemade port	226±66	Two conversions to open surgery	
Khanna et al. (2011) [17]	R-LESS NephU (N=3)	300	One conversion to Lap	

Donor nephrectomy

Ramasamy et al. (2011) [34]	Retrospective comparison: LESS DN (N=101) vs. LLDN (N=663)	157 (84–257) vs. 148 (79–355), p=0.02	Overall complication rate 7.9 vs. 7.1 %. No difference in major complications	LESS DN: longer operative time, lower EBL, and shorter LOS. Higher WIT, but no difference in graft function
Canes et al. (2010) [36]	Matched-pair comparison: LESS DN (N=17) vs. LDN (N=17)	240 (180–495) vs. 222 (150–331), p=0.3	One LESS-DN patient developed allograft thrombosis	Shorter recovery with LESS DN, but higher WIT. No difference in graft function
Kurien et al. (2011) [37]	Randomized control trial: LESS DN (N=25) vs. LLDN (N=25)	172 ± 38 vs. 176 ± 48	Two patients in the LESS group required additional ports There were no major complications	LESS DN associated with less postoperative pain and shorter LOS, but higher WIT

Pediatric LESS surgery

Koh et al. (2010) [41]	LESS NPX for nonfunctional hydronephrotic kidneys (N=11)	139 (85–205)	Two patients developed ipsilateral unilateral hydroceles	

LLDN laparoendoscopic living donor nephrectomy, *LESS* laparoendoscopic single-site surgery, *DN* donor nephrectomy, *NPX* nephrectomy, *RN* radical nephrectomy, *PN* partial nephrectomy, *R-LESS* robotic laparoendoscopic single-site surgery, *Lap* conventional laparoscopic, *NephU* nephroureterectomy

122.3 ± 34.1 ml, VAS on discharge was 1.9 ± 0.8, and LOS was 3.8 ± 0.8 days. All tumors were organ-confined and all surgical margins negative. The conversion rate to conventional laparoscopy was 3 %. The overall complication rate was 12.1 %. Major complications requiring surgical repair were an incisional hernia and a bowel injury [7].

Seo et al. compared LESS RN in 10 patients with conventional laparoscopic RN in 12 patients who underwent surgery during the same time period. No cases were converted to conventional laparoscopic or open surgery. There was no difference in ORT, time to oral intake, pain control, LOS, and complication rate. There was a trend toward decreased blood loss in the LESS RN group (185.7 ± 121.9 vs. 324.0 ± 187.0, $p = 0.065$), but it was not statistically significant [9].

Robotic LESS (R-LESS) Nephrectomy

Robotic LESS (R-LESS) radical nephrectomy (PN) can be performed similarly to LESS nephrectomy using a GelPort access platform [16]. In their institutional experience with R-LESS, Khanna et al. performed R-LESS RN in 11 patients. The mean ORT was 172 min and LOS was 2.5 days. All patients had negative surgical margins. Complications included a seroma requiring drainage and skin cellulitis treated with antibiotics. One patient required transfusion for cardiac disease [17]. White et al. described a retrospective review of R-LESS RN in ten patients compared to a matched control group of conventional laparoscopic RN in ten patients. There was no difference in ORT, EBL, VAS, or complication rate. The robotic group had lower narcotic requirements (25.3 vs. 37.5 mg morphine equivalent, $p = 0.049$) and a shorter LOS (2.5 vs. 3.0 days, $p = 0.03$). No cases required the placement of additional trocars or conversion to laparoscopic or open surgery.

Retroperitoneal LESS Nephrectomy

LESS nephrectomy has also been described through a retroperitoneal approach. While the retroperitoneal approach does not offer the benefit of "scarless" surgery, it does have some distinct advantages. The retroperitoneal approach allows more direct access to the kidney and renal hilum, has a reduced need for the retraction of internal organs, and poses less risk of peritoneal contamination by spillage of urinary contents [18]. In addition, the retroperitoneal approach maintains peritoneal integrity, which can be important in end-stage renal disease patients who wish to perform peritoneal dialysis [19, 20].

The retroperitoneal approach offers a different set of surgical challenges. It is more difficult to check anatomical landmarks than transperitoneal R-LESS, and there is more clashing of laparoscopic instruments due to the relatively smaller working space [18]. Bent instruments are often not suitable for the retroperitoneal space, and flexible instruments have been found to be insufficient for providing the robust retraction and dissection necessary in a retroperitoneal LESS nephrectomy [21].

White et al. reported their initial experience with retroperitoneal LESS. The series included cryoablation, partial nephrectomy, metastectomy, and cyst decortication. They reported that the retroperitoneal approach is superior to the transperitoneal approach in posterior lesions and patients who have undergone previous intraabdominal surgery. In addition, the authors commented that LESS is better than standard laparoscopic retroperitoneal surgery because of improved cosmesis and likely decreased risk of inadvertent peritonotomy and epigastric vessel or bowel injury [22].

Chen et al. performed retroperitoneal LESS nephrectomy in 16 patients for the management of benign nonfunctioning kidneys. The mean ORT was 85 min (75–140), EBL was 56 ml (20–110), the mean time to resuming oral diet 1.5 days, and LOS was 4 (3–5) days. One case was converted to open surgery for failure to progress in a patient with genitourinary tuberculosis resulting in severe adhesions surrounding the kidney. No major intraoperative or postoperative complications were observed. The authors found the removal of retroperitoneal fat and adjacent tissue outside Gerota's fascia helpful in overcoming the limitations of the working space. In addition, they recommended using one bent instrument and one straight instrument to achieve triangulation. This helps avoid clashing because of the different instrument lengths [23]. Similar findings were documented by Chueh et al. in their retrospective review of retroperitoneal LESS nephrectomies for a variety of indications [19].

The use of retroperitoneal LESS RN using a homemade port for the management of renal masses in six patients was reported by Chung et al. The mean ORT was 235 min (190–335), EBL was 42 ml (10–100 ml), the time to oral intake was 45.4 h (12–72), and LOS was 5.8 days (5–8). All procedures were performed using standard laparoscopic instruments, and no conversions or complications were noted [20]. Pak et al. also described their experience with retroperitoneal LESS nephrectomy using a homemade port in their clinical series. Four patients underwent RN, with a mean ORT of 227.5 ± 50 min, EBL of 170 ± 156.8 ml, and LOS of 3.7 ± 0.5 days. Ten patients underwent simple nephrectomy, with a mean ORT of 168.7 ± 29.2 min, EBL of 113 ± 149.8 ml, and LOS of 4.6 ± 1.5 days. One patient required a transfusion, but there were no major perioperative complications [21].

LESS Partial Nephrectomy

Partial nephrectomy (PN) has become the standard for the surgical management of localized renal masses. PN achieves oncologic outcomes comparable to RN, while maximizing preservation of renal function [24]. LESS PN, while technically demanding, is feasible in carefully selected patients.

Aron et al. reported their experience with LESS PN in five patients. PN was performed using renal hilar clamping and sutured renal reconstruction. The median tumor size was 3 cm (1–5.9), ORT was 270 min (240–345), EBL was 150 ml (100–600), VAS 48 h after surgery was 2 (0–6), and the median LOS was 3 days (3–22). The median WIT was 20 min (11–29). An additional 5-mm port was required in one case to aid in retraction of the liver. There were no intraoperative complications and all surgical margins were negative. The postoperative course of one patient was complicated by a pulmonary embolism and bleeding from a pseudoaneurysm. Based on their experience, the authors recommended avoiding LESS PN in (1) patients with enlarged livers because of difficult retraction; (2) obese/tall patients because of difficultly reaching the hilum and adequately mobilizing the upper pole of the kidney; and (3) patients with solitary kidneys or renal insufficiency if hilar clamping is necessary [25].

In an attempt to minimize the risk of ischemic renal injury, Kaouk et al. performed LESS PN in five patients without hilar clamping. Hemostasis was obtained using argon beam coagulation, surgicel, and various bioglues. The mean tumor size was 2.1 ± 1.1 cm, ORT was 160 ± 25 min, EBL was 420 ± 475 ml, VAS at discharge was 1.7 ± 1.2, and LOS was 3.2 ± 1.6 days. One case was converted to standard laparoscopy to control bleeding in a difficult location. The patient required transfusion with 2 units and underwent 16 min of WIT. One patient with a negative intraoperative frozen margin had a final positive pathology. Based on their experience, the authors concluded that LESS PN is best suited for small, exophytic, anterior, lower pole tumors [26].

More recently, Cindolo et al. reported their experience with LESS PN in six patients performed without hilar clamping. Hemostasis was obtained using electrocautery and a bolster. The mean renal size was 2.1 cm (1–3.5), ORT was 148 min (30–550), EBL was 201 ml (30–550), the time to oral intake was 2.6 days, and LOS was 6 days (3–10). One case was converted to standard laparoscopy because of excessive bleeding in a patient with a posterior tumor. No transfusions were necessary. One patient suffered a cerebrovascular accident postoperatively with subsequent transitory left hemiparesis [27].

R-LESS Partial Nephrectomy

The R-LESS approach has been used to manage small renal masses. The robotic platform improves surgeon ergonomics and aids in the steep learning curve associated with pure LESS.

Kaouk et al. reported on the feasibility of R-LESS PN in two patients. PN was performed without hilar clamping, and hemostasis was obtained using argon beam coagulation, surgicel, and various bioglues. The mean tumor size was 2.0 ± 1.2 cm, ORT was 170 ± 57 min, EBL was 100 ml, VAS was 1 ± 0.5, and LOS was 3.5 ± 0.7 days. There were no conversions. The authors found endophytic and upper pole tumors to be particularly challenging secondary to suboptimal exposure and access [26].

In their institutional experience with LESS, Khanna et al. reported their experience with R-LESS PN in five patients. PN was performed without hilar clamping and hemostasis was obtained similar to the Kaouk series. The mean tumor size 4.0 cm, ORT was 172 min, EBL was 242 ml, and LOS was 2.8 days. All patients had negative surgical margins. One case was converted to standard robotic PN due to impaired access to an upper pole lesion and difficulty with liver retraction [17].

More recently, Han et al. reported their experience with R-LESS PN in 14 patients using a homemade port. An additional 12- mm port was placed below the subxiphoid process or alongside the single port. The additional "hybrid" port was used during suturing of the renal defect in right-sided masses. Switching between the assistant port and robotic instrument ports was found to extend the instrument reach and decrease clashing. The mean tumor size was 3.2 cm (1.2–6.5), ORT was 233 min (140–365), EBL was 464 ml (30–1,850), LOS was 5.2 days (3–11), and the mean ischemia time was 30 min (16–43). There were no port-related complications and all surgical margins were negative. However, 11 patients required transfusions, and 2 cases were converted to open surgery [28].

LESS Nephroureterectomy

There are only a handful of studies evaluating LESS nephroureterectomy. Most comprise a small subset description in published operative series for LESS.

In their series of 100 patients who underwent LESS procedures, Desai et al. reported two patients who underwent LESS nephroureterectomy. The ORT were 90 and 200 min, EBL 75 and 300 ml, and LOS 5 and 1 days. There were no complications, or conversions, but an additional 5-mm port was added in one case. The distal ureter was managed by cystoscopic resection and laparoscopic EndoGIA™ stapling (Covidien, Dublin, Ireland) of the distal ureter [10].

Alternative techniques for management of the distal ureter have been published. Ponsky et al. described their technique for performing LESS nephroureterectomy completely through a Pfannenstiel incision in one patient. The kidney and ureter were mobilized through a Pfannenstiel single port, and an open bladder cuff was taken through the same incision to remove the distal ureter. The ORT was 409 min, EBL was 200 ml, and LOS was 4 days. The surgical margin was negative. The main challenge of operating through a Pfannenstiel incision was the extended distance from the incision to the kidney, which was overcome with the use of bariatric instruments [29].

Lee et al. published their experience with pure LESS nephroureterectomy for the surgical management of upper tract urothelial carcinoma using a homemade port in 10 patients. The distal ureter was managed by circumferentially dissecting around the ureteral orifice and resecting the ureter through an extravesical approach. The resulting bladder defect was closed in two layers. The mean ORT was 225.63 ± 65.87 min, but significantly decreased with increasing experience. The mean EBL was 187.50 ± 83.45 ml and the LOS was 4.75 ± 3.37 days. There was one positive surgical margin in a pT3N2 disease. An open incision was required to complete the renal hilar lymphadenectomy in one case, and an open Gibson incision was required due to severe adhesions around the distal ureter in a second case. There were no major complications [30].

Khanna et al. described their experience performing R-LESS nephroureterectomy in three patients. Each case in the series was performed differently. In the first case, the distal ureter was managed through an open Gibson incision. In the second case, the GelPort was placed through a Gibson incision, and the same incision was used to manage the distal ureter. In the third case, the nephrectomy was performed through the umbilicus using the GelPort. The robot was then reoriented toward the pelvis to perform the distal ureterectomy. The mean ORT was 300 min, EBL was 183 ml, and LOS was 3.3 days. There were no major complications. One case was converted to standard laparoscopy due to difficulty visualizing and accessing the upper pole of the kidney when the single port was placed through a Gibson. All surgical margins were negative. There was no evidence of disease recurrence at 17.8 months [17].

LESS Donor Nephrectomy

Laparoscopic living-donor nephrectomy (LDN) has been the standard of care since its introduction in 1995 [31]. This has led to decreased morbidity, improved cosmesis, and shorter recovery time. Studies have shown laparoscopic donor nephrectomy (DN) produces allografts of similar immediate and long-term function to open surgery [32, 33]. Efforts are constantly being made to further decrease the morbidity to the donor. LESS DN can be the potential next step, given the development of multichannel ports and articulating instruments. LESS can minimize the morbidity associated with extra trocar sites, such as hernias, pain, and bleeding due to epigastric vessel injury [34].

The first LESS DN was performed by Gill et al. in 2008 through an intraumbilical incision in four patients. The LESS DN technique otherwise duplicated the steps of a conventional laparoscopic donor nephrectomy. At the time the procedure was performed, it was called "embryonic natural orifice transumbilical endoscopic surgery" (E-NOTES) [35]. Since that time, multiple studies have demonstrated the feasibility and efficacy of LESS DN.

Ramasamy et al. retrospectively compared conventional LDN in 663 patients vs. LESS DN in 101 patients. LESS DN was found to have a longer mean ORT (156.8 vs. 148 min, $p=0.02$), lower EBL (91.3 vs. 121.9 ml, $p=0.003$), higher oral but lower intravenous hospital analgesic requirements ($p<0.001$ and 0.002, respectively), and shorter LOS (2.4 vs. 2.9 days, $p<0.001$). The LESS DN group had a higher WIT (3.9 vs. 4 min, $p=0.03$), but the graft function was similar to that of conventional LDN. There was no difference in the overall 30 days' complication rate (7.1 vs. 7.9 %, $p>0.05$). There was one major complication (Clavien grade 3–5) in the LESS DN group and eight major complications in LDN group. One LDN patient required conversion to open for a vascular complication [34].

Canes et al. performed a matched-pair comparison between 17 LESS DN and LDN patients. There was no difference in ORT, EBL, LOS, or VAS. After discharge,

LESS DN was associated with significantly fewer days on oral pain medication (6 vs. 20 days, $p=0.01$), days off work (18 vs. 46 days, $p=0.0009$), and days to 100 % physical recovery (29 vs. 83 days, $p=0.03$). WIT was higher in LESS (6.1 vs. 3 min, $p<0.0001$); however, graft function was immediate and comparable between groups. One allograft in the LESS group thrombosed postoperatively [36].

Kurien et al. reported the results of their randomized clinical trial comparing LESS DN ($N=25$) vs. LDN ($N=25$). There was no difference in ORT and EBL. The postoperative patient pain scores were significantly lower in the LESS DN after 48 h (1.24 ± 0.72 vs. 2.08 ± 0.91, $p=0.0004$). The LESS DN had a shorter LOS (3.92 ± 0.76 vs. 4.56 ± 0.82 days, $p=0.003$). The WIT in the LESS DN group (5.11 ± 1.01 vs. 7.15 ± 1.84 min, $p<0.0001$) was longer, but the total ischemia times in both groups were similar. There was no difference in intraoperative (16 vs. 8 %, $p=0.2$) and postoperative complications (16 vs. 20 %, $p=0.99$). One patient in the LDN group suffered sudden cardiac death, resulting in graft loss. There was no graft loss in the LESS DN group. The estimated glomerular filtration rates of recipients at 1 year were comparable for both groups. The donor's quality of life, body image, and cosmetic scores were comparable for both groups [37].

Afaneh et al. published a retrospective matched-pair comparison between LESS DN and LDN in 50 patients. The mean ORT was greater in LESS (166 ± 28.7 vs. 129 ± 29.8 min, $p<0.0001$), with a trend toward decreasing operative time with increasing case number. There was no difference in EBL, VAS, or LOS. Patients reported a shorter time to complete recovery in LESS DN patients (24.4 ± 5.3 vs. 27.0 ± 4.9 days, $p=0.01$). There was no difference in WIT or the number of complications. One LESS DN patient was converted to hand-assisted laparoscopy because of GelPort device leakage and failure to maintain a pneumoperitoneum. A second patient was converted to conventional laparoscopy to optimize hilar dissection. There was one major complication in the LESS DN group, a grade 3 laceration to the posterior midpole cortex during extraction. The allograft maintained normal function and the patient's creatinine was 1.08 at 15 months. One patient in the LPN group had one adrenal vein injury and another patient had a splenic laceration [33].

It is critical to ensure the safety of the donor and harvesting of the donor allograft in perfect condition. The largest concern is increased WIT, likely due to the extra time needed to create an adequate fascial incision for allograft extraction [34, 36, 37]. However, most available evidence suggests that the range of WIT reported in the literature has a negligible effect on both short- and long-term allograft function [33, 36].

LESS DN has much potential to minimize morbidity to the donor. LESS provides improved cosmesis and less morbidity from trocar-associated pain. A common complaint in LPN patients is lingering discomfort in the lower quadrant trocar incision. This is the main working port during LDN and is eliminated with the LESS technique [36].

LESS DN has a steep learning curve. However, with proper training, careful patient selection, and thorough planning, LESS DN has the potential to become the future gold standard procedure [38].

Pediatric LESS Surgery

Modifications to adult laparoscopic techniques for pediatric patients have resulted in the successful application of laparoscopic surgery in children [39]. LESS has been used for multiple procedures in children, such as nephrectomy, orchiectomy, and varicocelectomy [40]. Their well-defined tissue planes, minimal intraabdominal fat, and relatively thin abdominal walls make pediatric patients ideal for the application of laparoscopic techniques. However, their smaller internal working space and large equipment size relative to pediatric patients makes LESS challenging.

Koh et al. presented the largest series of LESS nephrectomy to date for poorly functioning hydronephrotic kidneys in patients ranging in age from infants to adolescents. The mean operative time was 139 min (85–205), EBL was 18 ml (5–150), and LOS was 1.5 days (1.0–2.1). A 3-mm needlescopic accessory port was used early in the experience in five cases. No intraoperative complications were noted. Postoperatively, two boys developed unilateral ipsilateral hydroceles. The mean operative times and LOS were comparable to that of conventional laparoscopy in children. Pediatric LESS procedures have been demonstrated to be feasible in multiple studies and warrant further study [40–42].

Conclusions

An increasing body of literature has shown LESS to be safe and effective with outcomes that may be comparable to conventional laparoscopic surgery. LESS offers the potential for improved cosmesis and faster rehabilitation, but is associated with increased cost and unique surgical challenges. As technique, experience, and equipment continue to improve for LESS, perioperative outcomes should continue to improve and patient demand can be expected to rise.

Patient safety is paramount. Patients' interest in "scarless" outcomes after surgery has been shown to be secondary to increased risk of complications and morbidity [43]. Careful patient selection is critical for the successful application of LESS. The current literature suggests that the ideal urologic LESS candidate is a nonobese (BMI < 30) patient of average height, without prior abdominal surgery, being treated for benign disease. The procedure must be performed by a surgeon proficient in standard laparoscopic techniques [44]. Surgeons should start with benign conditions, as malignant disease at pathology has been shown to be a predictive factor for complications after LESS [45]. Ultimately, future well-designed studies are necessary to determine the long-term safety, efficacy, and appropriate indication of LESS for urologic conditions.

References

1. Clayman R, Kavoussi LR, Soper N, et al. Laparoscopic nephrectomy: initial case report. J Urol. 1991;146:278.
2. Raybourn III JH, Rane A, Sundaram CP. Laparoendoscopic single-site surgery for nephrectomy as a feasible alternative to traditional laparoscopy. Urology. 2010;75:100.
3. Gill I, Advincula A, Aron M, et al. Consensus statement of the consortium for laparoendoscopic single-site surgery. Surg Endosc. 2010;24:762.
4. Rane A, Rao P, Rao P. Single-port-access nephrectomy and other laparoscopic urologic procedures using a novel laparoscopic port (R-port). Urology. 2008;72:260.
5. Raman JD, Bensalah K, Bagrodia A, et al. Laboratory and clinical development of single keyhole umbilical nephrectomy. Urology. 2007;70:1039.
6. Eisenberg MS, Cadeddu JA, Desai MM. Laparoendoscopic single-site surgery in urology. Curr Opin Urol. 2010;20:141.
7. Greco, F., Veneziano, D., Wagner, S. et al.: Laparoendoscopic Single-Site Radical Nephrectomy for Renal Cancer: Technique and Surgical Outcomes. European Urology, 2012;62:168.
8. Autorino R, Cadeddu JA, Desai MM, et al. Laparoendoscopic single-site and natural orifice transluminal endoscopic surgery in urology: a critical analysis of the literature. Eur Urol. 2011;59:26.
9. Seo I, Lee J, Rim J. Laparoendoscopic single-site radical nephrectomy: a comparison with conventional laparoscopy. J Endourol. 2011;25:465.
10. Desai MM, Berger AK, Brandina R, et al. Laparoendoscopic single-site surgery: initial hundred patients. Urology. 2009;74:805.
11. Haber G-P, White MA, Autorino R, et al. Novel robotic da Vinci instruments for laparoendoscopic single-site surgery. Urology. 2010;76:1279.
12. Joseph R, Goh A, Cuevas S, et al. "Chopstick" surgery: a novel technique improves surgeon performance and eliminates arm collision in robotic single-incision laparoscopic surgery. Surg Endosc. 2010;24:1331.
13. Raman JD, Bagrodia A, Cadeddu JA. Single-incision, umbilical laparoscopic versus conventional laparoscopic nephrectomy: a comparison of perioperative outcomes and short-term measures of convalescence. Eur Urol. 2009;55:1198.
14. Tugcu V, Ilbey Y, Mutlu B, et al. Laparoendoscopic single-site surgery versus standard laparoscopic simple nephrectomy: a prospective randomized study. J Endourol. 2010;24:1315.
15. Stolzenburg J-U, Kallidonis P, Ragavan N, et al. Clinical outcomes of laparo-endoscopic single-site surgery radical nephrectomy. World J Urol. 2011. doi:10.1007/s00345-011-0765-1 [Epub ahead of print].
16. Stein RJ, White WM, Goel RK, et al. Robotic laparoendoscopic single-site surgery using GelPort as the access platform. Eur Urol. 2010;57:132.
17. Khanna R, Stein R, White M, et al. Single institution experience with robotic laparoendoscopic single site renal procedures. J Endourol. 2012;26(3):230–4.
18. Hemal A. Laparoscopic retroperitoneal extirpative and reconstructive renal surgery. J Endourol. 2011;25:209.
19. Chueh S-CJ, Sankari BR, Chung S-D, et al. Feasibility and safety of retroperitoneoscopic laparoendoscopic single-site nephrectomy: technique and early outcomes. BJU Int. 2011; 108:1879.
20. Chung S-D, Huang C-Y, Tsai Y-C, et al. Retroperitoneoscopic laparo-endoscopic single-site radical nephrectomy (RLESS-RN): initial experience with a homemade port. World J Surg Oncol. 2011;9:138.
21. Pak C-H, Baik S, Kim CS. Initial experience with retroperitoneal laparoendoscopic single-site surgery for upper urinary tract surgery. Korean J Urol. 2011;52:842.

22. White, M.A., Autorino, R., Spana, G. et al.: Robotic Laparoendoscopic Single-Site Radical Nephrectomy: Surgical Technique and Comparative Outcomes. European Urology, 2011;59: 815.
23. Chen, Z., Chen, X., Luo, Y. et al.: Retroperitoneal Laparoscopic Single-Site Simple Nephrectomy: Initial Experience. J Endourol, 2012;26:647.
24. Patil MB, Lee DJ, Gill IS. Eliminating global renal ischemia during partial nephrectomy: an anatomical approach. Curr Opin Urol. 2012;22:83–7.
25. Aron M, Canes D, Desai MM, et al. Transumbilical single-port laparoscopic partial nephrectomy. BJU Int. 2009;103:516.
26. Kaouk JH, Goel RK. Single-port laparoscopic and robotic partial nephrectomy. Eur Urol. 2009;55:1163.
27. Cindolo L, Berardinelli F, Gidaro S, et al. Laparoendoscopic single-site partial nephrectomy without ischemia. J Endourol. 2010;24:1997.
28. Han WK, Kim DS, Jeon HG, et al. Robot-assisted laparoendoscopic single-site surgery: partial nephrectomy for renal malignancy. Urology. 2011;77:612.
29. Ponsky LE, Steinway ML, Lengu IJ, et al. A Pfannenstiel single-site nephrectomy and nephroureterectomy: a practical application of laparoendoscopic single-site surgery. Urology. 2009;74:482.
30. Lee J, Kim S, Moon H, et al. Initial experience of laparoendoscopic single-site nephroureterectomy with bladder cuff excision for upper urinary tract urothelial carcinoma performed by a single surgeon. J Endourol. 2011;25:1763.
31. Ratner L, Ciseck L, Moore R, et al. Laparoscopic live donor nephrectomy. Transplantation. 1995;60:1047.
32. Nicholson ML, Kaushik M, Lewis GRR, et al. Randomized clinical trial of laparoscopic versus open donor nephrectomy. Br J Surg. 2010;97:21.
33. Afaneh C, Aull MJ, Gimenez E, et al. Comparison of laparoendoscopic single-site donor nephrectomy and conventional laparoscopic donor nephrectomy: donor and recipient outcomes. Urology. 2011;78:1332.
34. Ramasamy R, Afaneh C, Katz M, et al. Comparison of complications of laparoscopic versus laparoendoscopic single site donor nephrectomy using the modified Clavien grading system. J Urol. 2011;186:1386.
35. Gill IS, Canes D, Aron M, et al. Single port transumbilical (E-NOTES) donor nephrectomy. J Urol. 2008;180:637.
36. Canes D, Berger A, Aron M, et al. Laparo-endoscopic single site (LESS) versus standard laparoscopic left donor nephrectomy: matched-pair comparison. Eur Urol. 2010;57:95.
37. Kurien A, Rajapurkar S, Sinha L, et al. Standard laparoscopic donor nephrectomy versus laparoendoscopic single-site donor nephrectomy: a randomized comparative study. J Endourol. 2011;25:365.
38. Desai M. Single-port surgery for donor nephrectomy: a new era in laparoscopic surgery? Nat Clin Pract Urol. 2009;6:1.
39. Lee DJ, Kim PH, Koh CJ. Current trends in pediatric minimally invasive urologic surgery. Korean J Urol. 2010;51:80.
40. Kocherov S, Lev G, Shenfeld OZ, et al. Laparoscopic single site surgery: initial experience and description of techniques in the pediatric population. J Urol. 2011;186:1653.
41. Koh CJ, De Filippo RE, Chang AY, et al. Laparoendoscopic single-site nephrectomy in pediatric patients: initial clinical series of infants to adolescents. Urology. 2010;76:1457.
42. Cabezalí Barbancho D, Gómez Fraile A, López Vázquez F, et al. Single-port nephrectomy in infants: initial experience. J Pediatr Urol. 2011;7:396.
43. Bucher P, Pugin F, Ostermann S, et al. Population perception of surgical safety and body image trauma: a plea for scarless surgery? Surg Endosc. 2011;25:408.
44. Gettman MT, White WM, Aron M, et al. Where do we really stand with LESS and NOTES? Eur Urol. 2011;59:231.
45. Greco F, Cindolo L, Autorino R, et al. Laparoendoscopic single-site upper urinary tract surgery: assessment of postoperative complications and analysis of risk factors. Eur Urol. 2012;61(3):510–6.

Chapter 22
LESS: Adrenal Surgery

Soroush Rais-Bahrami and Lee Richstone

Keywords Adrenalectomy•Laparoscopy•Retroperitoneoscopy•Pheochromocytoma Aldosteronoma • Adrenal cortical carcinoma

Introduction

History of Minimally Invasive Adrenal Surgery

Adrenal surgery has been an operative niche shared by urologists and general surgeons. Traditionally, adrenal surgery has provided extirpative options for adrenal tumors, including those suspicious for adrenal cortical carcinoma, functional adrenal adenomas, and cases where metastectomy of adrenal lesions were targeted. With the advent of laparoscopy, minimally invasive surgical access to the adrenal glands forged ahead, beginning with its first report in 1992 [1]. The anatomic position of the adrenals located within the upper retroperitoneum inspired surgeons to further expand upon traditional transperitoneal laparoscopy and explore the retroperitoneoscopic approach [2].

These minimally invasive approaches bear an inherent appeal especially for surgery on the adrenal glands as they are small and deeply seated, where exposure and visualization are of paramount importance. Moreover, given the typically small size of the adrenal specimen, there is an inherent opportunity to minimize the incision size, thereby providing better cosmesis. Additional goals include the improvement of postoperative pain and shortening of the convalescence period [3]. Some studies have also described fewer complications and reduced costs with the laparoscopic

S. Rais-Bahrami, M.D. (✉) • L. Richstone, M.D.
The Smith Institute for Urology, The Hofstra-North Shore LIJ School of Medicine,
450 Lakeville Road Suite M41, New Hyde Park 11040, NY, USA
e-mail: soroushraisbahrami@gmail.com; lrichsto@nshs.edu

A. Rane et al. (eds.), *Scar-Less Surgery*,
DOI 10.1007/978-1-84800-360-6_22, © Springer-Verlag London 2013

approach compared to open surgery in addition to improved convalescence [4, 5]. Currently, laparoscopic adrenalectomy has surpassed open surgery in many centers and serves as the gold standard for the treatment of most adrenal lesions [6, 7]. With added experience and more surgeons performing laparoscopy, the realm of laparoscopic adrenalectomy has since been expanded with attempts to provide organ-sparing surgery, minimize operative morbidity, and further improve cosmetic outcomes. To provide these outcome goals, laparoscopic partial adrenalectomy, robot-assisted laparoscopic approaches, and laparoendoscopic single-site (LESS) adrenalectomy have been reported and are beginning to take shape in high-volume centers.

Development of LESS for Adrenal Surgery

Hirano and colleagues reported the first series of patients undergoing a single-port adrenalectomy in 2005 [8]. This report predated the majority of LESS urologic surgery that emerged in the latter part of the same decade. It detailed a retroperitoneoscopic single-site approach successfully accomplished in 53 patients without insufflation performed via a single large port placed through a 4.5-cm flank incision.

Since this initial report, a number of case reports, retrospective series, and protocolled cohort and randomized studies have reported various techniques, operative feasibility, and comparative outcomes of LESS adrenalectomy as a new modality for extirpative adrenal surgery [9–13]. Also, the expansion to LESS adrenalectomy took shape with proof-of-concept investigations in porcine and human cadaver models with the goal of achieving "no visible scar" postoperatively [14]. Furthermore, descriptions of LESS partial adrenalectomy and LESS bilateral adrenalectomy have also been published as case reports [15, 16].

Largely, the data on this topic have presented a wide spectrum of operative approaches, all with the intended goals of minimizing apparent incisional scars and improving postoperative outcome measures, including convalescence. Also, they focus on the utmost goals of maintaining equivalent safety and surgical outcomes as measured by complication rates and pathologic outcomes.

Current State of LESS Adrenal Surgery

Instrumentation

LESS surgery is a natural extension of conventional laparoscopy further minimizing incisions to perform equivalent intracorporeal surgical operations. However, to facilitate the use of a single operative site traversed by the laparoscope and working instruments, novel access platforms and modified instruments have been developed specific to this field. The wide variety of unique ports, smaller, flexible fiber optic laparoscopes, and flexible or prebent working instruments specific to LESS surgery are discussed in greater detail in other chapters of this text. For access specific to the adrenal gland, depending on the approach, a host of access platforms can be employed, as outlined in Table 22.1.

Table 22.1 Access platforms specific to the adrenal gland, depending on the approach

R-Port®	Advanced Surgical Concepts; Dublin, Ireland
TriPort™	Two 5-mm ports, one 12-mm port, one insufflation channel
	Incision required: 1.0–2.5 cm
	Disposable
QuadPort™	Two configurations: (1) four 12-mm ports, one insufflation channel, (2) two 12-mm ports, one 5-mm port, and one 15-mm port, one insufflation channel
	Incision required: 2.5–6.0 cm
	Disposable
Uni-X™	Pnavel Systems; Brooklyn, NY
	Three 5-mm ports, one insufflation channel
	Incision required: 2 cm
	Disposable
UNO	Ethicon Endo-Surgery; Cincinnati, OH
	Two 5-mm ports, one 15-mm port with 5-mm reducer cap
	Incision required: 1.5 cm
	Disposable
X-Cone	Storz; Tuttlingen, Germany
	Four 5-mm ports, one 5–13-mm port
	Incision required: 2.5–3 cm
	Reusable with up to 20 sterilizations
Gel-Port®/Gel-POINT®	Applied Medical; Rancho Santa Margarita, CA
	Accepts multiple conventional trocars or direct insertion of instruments
	Incision required: 1.5–7 cm
	Disposable
SILS™ Access	Covidien; Hamilton HM FX, Bermuda
	Three foam insertion sites for passage of low-profile trocars
	Incision required: 2.5–3 cm
	Disposable
AirSeal®	Surgiquest; Orange, CT
	Uses recirculating CO_2 to create seal, may pass multiple instruments through ports of varying calibers
	Incision required: 1.5–2.5 cm
	Disposable
SPIDER® Platform	TransEnterix; Morrisville, NC
Regular	Two 6-mm flexible instrument delivery tubes and two 6-mm rigid channels
	Incision required: 1.7 cm
	Reusable components
Advanced	Two 6-mm flexible instrument delivery tubes, one 6-mm rigid channel, and one 13-mm rigid channel
	Incision required: 2.3 mm
	Reusable components

Surgical Approaches

Surgical approaches for LESS adrenal surgery are either transperitoneal or retroperitoneal, mimicking the surgical techniques used during conventional laparoscopy and open surgery. A transperitoneal approach can be achieved via a periumbilical or nonumbilical location [17–20]. The benefits of the transperitoneal approach include a wider working space within a pneumoperitoneum, allowing for more fascile instrument manipulation. For some surgeons, the transperitoneal approach allows for a more controlled dissection with clearly defined anatomic landmarks. However, the added bowel manipulation and retraction used may lead to longer operative times.

The incision within the umbilical ring postoperatively hides well within the skin folds of the umbilicus, providing essentially no visible scar. In cases of obese patients in which the periumbilical access incision must be lateralized, there is a small incisional scar resulting outside the umbilical ring postoperatively. Similarly, transperitoneal LESS surgery via a mini-Pfannenstiel incision provides a small postoperative scar, but this is commonly well masked by hair growth or clothing [21]. However, this suprapubic or mini-Pfannenstiel incision is not commonly used for LESS adrenal surgery compared to extirpative LESS renal surgery.

The retroperitoneoscopic technique has been described as either a lateral or posterior incision approach [8, 12, 22]. Those that prefer the retroperitoneoscopic technique for adrenal surgery largely elect to use this approach for its direct route to the adrenals and reduced manipulation of intraperitoneal structures, including the bowel and other organs that otherwise must be retracted to allow for visualization and dissection. Although the incision is minimized, the retropertoneoscopic approach through either a small flank or posterior incision will be in a visible area of the body.

Indications

The vast majority of adrenal lesions are amenable to laparoscopic adrenlaectomy as offered by many urologists and general surgeons. Functional adrenal neoplasms suspected to be benign lesions are the most common targets for adrenalectomy and present the largest body of laparoscopic and LESS adrenalectomy experience. Reports of LESS adrenalectomy have documented resection of pheochromocytomas, aldosterone-producing adenomas, and corticosteroid-producing adenomas.

Rarely, in select patients with lesions suspected to be metastases to the adrenal gland, they will be resected if they are a solitary focus and can render the patient with no evidence of residual disease. These cases of metastasectomy have been reported for a number of different primary cancer types [23–25]. Data on laparoscopic adrenalectomy and furthermore LESS adrenalectomy for resection of metastatic lesions are limited [26–28].

Lastly, laparoscopy, and now LESS surgery, enter a debated arena for the treatment of larger adrenal masses suspicious for adrenal cortical carcinoma. As with any oncologic operation, the goal is that of complete, intact resection, from which this debate stems. This controversy exists between open and laparoscopic surgeries for possible adrenal malignancy, but the current standard of care recommends that large adrenal masses or masses with other characteristics suspicious for adrenal cortical carcinoma should be approached via a traditional open surgical resection. Nevertheless, laparoscopic adrenalectomy for these larger masses has been reported with successful and durable results [29–31].

Special Techniques

The techniques employed for LESS adrenalectomy largely mirror the techniques used during conventional laparoscopic adrenalectomy, whether done via a transperitoneal or retroperitoneal approach. This section will highlight techniques and instrument use specific to the success of LESS surgery of the adrenal gland.

The patients are positioned in a modified flank or flank position as preferred for each of the approaches employed. For the transperitoneal procedure, it is essential to have complete colonic reflection, which frees an instrument from providing bowel retraction. For left-sided surgery, complete lateral dissection of the spleen for medial mobilization provides optimal visualization and operative access to the adrenal gland.

To overcome the challenge of liver retraction for right-sided LESS adrenal surgery, an independent instrument is often required to provide retraction or elevation of the liver edge. If the access platform being used does not provide an adequate number of ports to allow access for a liver retractor in addition to the laparoscope and working instruments used for dissection, a needlescopic instrument can be introduced without inserting additional trocars [32]. The use of these needlescopic instruments has been described and modifications specific to liver retraction have been reported whereby gauze was placed at the tips of these very narrow-tipped forceps to create a blunter retraction device [33].

Vascular control and hemostasis are essential principles of all surgical techniques. However, with more minimally invasive approaches being used that limit the number of instruments and the flexibility of reach, these principles are ever more important to maintain throughout the course of the operation. Depending on the trocar sizes of the access platform used, various sizes of coagulating devices, including the LigaSure™ device (Valleylab, Boulder, CO), and harmonic scalpels have been described [17]. The LigaSure™ device allows for a combination of blunt dissection, coagulation of vessels and tissue edges, and precise sharp incision through coagulated tissues.

Reported Experience

Currently, a wide range of reports exists in the literature supporting LESS adrenalectomy as a feasible surgical technique with reliable outcomes. Largely, the data are retrospective and descriptive in nature. However, there is a move toward prospective case-matched controls comparing LESS to conventional laparoscopy head to head.

To date, the body of literature on the subject of LESS adrenalectomy is representative of the experience of multiple institutions worldwide. This signifies a global adoption of these techniques to potentiate even more minimally invasive surgery in the future, and these efforts are instrumental in validating the value of LESS as a possible frontier to this end.

Postoperative convalescence is a major endpoint to consider with LESS surgery. A contemporary series of transperitoneal LESS adrenalectomies reported equivalent perioperative outcomes (operative time, blood loss, complication rates, and hospital stay) with significantly less postoperative pain compared to conventional laparoscopic adrenalectomies [13]. In this study, the patients were well matched in the two groups by preoperative parameters, including sex, age, tumor size, and indications for adrenalectomy. The LESS cohort of patients demonstrated lower analgesic requirements as measured by the duration of intravenous patient-controlled analgesia use. Also, a matched-pair comparison of retroperitoneal LESS adenalectomy compared to standard retroperiteoscopic adrenalectomy revealed similar results, albeit with a longer operative time in this early experience [12]. In this study, patients undergoing LESS were matched in a 1:2 ratio to conventional retroperitoneoscopic adrenalectomy performed by the same surgeon and were found to have significantly less in-hospital analgesic use. Walz and colleagues reported a case-control study of retroperitoneal LESS versus conventional retroperitoneoscopic adrenalectomy and found a significantly shorter hospital stay [34].

Limitations

The limitations of LESS adrenalectomy have been reported in a number of papers but mostly as isolated discussion points addressing complications encountered, the number of intraoperative conversions in early series, and suggestions of how to overcome the technical challenges inherent to the operative approach. Complications have been reported in the early series of LESS adrenalectomy in 0–10.5 % of cases, which includes major and minor complications combined [12, 32, 33]. Of note, the vast majority of complications reported were minor, requiring no operative or interventional treatments. However, major complications reported after LESS adrenalectomy include bleeding requiring transfusion, postoperative hypocortisolism, fulminant hepatitis, and pulmonary embolism.

A focus on technical difficulties was provided by Ishida and colleagues [33]. They reported on the challenges and technical difficulties specific to LESS adrenalectomy in comparison to conventional laparoscopic adrenalectomy performed by a single surgeon. They reported equal rates of complications and a statistically equivalent volume of estimated blood loss in the two patient cohorts. They did find that LESS adrenalectomy required more "one-handed manipulation" and "tissue regrasping" compared to the conventional laparoscopic approach with multiple tro-cars, allowing for improved instrument triangulation and complimentary functions. A temporal analysis did find that the duration of "one-handed manipulation" did decrease as surgeon experience with the LESS approach increased. This work is unique in quantitatively assessing these intraoperative parameters often described as the challenges to the single-site technique.

With any new advancement or modification in technique, rates of intraoperative conversion to the established, gold standard technique serve as a benchmark of feasibility. In one of the earliest LESS adrenalectomy series, 53 patients with adre-nal tumors were treated successfully with a retroperitoneoscopic adrenalectomy via a 4.5-cm trocar and one patient (1.9 %) required conversion to open surgery sec-ondary to excessive blood loss from an adrenal vein injury [8]. In subsequent reports, rates of conversion to open surgery as well as conversion to conventional laparoscopy, whereby additional ports are placed, have been reported. Overall, a conversion to multiple-incision laparoscopy and open adrenalectomy has been reported in 0–11 % and 0–1.9 % of cases, respectively [2, 13, 33, 35]. However, the rates of conversion may be underreported, as there are few prospective studies reporting LESS adrenalectomy in the literature. The vast majority of studies are retrospective in nature and occasionally report the conversion to conventional lap-aroscopy or open surgery as a discussion point rather than as a consistently reported parameter.

Future Directions

Advances in Technology

With continued efforts to minimize operative morbidity by developing minimally invasive surgical techniques, LESS adrenalectomy has proven its versatility and opened an arena of potential discovery and advancement. Since 2005, LESS adrena-lectomy has been performed through different incisions and with the use of numer-ous different access ports and instruments. As the field of LESS surgery expands for adrenal and nonadrenal surgery, so too will the multitude of options for different operative devices associated with the field.

Access platforms have evolved dramatically and are recognized as a fundamental underpinning of LESS surgery. There are advances underway to improve the cost-effectiveness and availability of ports, as most marketed designs are disposable and costly compared to conventional laparoscopic trocars. Several groups have reported their use of "homemade" ports and described these functional designs of LESS access platforms for potential widespread use [35–37]. Future iterations of access ports are also considering the maintenance of stable pneumoperitoneum pressures while considering the added torque applied to the trocar components during LESS surgery due to limited work space and challenges with triangulations inherent to the single-site approach.

Research efforts for improved laparoscopes and working instrumentation are also under way to facilitate the application and advancement of LESS surgery. Many surgeons largely use standard laparoscopic instruments, employing specialized articulating instruments designed for LESS surgery only when necessary [38]. Robotic LESS has been reported, describing the use of the da Vinci® Surgical System (Intuitive Surgical, Sunnyvale, CA) [39, 40]. Efforts are under way to develop smaller motorized robot systems either as an adjunct to the conventional laparoscopic tools or integrated into these working instruments to allow for articulation to overcome the inherent challenges of LESS [41].

Advances with optical imaging have provided for smaller, flexible laparoscopes allowing for LESS surgery. However, in the future, these technologies may be shrunk further to be incorporated into the access trocar or developed as intracorporeal robotic devices that are implanted at the beginning of the case and retrieved prior to closure, to further minimize the size of the operative incision and eliminate an instrument in the limited operative workspace [42–44].

Expanding Experience

LESS urologic surgery has been demonstrated as the next evolutionary step, expanding upon conventional laparoscopy. Developed and supported for its proposed benefits of improved convalescence and cosmesis, this modified extension of laparoscopy has been reported as a feasible and safe operation for adrenal surgery. However, as with all surgical advances, the dissemination of LESS surgery is dependent upon the realized value of its use. Furthermore, it must prove reproducible beyond selected innovative centers of excellence that have reported their early experiences to date, in order to be a widespread option for patients.

As the experience and acceptance of LESS increases, trainees of minimally invasive surgery will have increased exposure to the unique techniques used to overcome the challenges of single-site surgery and then will be able to propagate these skills into their respective practices, both private and academic-based worldwide [45]. As LESS diffuses throughout the experience of more residents and fellows in training and enters the realm of private community practices, the number of cases will inevitably increase. With further development of LESS-designed access platforms, instrumentation, and robotic compatibility, this evolutionary step may provide a growing niche for urologic surgery with expanding indications.

Series of LESS adrenalectomy have begun to provide matched-cohort and prospective comparative studies. However, in the future, more prospective and preferably randomized studies are required to provide high-level evidence to support LESS surgery for all the benefits over its foundational techniques of conventional laparoscopy and endoscopy from which it stems [46].

Conclusions

LESS adrenalectomy has been reported as a safe and feasible extension of conventional laparoscopy to minimize incisions as well as decrease postoperative pain and convalescence time without significantly compromising other operative parameters. This technique has been used in a variety of centers for extirpative surgery for a wide range of adrenal pathologies. In the future, LESS adrenal surgery will likely be provided as a viable surgical option by more urologists, providing a more minimally invasive approach than the current gold standard laparoscopic adrenalectomy for most adrenal masses.

References

1. Gagner M, Lacroix A, Bolté E. Laparoscopic adrenalectomy in Cushing's syndrome and pheochromocytoma. N Engl J Med. 1992;327(14):1033.
2. Zhang X, Fu B, Lang B, Zhang J, Xu K, Li HZ, Ma X, Zheng T. Technique of anatomical retroperitoneoscopic adrenalectomy with report of 800 cases. J Urol. 2007;177(4):1254–7.
3. Hansen P, Bax T, Swanstrom L. Laparoscopic adrenalectomy: history, indications, and current techniques for a minimally invasive approach to adrenal pathology. Endoscopy. 1997;29(4):309–14.
4. Guazzoni G, Montorsi F, Bocciardi A, Da Pozzo L, Rigatti P, Lanzi R, Pontiroli A. Transperitoneal laparoscopic versus open adrenalectomy for benign hyperfunctioning adrenal tumors: a comparative study. J Urol. 1995;153(5):1597–600.
5. Schell SR, Talamini MA, Udelsman R. Laparoscopic adrenalectomy for nonmalignant disease: improved safety, morbidity, and cost-effectiveness. Surg Endosc. 1999;13(1):30–4.
6. Smith CD, Weber CJ, Amerson JR. Laparoscopic adrenalectomy: new gold standard. World J Surg. 1999;23(4):389–96.
7. Vargas HI, Kavoussi LR, Bartlett DL, Wagner JR, Venzon DJ, Fraker DL, Alexander HR, Linehan WM, Walther MM. Laparoscopic adrenalectomy: a new standard of care. Urology. 1997;49(5):673–8.
8. Hirano D, Minei S, Yamaguchi K, Yoshikawa T, Hachiya T, Yoshida T, Ishida H, Takimoto Y, Saitoh T, Kiyotaki S, Okada K. Retroperitoneoscopic adrenalectomy for adrenal tumors via a single large port. J Endourol. 2005;19(7):788–92.
9. Tunca F, Senyurek YG, Terzioglu T, Sormaz IC, Tezelman S. Single-incision laparoscopic left adrenalectomy. Surg Laparosc Endosc Percutan Tech. 2010;20(4):291–4.
10. Ryu DS, Park WJ, Oh TH. Retroperitoneal laparoendoscopic single-site surgery in urology: initial experience. J Endourol. 2009;23(11):1857–62.
11. Perretta S, Allemann P, Asakuma M, Dallemagne B, Marescaux J. Adrenalectomy using natural orifice translumenal endoscopic surgery (NOTES): a transvaginal retroperitoneal approach. Surg Endosc. 2009;23(6):1390.
12. Shi TP, Zhang X, Ma X, Li HZ, Zhu J, Wang BJ, Gao JP, Cai W, Dong J. Laparoendoscopic single-site retroperitoneoscopic adrenalectomy: a matched-pair comparison with the gold standard. Surg Endosc. 2011;25:2117–24. Epub 2010 Dec 18.
13. Jeong BC, Park YH, Han DH, Kim HH. Laparoendoscopic single-site and conventional laparoscopic adrenalectomy: a matched case-control study. J Endourol. 2009;23(12):1957–60.
14. Allemann P, Perretta S, Marescaux J. Surgical access to the adrenal gland: the quest for a "no visible scar" approach. Surg Oncol. 2009;18(2):131–7.

15. Yuge K, Miyajima A, Hasegawa M, Miyazaki Y, Maeda T, Takeda T, Takeda A, Miyashita K, Kurihara I, Shibata H, Kikuchi E, Oya M. Initial experience of transumbilical laparoendoscopic single-site surgery of partial adrenalectomy in patient with aldosterone-producing adenoma. BMC Urol. 2010;10:19.

16. Jeong CW, Park YH, Shin CS, Kim HH. Synchronous bilateral laparoendoscopic single-site adrenalectomy. J Endourol. 2010;24(8):1301–5.

17. Nozaki T, Ichimatsu K, Watanabe A, Komiya A, Fuse H. Longitudinal incision of the umbilicus for laparoendoscopic single site adrenalectomy: a particular intraumbilical technique. Surg Laparosc Endosc Percutan Tech. 2010;20(6):e185–8.

18. Castellucci SA, Curcillo PG, Ginsberg PC, Saba SC, Jaffe JS, Harmon JD. Single port access adrenalectomy. J Endourol. 2008;22(8):1573–6.

19. Cindolo L, Gidaro S, Tamburro FR, Schips L. Laparo-endoscopic single-site left transperitoneal adrenalectomy. Eur Urol. 2010;57(5):911–4.

20. Rais-Bahrami S, Montag S, Atalla MA, et al. Laparoendoscopic single-site surgery of the kidney with no accessory trocars: an initial experience. J Endourol. 2009;23(8):1319–24.

21. Andonian S, Herati AS, Atalla MA, Rais-Bahrami S, Richstone L, Kavoussi LR. Laparoendoscopic single-site pfannenstiel donor nephrectomy. Urology. 2010;75(1):9–12.

22. Walz MK, Alesina PF. Single access retroperitoneoscopic adrenalectomy (SARA) – one step beyond in endocrine surgery. Langenbecks Arch Surg. 2009;394(3):447–50.

23. Collinson FJ, Lam TK, Bruijn WM, de Wilt JH, Lamont M, Thompson JF, Kefford RF. Long-term survival and occasional regression of distant melanoma metastases after adrenal metastasectomy. Ann Surg Oncol. 2008;15(6):1741–9.

24. Ambrogi V, Tonini G, Mineo TC. Prolonged survival after extracranial metastasectomy from synchronous resectable lung cancer. Ann Surg Oncol. 2001;8(8):663–6.

25. Kohli M, Viswamitraa S, Schaefer R, Faas FH, Kumar U. Metastasectomy for isolated bilateral adrenal metastases in hormone-refractory prostate cancer. Clin Adv Hematol Oncol. 2006;4(10):754–5.

26. Mazzaglia PJ, Vezeridis MP. Laparoscopic adrenalectomy: balancing the operative indications with the technical advances. J Surg Oncol. 2010;101(8):739–44.

27. Asbun HJ, Straznicka M, Strong VE. The role of minimal access surgery for metastasectomy and cytoreduction. Surg Oncol Clin N Am. 2007;16(3):607–25, ix.

28. Cindolo L, Gidaro S, Neri F, Tamburro FR, Schips L. Assessing feasibility and safety of laparoendoscopic single-site surgery adrenalectomy: initial experience. J Endourol. 2010;24(6): 977–80.

29. Fassnacht M, Allolio B. What is the best approach to an apparently nonmetastatic adrenocortical carcinoma? Clin Endocrinol (Oxf). 2010;73(5):561–5.

30. Brix D, Allolio B, Fenske W, Agha A, Dralle H, Jurowich C, Langer P, Mussack T, Nies C, Riedmiller H, Spahn M, Weismann D, Hahner S, Fassnacht M, German Adrenocortical Carcinoma Registry Group. Laparoscopic versus open adrenalectomy for adrenocortical carcinoma: surgical and oncologic outcome in 152 patients. Eur Urol. 2010;58(4):609–15.

31. Sharma R, Ganpule A, Veeramani M, Sabnis RB, Desai M. Laparoscopic management of adrenal lesions larger than 5 cm in diameter. Urol J. 2009;6(4):254–9.

32. Gill IS, Advincula AP, Aron M, Caddedu J, Canes D, Curcillo 2nd PG, Desai MM, Evanko JC, Falcone T, Fazio V, Gettman M, Gumbs AA, Haber GP, Kaouk JH, Kim F, King SA, Ponsky J, Remzi F, Rivas H, Rosemurgy A, Ross S, Schauer P, Sotelo R, Speranza J, Sweeney J, Teixeira J. Consensus statement of the consortium for laparoendoscopic single-site surgery. Surg Endosc. 2010;24(4):762–8.

33. Ishida M, Miyajima A, Takeda T, Hasegawa M, Kikuchi E, Oya M. Technical difficulties of transumbilical laparoendoscopic single-site adrenalectomy: comparison with conventional laparoscopic adrenalectomy. World J Urol. 2010 [Epub ahead of print].

34. Walz MK, Groeben H, Alesina PF. Single-access retroperitoneoscopic adrenalectomy (SARA) versus conventional retroperitoneoscopic adrenalectomy (CORA): a case-control study. World J Surg. 2010;34(6):1386–90.

35. Chung SD, Huang CY, Wang SM, Tai HC, Tsai YC, Chueh SC. Laparoendoscopic single-site (LESS) retroperitoneal adrenalectomy using a homemade single-access platform and standard laparoscopic instruments. Surg Endosc. 2011;25(4):1251–6.
36. Jeon HG, Jeong W, Oh CK, Lorenzo EI, Ham WS, Rha KH, Han WK. Initial experience with 50 laparoendoscopic single site surgeries using a homemade, single port device at a single center. J Urol. 2010;183(5):1866–71.
37. Lee SW, Lee JY. Laparoendoscopic single-site urological surgery using a homemade single port device: the first 70 cases performed at a single center by one surgeon. J Endourol. 2011;25(2):257–64.
38. Zhang X, Shi TP, Li HZ, Ma X, Wang BJ. Laparo-endoscopic single site anatomical retroperitoneoscopic adrenalectomy using conventional instruments: initial experience and short-term outcome. J Urol. 2011;185(2):401–6.
39. Kaouk JH, Goel RK, Haber GP, Crouzet S, Stein RJ. Robotic single-port transumbilical surgery in humans: initial report. BJU Int. 2009;103(3):366–9.
40. Stein RJ, White WM, Goel RK, Irwin BH, Haber GP, Kaouk JH. Robotic laparoendoscopic single-site surgery using GelPort as the access platform. Eur Urol. 2010;57(1):132–6.
41. Göpel T, Härtl F, Schneider A, Buss M, Feussner H. Automation of a suturing device for minimally invasive surgery. Surg Endosc. 2011;25:2100–4. Epub 2011 Feb 7.
42. Terry BS, Ruppert AD, Steinhaus KR, Schoen JA, Rentschler ME. An integrated port camera and display system for laparoscopy. IEEE Trans Biomed Eng. 2010;57(5):1191–7.
43. Swain P, Austin R, Bally K, Trusty R. Development and testing of a tethered, independent camera for NOTES and single-site laparoscopic procedures. Surg Endosc. 2010;24(8): 2013–21.
44. Raman JD, Scott DJ, Cadeddu JA. Role of magnetic anchors during laparoendoscopic single site surgery and NOTES. J Endourol. 2009;23(5):781–6.
45. Kaouk JH, Autorino R, Kim FJ, Han DH, Lee SW, Yinghao S, Cadeddu JA, Derweesh IH, Richstone L, Cindolo L, Branco A, Greco F, Allaf M, Sotelo R, Liatsikos E, Stolzenburg JU, Rane A, White WM, Han WK, Haber GP, White MA, Molina WR, Jeong BC, Lee JY, Linhui W, Best S, Stroup SP, Rais-Bahrami S, Schips L, Fornara P, Pierorazio P, Giedelman C, Lee JW, Stein RJ, Rha KH. Laparoendoscopic single-site surgery in urology: worldwide multi-institutional analysis of 1076 cases. Eur Urol. 2011;60(5):998–1005.
46. Tracy CR, Raman JD, Cadeddu JA, Rane A. Laparoendoscopic single-site surgery in urology: where have we been and where are we heading? Nat Clin Pract Urol. 2008;5(10):561–8.

Chapter 23
LESS: Pelvic Reconstructive Urological Surgery

André Luis de Castro Abreu and Monish Aron

Keywords LESS • Laparoendoscopic single-site surgery • Reconstructive surgery
Pelvic urological surgery • Reconstructive urological surgery • Single port • LESS
urology • Pelvic reconstructive urological surgery

Abbreviations

EBL   Estimated blood loss
LOS   Length of stay
OR   Operating room
VAPS   Visual analog pain scale
LESS   Laparoendoscopic single-site surgery
BMI   Body mass index

Introduction

Over the last two decades, laparoscopic urologic surgery has become an established
approach for the treatment of various urological diseases [1, 2]. Since the very
beginning, pioneers in laparoscopic urology were at a disadvantage not just from the
viewpoint of defining and learning a new procedure, but also from the lack of appropriate instruments [3]. In the early days, laparoscopic urological procedures were
primarily extirpative. With increasing experience and the development of new tools,
laparoscopic surgery became more widespread. Nowadays, even complex

A.L. de Castro Abreu, M.D. (✉) • M. Aron, M.D., MCh, FRCS
Department of USC Institute of Urology, Center for Advanced Robotic and Laparoscopy
Surgery, USC Institute of Urology, Keck Medical Center of USC, University of Southern
California, 1411 East Lake Avenue, Suite 7416, Los Angeles, CA 90089-2211, USA
e-mail: andreluisabreu@gmail.com; monisharon@hotmail.com

A. Rane et al. (eds.), *Scar-Less Surgery*,
DOI 10.1007/978-1-84800-360-6_23, © Springer-Verlag London 2013

reconstructive urological procedures can be performed laparoscopically that compare favorably to conventional open surgery [4].

The fundamental rationale behind the success of laparoscopy is the reduced trauma of access while reproducing the excellent outcomes of open surgery with the benefits of a quicker recovery, decreased blood loss, decreased postoperative pain, and superior cosmesis, among others. Conventional laparoscopic procedures are performed using multiple ports placed in different parts of the abdomen, which allows triangulated access to the organ of interest. The triangulation between the ports allows excellent visualization of the operative field and facilitates the optimal angles to retract structures and perform a variety of surgical maneuvers.

Most recently, laparoendoscopic single-site surgery (LESS) emerged as an evolution of conventional laparoscopy to further improve cosmesis and provide a potentially "scarless" surgery [5, 6].

LESS most commonly uses a multichannel device through a single skin incision to perform laparoscopic interventions [7]. Despite the "loss" of traditional triangulation between ports, a wide variety of extirpative and reconstructive urinary tract surgeries have been performed using the LESS platform [8].

In this chapter, we present a review of the literature pertaining to the use of LESS in reconstructive pelvic urologic surgery.

Materials and Methods

A comprehensive electronic literature review was performed using PubMed as the source, for papers published in the English language between and including January 2001 and June 2011. The keywords used for the search were "LESS," "single port," "laparoendoscopic single-site surgery," "reconstructive urologic surgery," and "pelvic reconstructive urologic surgery" [9].

Results

A total of eight original articles met the criteria of LESS for pelvic reconstructive urological surgery although there was some overlap of cases among the case series reported [10–17].

The results are summarized in Tables 23.1, 23.2, and 23.3. Overall, reconstructive pelvic urological surgeries were performed in 27 patients, encompassing six different types of procedures. The most common procedure ($n=14$, 52 %) was abdominal sacrocolpopexy. In three cases (11.1 %), the da Vinci® (Intuitive Surgical, Sunnyvale, CA) robot assisted LESS sacrocolpopexy. The mean age of the patients ranged from 20 to 77 years, and the mean BMI ranged from 26 to 31.5 kg/m². In 92 % ($n=24$) of the cases, the approach was transperitoneal with the single port

Table 23.1 Demographics of LESS reconstructive urological pelvic surgery series

Author	Procedure	n	Indication	Technique	Age (year)[a]	BMI (kg/m^2)[a]	Previous surgery
White[b] [10, 11]	ASC[c]	10	POP I (1), POP II (9)	Retroperitoneal mesh	59.5	25.8	Pelvic surgery for prolapse in five patients
White[b] [11]	Ureteral reimplant	1	NA	Psoas hitch	NA	NA	NA
Tome [12]	ASC	1	POP 4	Retroperitoneal mesh	52	NA	Vaginal hysterectomy, TOT, perineoplasty
Ingber [13]	Excision of foreign body in the bladder	2	Sling mash inside bladder	Sling mesh excision	77	31.5	Midurethral sling
Stolzenburg [14]	Bladder diverticulectomy	4	8.5 (4–9) cm bladder diverticulum	Bladder diverticulectomy	51	26	NA
Desai[d] [15, 16]	Ureteral reimplant	2	Ureteral stricture	Psoas hitch[d]	42, 22	25, 20	Vaginal hysterectomy
Desai[d] [15, 16]	Ileal ureter	3	Ureteral stricture	Ileal ureter replacement	49 (25)	26 (2)	Ureteral instrumentation for recurrent stone disease
Nogueira [17]	Augmentation enterocystoplasty	1	Neurogenic bladder	Subtotal cystectomy + enterocystoplasty	20	NA	NA

ASC abdominal sacral colpopexy, n number of patients, POP pelvic organ prolapse, BMI body mass index, TOT transobturatory sling, NA not available

[a]Results in mean (standard deviation)

[b]The same group published 13 ASC in the same year, including two robotic LESS cases. We assume that it was the same cohort of patients with the addition of three new cases

[c]Concomitant procedures were performed: tension-free vaginal tape (1), trans-obturator tape (5), and vaginal cystocele repair (1) were performed

[d]The same author published in the same year a ureteral reimplant using a Psoas hitch ($n = 1$) technique; in the other case the technique was not mentioned

Table 23.2 Instruments used for LESS reconstructive urological pelvic surgery

Procedure	Port type	Instrument type	Camera type
ASC [10, 11]	Uni-X	Standard and articulating	5-mm flexible; 0°
Ureteral reimplant [11]	NA	da Vinci platform	da Vinci platform
ASC [12]	Alexis + hand-made	Conventional laparoscopic	10-mm rigid; 0°
Excision of foreign body in the bladder [13]	TriPort	Standard and articulating	NA
Bladder diverticulectomy [14]	TriPort	Straight and prebent	5-mm HD 30°
Ureteral reimplant [15, 16]	R-Port	Straight and prebent	5-mm 30° rigid or 0° flexible-tip
Ileal ureter [15, 16]	R-Port	Straight and prebent	5-mm 30° rigid or 0° flexible-tip
Augmentation enterocysto-plasty [17]	QuadPort	Standard and articulating	5-mm flexible; 0°

ASC abdominal sacral colpopexy, *NA* not available

placed at the umbilicus, and the mean skin incision length ranged from 1.5 to 5 cm (Table 23.1). In 25 (96 %) procedures, commercial ports available in the market were used with or without articulating or prebent instruments and flexible-tip cameras specifically designed for LESS (Table 23.2).

The mean operative time ranged from 113 to 300 min, and the mean estimated blood loss ranged from 47.5 to 250 ml. Blood transfusion was not required in any case. Except for one series of abdominal sacrocolpopexy, all other series employed additional maneuvers such as percutaneous placed sutures, additional transperitoneal needlescopic grasper, transurethral grasper, extracorporeal knots, or exteriorization of the bowel, to expose the operative field or to facilitate retraction or suturing.

There were no conversions to standard laparoscopic, robotic, or open surgery. There were no intraoperative complications. Only one (3.7 %) postoperative complication occurred. It was anastomotic urine leak requiring nephrostomy tube in one patient that underwent ileal ureter replacement. No patient died. In three series, the visual analog pain scale (VAPS, minimum 1 and maximum 10) scores were evaluated; the mean VAPS ranged from 0.7 to 3. The mean hospital stay ranged from 19.25 h to 6 days. Cosmesis was not evaluated by any validated questionnaires in any series. There was no recurrence or treatment failure during the short follow-up (Table 23.3).

Discussion

With the evolution of laparoscopy in the last two decades and with increasing experience, even advanced reconstructive surgeries can be performed laparoscopically [4]. Although feasible, complex reconstructive urological procedures requiring

Table 23.3 Intraoperative and follow-up of LESS reconstructive urological pelvic surgery

Procedure	Access	Incision (cm)[a]	Additional port or maneuver	VAPS[a]	OR time (min)[a]	EBL (ml)[a]	LOS (days)[a]	Conversion/ complication	Follow-up
ASC [10, 11]	Umbilicus; transperitoneal	1.8	None	0.7/10	162 (25)	47.5	1.5	No/no	6 months; one vaginal cystocele repair and two TVT
Ureteral reimplant [11]	NA	NA	NA	3/10	180	100	3	No/no	MAG3 normal
ASC [12]	Umbilicus; transperitoneal	3.5	None[b] (external sutures, knotless)	NA	150	100	<1	No/no	3 months, apical anatomic success
Excision of foreign body in the bladder [13]	Transvesical	1.5	None[c] (transurethral grasper)	3/10	113	100	<1	No/no	7 months; no mesh erosion recurrence
Bladder diverticulectomy [14]	Umbilicus; transperitoneal	NA	None[d] (external sutures)	1.25	130 (median)	<150	NA	No/no	1, 3, and 6 months; not detailed
Ureteral reimplant [15, 16]	Umbilicus; transperitoneal	2	2-mm grasper	NA	210, 140	100, 250	2	No/no	Unobstructed drainage
Ileal ureter [15, 16]	Umbilicus; transperitoneal	3	2-mm grasper[e] (exteriorized bowel)	NA	330 (42)	170 (113)	4	No/1[f]	Unobstructed drainage
Augmentation enterocystoplasty [17]	Umbilicus; transperitoneal	5	None[e] (exteriorized bowel)	NA	300	<100	6	No/no	1-month improvement in bladder capacity

ASC abdominal sacral colpopexy, *NA* not available, *TVT* tension-free vaginal tape, *VAPS* visual analog pain scale, *OR* operating room, *EBL* estimated blood loss, *LOS* hospital stay

[a]Results in mean (standard deviation)

[b]Two external (percutaneous) sutures were used to retract the sigmoid colon (laterally) and the vagina (anteriorly) and weck clips were applied at the end of the stitch to avoid intracorporeal knots

[c]In one patient a transurethral Maryland grasper was used to aid suturing and hemostasis

[d]External (percutaneous) suture was used to retract the diverticulum

[e]Bowel was exteriorized to prepare the ileal graft and to reconstruct the bowel

[f]Anastomotic urine leak requiring nephrostomy drainage in one patient

[g]Bowel was exteriorized to prepare the graft and to reanastomose the bowel. A combination of intracorporeal and extracorporeal knot tying was used to facilitate the anastomosis

extensive intracorporeal suturing remain challenging. With an aim to further improve cosmesis and decrease surgical morbidity, LESS emerged as an evolution of the conventional laparoscopic procedure.

In this chapter we reviewed the LESS literature pertaining to pelvic reconstructive urological surgery. LESS is still in its infancy; many surgeons are still on the learning curve, and the development of specialized instruments is still lagging behind surgical needs. Pelvic reconstructive urological LESS poses multiple challenges, and this is one of the reasons behind the paucity of publications in this area. In fact, a recent multiinstitutional analysis showed that 86 % of LESS urological procedures were performed in the upper urinary tract and 84 % were extirpative or ablative [18]. To our knowledge, there are no urinary diversions performed by LESS yet, but complex procedures like bladder augmentation and ileal ureteral replacement have been safely performed through single-port techniques [15, 16]. Kaouk et al. [19] performed LESS radical cystectomy in three patients, but the urinary diversions were performed extracorporeally.

Certainly, the most challenging issues with LESS come from its use of a single incision to perform major laparoscopic procedures. As such, the instruments and camera are in close proximity to each other. This makes the operative field crowded, externally and internally, and hence instrument clashing is common both externally and internally. Another major technical challenge of LESS is the lack of triangulation between the instruments. Therefore, retraction and countertraction as well as achieving optimum angles for intracorporeal suturing are difficult. In the series reviewed in this chapter, additional 2-mm needlescopic instruments, percutaneous sutures, or exteriorizing the bowel were some of the maneuvers employed to improve visualization, optimize retraction and countertraction, as well as facilitate suturing and knotting.

Indeed, Desai et al. [15, 16] and Noguera et al. [17] exteriorized the bowel during LESS ileal ureter and bladder augmentation, respectively. This was reported to facilitate either ileal graft preparation as well as bowel reconstruction, thereby decreasing the operative time. The use of ancillary needlescopic instruments during LESS does not invalidate the surgery as a LESS procedure [7]. Desai et al. [15, 16] have reported the use of needlescopic instruments to perform ureteral reimplantation and ileal ureter replacement directly through a skin puncture without using an additional port.

The surgical device industry is actively developing new instruments, cameras, and robotic systems to assist LESS. In fact, the majority of the series in this review used articulating instruments and flexible-tip cameras as well as prebent instruments to improve the feasibility of LESS, especially for reconstructive procedures. White et al. [10, 11] successfully used robotic technology to assist LESS in three cases. Indeed, the use of robots can be the link to facilitate LESS, improve ergonomics and visualization, and increase degrees of freedom of the surgical instruments, thereby facilitating dissection and suturing [20, 21].

There is a lack of randomized studies comparing different approaches such as LESS, conventional laparoscopy, robotics, or open surgery for pelvic reconstructive urological surgeries. White et al. [10] compared 30 patients who underwent abdominal sacrocolpopexy according to the approach: 10 laparoscopic, 10 robotic, and 10 LESS. They reported no significant difference in terms of OR time, EBL, VAPS, or LOS among the groups. Performing LESS ureteral reimplant in two cases, Desai et al. [15] reported an OR time of 240 and 140 min, EBL of 100 and 250 cc, and LOS of 2 days. These results are comparable to those reported by Seideman et al. [22] performing conventional laparoscopic reimplantation, although this group performed Boari flap in 21 patients (47 %). For ileal ureter replacement, again, OR time (470 vs. 330 min), EBL (375 vs. 170 cc), and LOS (5 vs. 4 days) are comparable when performed by conventional laparoscopy or LESS, respectively [15, 23]. Noguera et al. [17] performing LESS enterocystoplasty reported similar results as Gill et al. [24], who reported the initial cases of conventional laparoscopic enterocystoplasty. Both exteriorized the bowel to prepare the ileal graft as well as complete the bowel anastomosis. The OR time, EBL, and LOS were 5 versus 5.3 h, <100 versus 50 cc, 6 versus 7 days, respectively, for LESS versus standard laparoscopic bladder augmentation.

There was only one complication reported in the series reviewed in this paper. It was an anastomotic urine leak requiring drainage. Also, there were no conversions to standard laparoscopy, or to open surgery. In the largest series reported with LESS so far, the overall intraoperative and postoperative complications were 3.3 % and 9.5 %, respectively, and the rate of conversion was 20.8 % [18]. The very low complication rate noted in this review of LESS pelvic reconstruction could be attributed to the small number of patients, careful case selection, and surgeon/team experience with standard laparoscopic as well as LESS procedures [7].

Conclusions

LESS pelvic reconstruction is still in its infancy, although complex reconstructive procedures have been reported with gratifying results. Additional studies with larger numbers of patients as well as prospective randomized studies are still needed to evaluate the real benefits of LESS over conventional laparoscopy or robotic surgery. The use of appropriate tools specifically designed for LESS seems to facilitate these complex procedures, although they are not essential. The use of robotic platforms to assists LESS appears to be the future.

References

1. http://www.auanet.org/content/media/renalmass09.pdf.
2. http://www.uroweb.org/fileadmin/guidelines/2012_Guidelines_large_text_print_total_file.pdf.
3. Clayman RV, Kavoussi LR, Soper NJ, et al. Laparoscopic nephrectomy. N Engl J Med. 1991;324(19):1370–1.

4. Rassweiler J, Pini G, Gözen AS, et al. Role of laparoscopy in reconstructive surgery. Curr Opin Urol. 2010;20(6):471–82.
5. Rane A, Kommu S, Eddy B, et al. Clinical evaluation of a novel laparoscopic port (R-port) and evolution of the single laparoscopic port procedure (SliPP). J Endourol. 2007;21 Suppl 1: A22–3.
6. Raman JD, Bensalah K, Bagrodia A, et al. Laboratory and clinical development of single key-hole umbilical nephrectomy. Urology. 2007;70:1039–42.
7. Gill IS, Advincula AP, Aron M, et al. Consensus statement of the consortium for laparoendo-scopic single-site surgery. Surg Endosc. 2010;24(4):762–8.
8. Desai MM, Rao PP, Aron M, et al. Scarless single port transumbilical nephrectomy and pyelo-plasty: first clinical report. BJU Int. 2008;101(1):83–8.
9. http://www.ncbi.nlm.nih.gov/pubmed/.
10. White WM, Goel RK, Swartz MA, et al. Single-port laparoscopic abdominal sacral colpopexy: initial experience and comparative outcomes. Urology. 2009;74(5):1008–12.
11. White WM, Haber GP, Goel RK, et al. Single-port urological surgery: single-center experience with the first 100 cases. Urology. 2009;74(4):801–4.
12. Tome AL, Tobias-Machado M, Correa WF. Laparoendoscopic single-site (LESS) sacrocol-popexy: feasibility and efficacy of knotless procedure performed with conventional instru-ments. Int Urogynecol J Pelvic Floor Dysfunct. 2011;22(7):885–7.
13. Ingber MS, Stein RJ, Rackley RR, et al. Single-port transvesical excision of foreign body in the bladder. Urology. 2009;74(6):1347–50.
14. Stolzenburg JU, Do M, Kallidonis P, et al. Laparoendoscopic single-site bladder diverticulec-tomy: technique and initial experience. J Endourol. 2011;25(1):85–90.
15. Desai MM, Berger AK, Brandina R, et al. Laparoendoscopic single-site surgery: initial hun-dred patients. Urology. 2009;74(4):805–12.
16. Desai MM, Stein R, Rao P, et al. Embryonic natural orifice transumbilical endoscopic surgery (E-NOTES) for advanced reconstruction: initial experience. Urology. 2009;73(1):182–7.
17. Noguera RJ, Astigueta JC, Carmona O, et al. Laparoscopic augmentation enterocystoplasty through a single trocar. Urology. 2009;73(6):1371–4.
18. Kaouk JH, Autorino R, Kim FJ, et al. Laparoendoscopic single-site surgery in urology: world-wide multi-institutional analysis of 1076 cases. Eur Urol. 2011;60(5):998–1005.
19. Kaouk JH, Goel RK, White MA, et al. Laparoendoscopic single-site radical cystectomy and pelvic lymph node dissection: initial experience and 2-year follow-up. Urology. 2010;76(4): 857–61.
20. Rane A, Autorino R. Robotic natural orifice translumenal endoscopic surgery and laparoendo-scopic single-site surgery: current status. Curr Opin Urol. 2011;21(1):71–7.
21. Rane A, Tan GY, Tewari AK. Laparo-endoscopic single-site surgery in urology: is robotics the missing link? BJU Int. 2009;104(8):1041–3.
22. Seideman CA, Huckabay C, Smith KD, et al. Laparoscopic ureteral reimplantation: technique and outcomes. J Urol. 2009;181(4):1742–6.
23. Stein RJ, Turna B, Patel NS, et al. Laparoscopic assisted ileal ureter: technique, outcomes and comparison to the open procedure. J Urol. 2009;182(3):1032–9.
24. Gill IS, Rackley RR, Meraney AM, et al. Laparoscopic enterocystoplasty. Urology. 2000;55(2): 178–81.

Chapter 24
LESS: Radical Prostatectomy

Humberto Kern Laydner and Jihad H. Kaouk

Keywords Prostatic neoplasms • Prostate cancer • Prostatectomy • Radical prostatectomy • LESS • Single port • R-LESS • Robotics • NOTES

Introduction

Prostate cancer is the most commonly diagnosed nonskin cancer and the second leading cause of cancer-related death in men in the United States [1]. The anatomical approach to radical retropubic prostatectomy was developed by Walsh et al. in the early 1980s [2]. It rapidly became the standard surgical procedure for radical prostatectomy. In 1997, Schuessler et al. performed the first laparoscopic radical prostatectomy [3]. After Guillonneau et al. reported their technique in 1998, the laparoscopic approach started to receive more acceptance for the treatment of prostate cancer [4].

Two decades ago, the desire to offer patients a reduced morbidity and improved cosmesis was the driving force for the development of laparoscopy and is once again what motivates surgeons to perform laparoscopic surgery through a small single incision [5]. The use of laparoendoscopic single-site

H.K. Laydner, M.D.
Laparoscopic and Robotic Surgery, Glickman Urological and Kidney Institute,
Cleveland Clinic, 9500 Euclid Avenue, Glickman Urological and Kidney Institute,
Q9/100A, Cleveland, OH 44195, USA
e-mail: laydneh@ccf.org, dr.1berto@terra.com.br

J.H. Kaouk, M.D. (✉)
Director, Laparoscopic and Robotic Surgery, Glickman Urological and Kidney Institute,
Cleveland Clinic, 9500 Euclid Avenue, Glickman Urological and Kidney Institute, Q10-1,
Cleveland, OH 44195, USA
e-mail: kaoukj@ccf.org

A. Rane et al. (eds.), *Scar-Less Surgery*,
DOI 10.1007/978-1-84800-360-6_24, © Springer-Verlag London 2013

surgery (LESS) has increased rapidly, and nearly the entire spectrum of urologic laparoscopic surgery has been demonstrated to be feasible with this approach [6–8]. We started the application of this technique for the treatment of adenocarcinoma of the prostate in 2007, when it was still named "single-port laparoscopic radical prostatectomy" [9]. In 2008, the terminology LESS was consensually adopted, replacing the term "single-port laparoscopy," among others [10].

Our group introduced the da Vinci Surgical System to several LESS procedures, including radical prostatectomy, and named it robotic LESS (R-LESS) [11].

R-LESS Radical Prostatectomy

In the past 10 years, robotic surgery has revolutionized the way laparoscopic surgery is performed in the United States. Radical prostatectomy is probably the best example of this shift. Currently, the majority of radical prostatectomies in the United States are performed using the robot [12]. Much of the acceptance of this trend among surgeons can be credited to the dramatic improvements enabled by the robotic system to ergonomics and shortening of the learning curve. Present in LESS and NOTES, the idea of surgery with an invisible scar and minimal morbidity is fascinating for both patients and surgeons. However, it was made possible only at the expense of the surgeon's physical comfort, with a learning curve even steeper than standard laparoscopy.

Both robotic surgery and the pursuit of scarless surgery seem to be a no-way-back tendency. We have been trying to combine the best of both worlds in the clinical setting since May 2008. The robot notably improves the ergonomics of LESS, reduces instrument crossing, and adds instrument tip articulation, which facilitates suturing.

Patient Selection

Ideal candidates for LESS or R-LESS radical prostatectomy are patients with a life expectancy of 10 years or more, early-stage prostate cancer (T1c), no previous history of surgery or radiation to the lower abdomen or pelvic region, a medium-sized prostate (>20 and <60 g), few or no comorbidities, and a body mass index ≤ 35 kg/m^2. The appropriate patient selection is essential to warrant the safety of LESS radical prostatectomy; this is especially true during the initial learning curve. As the surgeon gains experience and confidence with the technique, these limits can be cautiously expanded.

The contraindications are the same as for standard laparoscopy, including uncorrected coagulopathy, significant conditions affecting cardiac output or pulmonary gas exchange, intestinal obstruction, abdominal wall infection, and peritoneal inflammatory process.

Fig. 24.1 Separate placement of SILS port and robotic trocars through the same skin incision

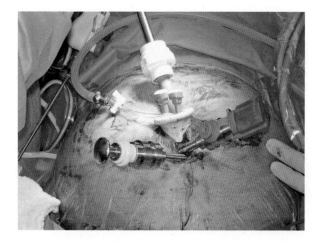

Surgical Technique

In this section, we'll describe the technique of R-LESS, which became our preferred approach when a patient is considered suitable for radical prostatectomy through a single skin incision.

Positioning

Under general anesthesia and endotracheal intubation, the patient is placed in the low lithotomy position with his legs on spreader bars, and the abdomen and genital area are prepped. Pneumatic compression is used to prevent deep vein thrombosis. The patient is secured to the table, with arms alongside the body. Strapping must be tight enough to avoid patient dislodgement during surgery, but breathing should not be limited. Abundant foam is used in pressure points. The robot is introduced into the field between the legs of the patient.

Access

An umbilical 2–5-cm skin incision is made. The size of the fascial incision varies according to the selected access device. When the SILS® port (Covidien, Norwalk, CT) is used, a finger is placed to guide the introduction of two robotic trocars adjacent to the fascial incision through two separate fascial stab incisions (Fig. 24.1). If using a GelPort® (Applied Medical, Rancho Santa Margarita, CA), the access device is placed through the fascial incision and the robot is docked in a three-arm approach. Alternatively, four trocars can be placed through separate fascial incisions in a diamond-shaped configuration.

Bladder Mobilization

Using the 8-mm EndoWrist® (Intuitive Surgical, Sunnyvale, CA) monopolar shears in the right arm, a 5-mm EndoWrist Schertel Grasper in the left, and a 30° lens looking upward, the parietal peritoneum is widely incised high on the anterior abdominal wall, and the bladder is dissected.

Incision of the Endopelvic Fascia

The endopelvic fascia is exposed and sharply incised, using the 8-mm EndoWrist monopolar shears in the right hand and a 5-mm EndoWrist Schertel Grasper or 8-mm EndoWrist ProGrasp forceps in the left. The prostate is mobilized off the levator muscle fibers.

Ligation of the Dorsal Venous Complex

The penile dorsal venous complex is ligated with a 2.0 polyglactin suture (Vicryl), using an 8- and 5-mm EndoWrist robotic needle driver. The dorsal vein stitch is secured to the pubic symphysis in an attempt to improve the early continence recovery rate [13]. Cranially, a back-bleeding stitch is placed across the anterior surface of the prostate.

Bladder Neck Dissection

A marionette suture is passed through the distal bladder neck or prostatic base to serve as a retractor. The anterior bladder neck is transected. The urethral catheter is suspended from the abdominal wall with a 2-0 suture and the posterior bladder neck is dissected away from the prostate (Fig. 24.2).

Seminal Vesicle Dissection

After incision of the anterior layer of the Denonvillier's fascia, the vas deferens and seminal vesicles are mobilized athermally with Hem-o-lok® clips (Teleflex Medical, Research Triangle Park, NC) in a nerve-sparing approach and with the 5-mm harmonic scalpel in a nonnerve-sparing approach.

Fig. 24.2 Urethral catheter suspended with marionette suture

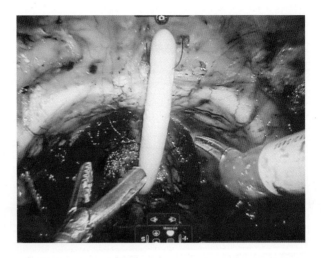

Prostatic Dissection

The use of the 8-mm robotic clip applier enables us to replicate the nerve-sparing technique used in RALP. With a combination of robotically applied Hem-o-lok clips and sharp dissection, an interfascial nerve-sparing approach is accomplished. Assistant retraction with the suction device and/or marionette sutures allows for placement of Hem-o-lok clips. A 5-mm harmonic scalpel can be used in the right arm, in a non-nerve-sparing surgery, to cauterize the lateral pedicles bilaterally. However, it can be difficult sometimes, as this instrument does not deflect or articulate.

Urethral Dissection and Division

The ligated dorsal vein complex is incised with the 8-mm monopolar shears. The underlying urethra is exposed and transected sharply, without electrocautery. The prostate apex is dissected in a retrograde fashion; the specimen is released and placed in a 10-mm laparoscopic bag.

Specimen Extraction

Some LESS procedures often require an extended skin incision to allow the retrieval of a large specimen inside the laparoscopic bag. Usually, this is not required in R-LESS radical prostatectomy (Fig. 24.3).

Fig. 24.3 Late postoperative
aspect of the incision

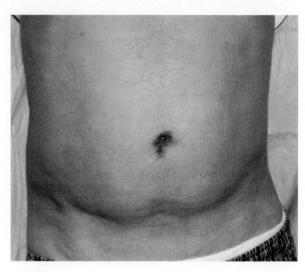

Pelvic Lymph Node Dissection

The lymph node dissection is performed in the same manner as in our RALP technique. External iliac and obturator fossa nodal tissues are removed with a laparoscopic spoon.

Urethrovesical Anastomosis

The urethrovesical anastomosis is performed with robotic needle drivers in both arms. Two sutures of 2-0 poliglecaprone 25 (Monocryl) on an RB-1 needle are placed in a semicircular "running" fashion starting from the 6 o'clock position toward the 12 o'clock position and then tied together. Before completion of the anastomosis, a 20 Fr Foley catheter is inserted into the bladder. The anastomosis is tested by instilling 100 ml of saline into the bladder to ensure water tightness. A Jackson–Pratt drain is placed in the pelvis and exited through a separate fascial stab but via the same skin incision.

Outcomes

At Cleveland Clinic, we initially performed four LESS radical prostatectomies without intraoperative complications [9]. One patient developed a rectourethral fistula, treated with a mucosal advancement flap. The mean operative time was 4.75 h. The mean hospital stay was 2–3 days. A Foley catheter and Jackson–Pratt drain were removed 2 weeks after surgery. Three patients used one or no pads daily for continence at 18 weeks of follow-up. Although the initial clinical disease stage for all patients was T1c, it was upstaged on final pathologic examination, with Gleason score $3+4=7$ and extracapsular extension (T3a). Two patients had positive margins located at the site of the extracapsular penetration. One of these patients has an undetectable prostate-specific antigen (PSA) level (<0.03 ng/dl) at 33 months of follow-up. After PSA recurrence (3.55 ng/dl), the other patient with a surgical positive margin had benign prostatic and seminal vesicle tissue demonstrated at biopsy of a prostate fossa nodule, with no evidence of carcinoma. PSA immunostains were used to evaluate the case and a senior pathologist was consulted. The remaining patients persist with undetectable levels of PSA.

Rabenalt et al. reported one case of a 74-year-old man, with a clinically localized prostate cancer Gleason score $3+3=6$, who underwent extraperitoneal LESS radical prostatectomy. The operative time was 290 min. The estimated blood loss was 100 ml. There were no intra- or postoperative complications, and no additional ports were used. Histopathology showed bilateral adenocarcinoma without extracapsular extension, Gleason $3+4=7$, with negative margins. Two weeks after surgery, the patient reported only mild urinary incontinence [14].

Since May 2008, we have abandoned standard LESS radical prostatectomy and switched our approach to R-LESS. Recently, we reported our initial experience of 20 R-LESS radical prostatectomies [15]. The mean operative time was 187.6 min, and the mean estimated blood loss was 128.8 ml. The visual analog pain score at discharge was 1.6 of 10. The mean hospital stay was 2.5 days. There was one conversion to standard RALP due to a large median lobe, which required better retraction. Conversion to hybrid R-LESS was necessary in two cases due to clashing and CO_2 leakage from the port, with the addition of an 8-mm robotic port placed. We had four complications, including an ileus in one patient, managed conservatively (Clavien grade 1), a transfusion in a patient on postoperative day 1 due to blood loss anemia (Clavien grade 2), a pulmonary embolus manifested 2 weeks after surgery and managed with 6 months of oral anticoagulation (Clavien grade 2), and one case of urosepsis that occurred 45 days after surgery, which required intensive care support and resolved with intravenous antibiotics (Clavien grade 4).

Pathology revealed four focal positive margins (three in T2 and one in T3a disease), with two occurring during the first three cases. Three of the four margins occurred at the apex; one occurred laterally. All of the positive margins were in nonnerve-sparing cases. The Gleason score was of $3+3=6$ in 3 patients, $3+4=7$ in 11 patients, $4+3=7$ in 4 patients, and $4+4=8$ in 2 patients. Lymph nodes were negative in all cases [15]. Currently, the PSA levels of all patients are undetectable, with a mean follow-up of 16 months.

A trend toward improved urinary continence was observed over the follow-up period. Three patients underwent an athermal nerve-sparing technique, and at 3 months postoperatively, one had an SHIM$\geq$21. Seventy-one percent of patients had their Foley catheters removed 1 week after surgery. Five patients who were found to have an anastomotic leak on cystogram required an additional week before removal of the catheter.

Barret et al. reported their experimental and clinical experience with hybrid R-LESS radical prostatectomy [16]. A 5-mm port was added at the right lower abdomen for suction and drain placement. There were no intraoperative complications, and margins were negative. Later, the same authors reported a complete R-LESS radical prostatectomy, with an operative time of 210 min and an estimated blood loss of 300 ml. There were no complications and prostatic margins were negative [17].

In 2010, Leewansangtong et al. from Thailand reported the first R-LESS radical prostatectomy in Asia [18]. A 71-year-old man with a clinical T3 adenocarcinoma of the prostate, Gleason score 4+4=8 on biopsy, received androgen deprivation for 3 months followed by R-LESS radical prostatectomy. The operative time was 335 min, the estimated blood loss was 250 ml, and no blood transfusion was required. There were no postoperative complications. The hospital stay was 4 days. Pathology exam showed T3c adenocarcinoma Gleason 9 with tumor regression after hormonal therapy, which was continued.

Fortunately, initial series were successful; however, we still advocate that LESS or R-LESS radical prostatectomy should be reserved only for highly selected cases, especially during the initial learning curve.

Limitations

Although the enthusiasm among surgeons and patients caused by promising early results, LESS still has several technical constraints that limit its applicability to a very selected number of patients and surgical centers. The restricted space available causes significant instrument clashing, which impairs adequate tissue retraction. The limited triangulation can be partially restored with prebent or articulating instruments. However, they often cause force dissipation and have counterintuitive maneuverability due to crossing.

Even though the robotic system added important benefits to LESS, R-LESS is not free of limitations. When a reduction in the range of motion of the robotic instruments is experienced, it is useful to switch the 8-mm robotic instruments to the 5-mm pediatric set. The 5-mm instruments deflect instead of articulate. Because the da Vinci® robot (Intuitive Surgical, Sunnyvale, CA) is bulky, an important adjustment is to set the system to fine-tuning, slowing the movement of the robotic arms and reducing external collisions [19]. Another helpful strategy is to identify in the surgical field the points where clashing starts to occur and attempt to stay inside these boundaries, keeping movements within a mentally delineated "clashing-free" area. If the surgeon needs to work in another area, he or she does it, moving all the instruments en bloc.

The possibility to obtain mid- and long-term oncological results equivalent to open surgery with standard laparoscopy has been well demonstrated for several different urological malignancies [20]. As the nature of standard laparoscopy and LESS is essentially the same, at least in theory, oncological outcomes should not be

Fig. 24.4 Robotic Single-Site™ platform and instruments

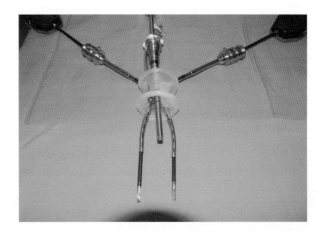

different between the two approaches. For LESS and R-LESS radical prostatectomy, the initial step of feasibility has already been demonstrated, yet the oncological efficacy has not been directly addressed. Certainly, longer-term results would be ideal in order to bolster the proof of oncologic equivalence, yet thus far only short- to mid-term follow-up is available due to the novelty of these techniques.

Future Directions

The application of robotic technology to the LESS approach solved some of the limitations inherent to this technique. However, the currently available robotic platform and its instruments were not designed specifically for LESS. Novel robotic instruments (Single-Site™; Intuitive Surgical, Sunnyvale, CA) were evaluated in a porcine model (Fig. 24.4) [21]. Recently, we evaluated in the cadaver model the second generation of this new robotic system specifically designed for R-LESS, which is now available for clinical use [22]. The configuration of the da Vinci Si® Surgical System (Intuitive Surgical) was specially adapted to perform R-LESS surgery. Only the robotic arms 1 and 2 and the camera arm are used, while the console and the slave remain the same. Two crossing curved cannulae for the robotic instruments, an 8.5-mm scope, and a 12-mm cannula are inserted through a multichannel port (Intuitive Surgical), which can be deployed through a single skin and fascial incision. The biggest limitation is the lack of articulation at the tip, which makes suturing more difficult than with the use of EndoWrist instruments. Some potential advantages of this system in comparison to standard LESS are improved range of motion, dexterity, instrument and scope stability, ergonomics, and decreased instrument collisions.

The convergence between robotic and LESS techniques is already bringing benefits. With further technological development, a better integration of robotic systems to the restricted space imposed by LESS is expected. If the full range of movements currently allowed by the standard robotic instruments becomes available for LESS, this technique will be certainly made accessible to a much higher number of patients and surgeons.

Conclusions

LESS and R-LESS radical prostatectomy are feasible and safe at the short-term evaluation in terms of perioperative outcomes. Longer follow-up is awaited to determine oncological safety. Prospective comparisons between these and more established techniques are also needed. R-LESS radical prostatectomy is ergonomically much superior when compared to conventional LESS radical prostatectomy.

Although it can sound obvious, it is worth mentioning that prudence (not fear) and the ability to recognize the limits of laparoscopic skills should always accompany surgeons. This is particularly important to have in mind before embracing new technologies and during challenging procedures, such as LESS and R-LESS radical prostatectomy.

References

1. American Cancer Society: Cancer Facts and Figures 2012. Atlanta, Ga: American Cancer Society, 2012. Accessed June 18, 2012. http://www.cancer.org/acs/groups/content/@epidemiologysurveilance/documents/document/acspc-031941.pdf.
2. Walsh PC, Lepor H, Eggleston JC. Radical prostatectomy with preservation of sexual function: anatomical and pathological considerations. Prostate. 1983;4:473–85.
3. Schuessler WW, Schulam PG, Clayman RV, Kavoussi LR. Laparoscopic radical prostatectomy: initial short-term experience. Urology. 1997;50:854–7.
4. Guillonneau B, Cathelineau X, Barret E, et al. Laparoscopic radical prostatectomy. Preliminary evaluation after 28 interventions. Presse Med. 1998;27:1570–4.
5. Autorino R, Cadeddu JA, Desai MM, et al. Reply from authors re: Jens J. Rassweiler. Is LESS/NOTES really more? Eur Urol. 2011;59:48–50.
6. Autorino R, Cadeddu JA, Desai MM, et al. Laparoendoscopic single-site and natural orifice transluminal endoscopic surgery in urology: a critical analysis of the literature. Eur Urol. 2011;59(1):26.
7. Khanna R, Autorino R, White M, et al. Laparoendoscopic single-site surgery: current clinical experience. BJU Int. 2010;106:897–902.
8. Kaouk JH, Autorino R, Kim FJ, et al. Laparoendoscopic single-site surgery in urology: worldwide multi-institutional analysis of 1076 cases. Eur Urol. 2011;60(5):998–1005.
9. Kaouk JH, Goel RK, Haber GP, et al. Single-port laparoscopic radical prostatectomy. Urology. 2008;72:1190–3.
10. Box G, Averch T, Cadeddu J, et al. Urologic NOTES Working Group. Nomenclature of natural orifice translumenal endoscopic surgery (NOTES) and laparoendoscopic single-site surgery (LESS) procedures in urology. J Endourol. 2008;22:2575–81.
11. Kaouk JH, Goel RK, Haber GP, et al. Robotic single-port transumbilical surgery in humans: initial report. BJU Int. 2009;103:366–9.

12. Lowrance WT, Eastham JA, Savage C, et al. Contemporary open and robotic radical prostatectomy practice patterns among urologists in the United States. J Urol. 2012;187(6):2087–93.
13. Patel VR, Coelho RF, Palmer KJ, Rocco B. Periurethral suspension stitch during robot-assisted laparoscopic radical prostatectomy: description of the technique and continence outcomes. Eur Urol. 2009;56:472–8.
14. Rabenalt R, Arsov C, Giessing M, et al. Extraperitoneal laparo-endoscopic single-site radical prostatectomy: first experience. World J Urol. 2010;28:705–8.
15. White MA, Haber GP, Autorino R, et al. Robotic laparoendoscopic single-site radical prostatectomy: technique and early outcomes. Eur Urol. 2010;58:544–50.
16. Barret E, Sanchez-Salas R, Kasraeian A, et al. A transition to laparoendoscopic single-site surgery (LESS) radical prostatectomy: human cadaver experimental and initial clinical experience. J Endourol. 2009;23:135–40.
17. Barret E, Sanchez-Salas R, Cathelineau X, et al. Re: initial complete laparoendoscopic single-site surgery robotic assisted radical prostatectomy (LESS-RARP). Int Braz J Urol. 2009;35:92–3.
18. Leewansangtong S, Vorrakitkatorn P, Amornvesukit T, et al. Laparo-endoscopic single site (LESS) robotic radical prostatectomy in an Asian man with prostate cancer: an initial case report. J Med Assoc Thai. 2010;93:383–7.
19. White MA, Haber GP, Autorino R, et al. Robotic laparoendoscopic single-site surgery. BJU Int. 2010;106:923–7.
20. Rassweiler J, Tsivian A, Kumar AV, et al. Oncological safety of laparoscopic surgery for urological malignancy: experience with more than 1,000 operations. J Urol. 2003;169:2072–5.
21. Haber GP, White MA, Autorino R, et al. Novel robotic da Vinci instruments for laparoendoscopic single-site surgery. Urology. 2010;76:1279–82.
22. Kaouk JH, Autorino R, Laydner H, et al. Robotic single-site kidney surgery: evaluation of second-generation instruments in a cadaver model. Urology. 2012;79(5):975–9.

Chapter 25
Single-Port Laparoscopy: Issues and Complications

Jay D. Raman

Keywords Single-site surgery • Laparoendoscopic single site surgery (LESS) Minimally invasive surgery • Complications • Modified Clavien system

Introduction

Minimally invasive surgical techniques have assumed a greater role in the management of benign and malignant urologic diseases. Numerous studies regarding various different pathologies have underscored that laparoscopic and/or robotic platforms can provide equivalent surgical outcomes with reduced morbidity when compared to their open counterparts. Nonetheless, a continuous impetus within the minimally invasive surgical community is exploring means to decrease surgical morbidity and improve perioperative convalescence. Such considerations have fueled the early experience with single-port laparoscopy (SPL), also known as laparoendoscopic single-site (LESS) surgery, whereby entire surgical procedures are performed via a single abdominal wall incision [1]. Early studies have suggested that the potential benefits of SPL (as compared to conventional laparoscopy) include decreased pain, lower blood loss, shorter convalescence, and improved cosmesis [2, 3].

Successful incorporation of SPL into a surgical practice requires an understanding of the various issues and complications related to this novel technique. In particular, preoperative issues that warrant consideration include appropriate patient and lesion selection, familiarity with available instrumentation, surgical training prior to actual cases, and incorporation of robotic platforms. Similarly, recognizing potential complications unique to SPL as well as management and prevention methodologies is crucial for early success.

J.D. Raman, M.D.
Department of Surgery, Penn State Milton S. Hershey Medical Center,
500 University Drive, C48308, Hershey, PA 17033, USA
e-mail: jraman@hmc.psu.edu

A. Rane et al. (eds.), *Scar-Less Surgery*,
DOI 10.1007/978-1-84800-360-6_25, © Springer-Verlag London 2013

In this chapter, some of the issues and complications highlighted above are discussed in greater detail to better prepare the reader for subsequent cases.

Issues of SPL

Patient Selection

There are no specific absolute contraindications to SPL beyond those related to the physiologic impact of pneumoperitoneum experienced in the setting of abdominal insufflation. Therefore, in theory, any patient who is deemed suitable for a conventional laparoscopic approach can be a potential candidate for SPL. However, appropriate patient selection is crucial to contribute to the ease (or lack thereof) for SPL cases.

Perhaps the ideal SPL patient is one with a relatively low body mass index (BMI) ($\leq$25) with limited (or no) prior abdominal surgery and a strong interest in the potential cosmesis benefit of single-incision surgery. In particular, a recent series from Mir and colleagues highlighted that since 2007, almost 50 % of nephrectomies at their institution were performed by SPL, with such patients having a younger median age (47 vs. 64 year, $p=0.004$) and lower BMI (24 vs. 28, $p=0.001$) compared to their conventional laparoscopy counterparts [4]. While a history of abdominal surgery is a consideration for patient selection, the actual anatomic site of prior abdominal surgery is likely more significant. For example, a prior appendectomy may minimally impact an SPL nephrectomy, although a history of splenectomy or cholecystectomy may increase the challenge of upper retroperitoneal SPL.

Although BMI is often commonly cited as a means to determine selection criteria for SPL, one can argue that the actual distribution of intraabdominal fat may be a more valuable metric to use. Figure 25.1 highlights axial imaging from two women with a BMI of 31 presenting for surgical management of left-enhancing renal lesions. The distribution of intraabdominal fat (i.e., Gerota's fat), however, is dramatically different. Specifically, the patient in Fig. 25.1a has minimal perirenal fat, while the one depicted in Fig. 25.1b has a dense amount of retroperitoneal fat with some inflammatory stranding. Surgical experience highlighted the latter case to be far more challenging for SPL. Therefore, it is this author's belief that the intraabdominal fat distribution surrounding the target organ of interest is far more important than the overall patient BMI for selection of SPL cases.

Lesion Selection

Target Organ

Appropriate lesion selection is paramount for the success of SPL cases. There are several key considerations in this regard. First, the target organ of choice warrants

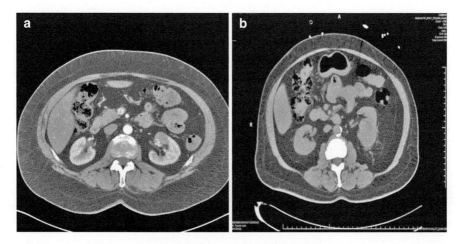

Fig. 25.1 (**a, b**) Differential perinephric fat distributions in two patients with a similar body mass index

consideration, with the broad distinction for urologists being upper retroperitoneal versus pelvic surgery. In general, upper tract pathologies appear to be far more commonly tackled with particular organs of interest, including the adrenal gland and kidney (nephrectomy, partial nephrectomy, renal ablation, and pyeloplasty) [5]. However, SPL procedures for prostate (prostatectomy, STEP), bladder (cystectomy, diverticulectomy, ureteral reimplant), and uterine (sacrocolpopexy) pathology have been described with success in the literature [6]. Familiarity with target organ anatomy and an extensive array of conventional laparoscopic cases as a foundation portends well for subsequent success.

Benign Versus Malignant Pathology

A broad categorization with respect to surgical lesions is the delineation between benign and malignant pathologies. While there are no firm guidelines regarding the use of SPL, it is essential for practicing urologists to understand salient considerations when managing each of these entities. With respect to benign diseases, the spectrum of difficulty ranges from facile to extremely challenging. The preoperative recognition of such differences is crucial to avoid intraoperative or postoperative complications. A prime example of this is SPL nephrectomy for a poorly functioning renal unit. Figure 25.2b (hydronephrotic kidney secondary to long-standing undiagnosed UPJ obstruction) and Fig. 25.2a (small atrophic right kidney causing renin-mediated hypertension) demonstrate two fairly straightforward simple nephrectomy SPL cases. Conversely, Fig. 25.2c demonstrates preoperative CT imaging for a poorly functioning kidney due to distal stricture disease with perinephric stranding and a history of a splenectomy (see surgical clip in left upper quadrant).

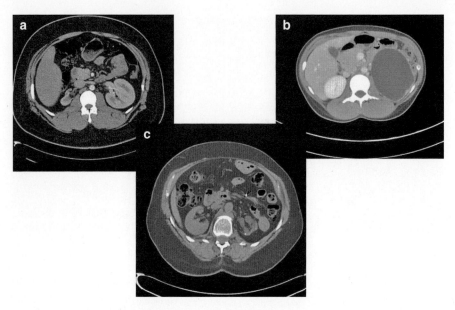

Fig. 25.2 (**a**) small atrophic right kidney causing renin-mediated hypertension; (**b**) hydronephrotic kidney secondary to longstanding undiagnosed UPJ obstruction; (**c**) poorly functioning kidney due to distal stricture disease with perinephric stranding and a history of a splenectomy

In this latter case, "simple nephrectomy" is a misnomer and management is best suited to a multitrocar laparoscopic or open approach. Thus, benign pathologies are not always best suited for SPL.

A central consideration when tackling SPL for malignancy is ensuring the adherence to oncologic and functional standards of care. With respect to prostate-ctomy, these standards include margin status as well as return of continence and sexual function [7]. In that regard, White and colleagues recently highlighted their initial series of robotic SPL prostatectomy by a single high-volume surgeon and noted a positive margin rate of 20 % (4 of 20 cases) [8]. Therefore, an inherent learning curve still exists for experienced SPL surgeons. When considering radi-cal cystectomy, a central consideration is not only the safe removal of the bladder, but also the quality of lymph node dissection. Abundant literature now under-scores the diagnostic but also therapeutic role of a lymphadenectomy for transi-tional cell carcinoma malignancies [9]. Finally, for renal pathology, a key point is to adhere to the oncologic principles of renal preservation. An increasing number of studies emphasize the benefit of partial versus radical nephrectomy for the prevention of chronic kidney disease [10]. Therefore, it is essential for minimally invasive surgeons to avoid the seduction of SPL nephrectomy due to ease over partial nephrectomy. Indeed, despite the inherently higher skill set, several groups have reported successful completion of such SPL cases, underscoring the feasibility [11, 12].

Instrumentation and Learning Curve

Familiarity with instrumentation is essential to avoid intraoperative issues during SPL cases. While most surgeons undertaking SPL are experienced laparoscopists, there is an inherent array of novel instruments unique to SPL. Access devices range from multiple distinct trocars inserted via a single incision to custom-made multiport disposable devices. Central considerations when choosing different modes of abdominal access include cost of the device, number of ports afforded by different access devices, size of access incision, ease of insertion, issues with procedural dislodgement, and wound-related complications.

Working instrumentation and camera optics similarly present potential issues that warrant consideration prior to SPL cases. A host of different tools, including bent and articulating devices as well as variable-length rigid instruments, all are available in the armamentarium. However, each presents inherent challenges, particularly when incorporating such tools in an effort to minimize extracorporeal and intracorporeal clashing. Finally, adequate optics is crucial for successful SPL while limiting iatrogenic complications due to poor visualization. There is no perfect solution, with success demonstrated with deflectable-tip and rigid cameras with differing angle lenses. Many of these issues are discussed in other chapters in greater detail. Collectively, however, it is likely that all of these considerations heighten the inherent learning curve of SPL, which may be the biggest contributor to surgical complications.

Transitioning to SPL, therefore, may be best suited via a stepwise progression with regards to both the number of ports utilized and the extent of operative procedures. A plausible training algorithm may involve steadily decreasing the number of operative ports from multitrocar laparoscopy to SPL as familiarity and comfort level increase Alternatively, multiple groups have encouraged the use of accessory 2- and 3-mm instruments to facilitate retraction, dissection, and intracorporeal suturing during SPL cases [5, 6, 13]. A graduated approach in surgical procedures further bodes well for integrating SPL into the surgical armamentarium. For example, renal ablation, cyst decortication, and varicocelectomy represent fairly simple cases well suited for early SPL cases. Thereafter, more challenging extirpative and reconstructive cases can be targeted as the learning curve flattens.

Incorporation of Robotic Platforms

As with many other urologic procedures, the incorporation of robotic platforms is assuming a greater role in SPL. However, even for facile robotic surgeons, the use of robotics for SPL presents novel challenges. Principally among this includes minimizing clashing of the robotic arms. Experimentation both with varying single-access devices as well as with differing trocar configurations may contribute to the ease of completion of cases. Additional modifications, including crossing the handedness at the robotic console as well as the usage of smaller trocars (8.5-mm camera, 5-mm working instruments), can further aid in minimizing collision of robotic arms. Indeed, incorporation of the VeSPA® surgical instruments (Intuitive Surgical, Sunnyvale, CA) may increase the range of motion, provide instrument and scope stability, and improve ergonomics while decreasing instrument clashing. Early porcine pilot series highlight the potential benefits of such purpose-built robotic single-port instrumentation [14].

Complications of SPL

An understanding of the key issues and potential barriers for SPL as highlighted above is essential to limit the potential for complications of SPL. Nonetheless, with enough surgical volume, complications will inevitably occur and therefore warrant discussion. A solid understanding of the potential complications, management, and prevention strategies is likely to limit the scope of sequelae when complications do occur.

Experience to Date

Learning from the surgical experience of others often provides an ideal forum to review potential complications. In that regard, some contemporary series from high-volume SPL surgeons are reviewed below.

In 2009, Desai and colleagues reported on their initial 100 patients undergoing SPL procedures for a variety of different indications [5]. All procedures were performed using a purpose-built SPL access device with a combination of articulating and bent instrumentation. The authors noted a 7 % conversion rate either to conventional laparoscopy ($n=3$) or open surgery ($n=4$). The overall complication rate from this series was 14 %, with five intraoperative (four bleeding, one bowel injury) and nine postoperative (bleeding, corneal abrasion, drug induced dyskinesia, urinary tract infection, and urinary leak) cases. The authors did note one mortality in their series in a Jehovah's Witness patient who bled following an SPL simple prostatectomy and refused transfusion products.

White and colleagues similarly reported on perioperative outcomes in an observational cohort of 100 patients who underwent SPL surgery at a single academic center between September 2007 and February 2009 [6]. As in the previous series described above, procedures were varied, ranging between upper and lower tract urologic pathologies. These authors noted no intraoperative complications, although six patients required conversion to standard laparoscopy. In this series, 11 % of patients had postoperative complications. When classified using the modified Clavien grading system (Table 25.1), complications include nine Grade II (seven transfusions, one urinary tract infection, and one deep venous thrombosis) and two

Grade IIIb (recto-urethral fistula, angioembolization). This group concluded that complications from their early experience were consistent with those published in historical data. Similar outcomes were noted by Choi et al. in a series of 171 consecutive SPL cases performed for a variety of indications at a single institution [15]. This series included both robotic ($n=73$) and pure laparoscopic ($n=98$) SPL cases. The authors observed that seven patients (4 %) required conversion to mini-incision open surgery. Furthermore, intraoperative complications occurred in seven cases (4 %), while postoperative complications (all Clavien Grade IIIa or lower) occurred in nine patients (5 %).

While these experiences highlighted above focus on a cohort of patients undergoing SPL, several series have focused attention on complications following specific indications. Permpongkosol and colleagues recently reviewed 18 cases over a 1-year period for patients undergoing SPL for benign kidney diseases (seven simple nephrectomies, ten cyst decortications, and one redo-dismembered pyeloplasty) [16]. Of the simple nephrectomies, two cases noted xanthogranulomatous pyelonephritis (XGP) on final pathology. These authors observed that SPL was completed in just over three quarters of cases, with the four conversions to standard laparoscopy occurring due to failure to progress ($n=2$), bleeding ($n=1$), and instrument error ($n=1$). One patient in this series developed a postprocedural incisional hernia. This group concluded that in select patients with benign renal pathology, SPL is a viable and safe treatment strategy. With regards to reconstructive urology, Best et al. reviewed 30-day complication rates following their initial series of SPL for adult pyeloplasty cases [17]. This study highlighted outcomes from 28 consecutive patients who underwent SPL pyeloplasty by a single experienced minimally invasive surgeon. These authors noted that seven patients (25 %) experienced a total of eight complications. In particular, four patients required additional nephrostomy tube drainage during the early postoperative period, one had an anastomotic leak requiring prolonged surgical drainage, one had a retroperitoneal hematoma necessitating a blood transfusion, and one had hematuria requiring a prolonged hospital duration by 48 h. Interestingly, of the patients experiencing complications, 71 %

Table 25.1 Modified Clavien complications scale

Complication grade	Description
I	Deviation from the normal postoperative course without the need for pharmacologic, radiologic, or surgical intervention
II	Minor complications requiring pharmacologic intervention, including blood transfusion, intravenous antibiotics, and total parenteral nutrition
IIIa	Intervention without general anesthesia
IIIb	Intervention with general anesthesia
IV	Life-threatening complications requiring intensive care unit management
V	Death due to complications

occurred during the first ten cases. This group therefore concluded that the SPL pyeloplasty procedure is a technically challenging operation even for an experienced laparoscopic surgeon. Furthermore, they highlight that the technical challenges of intracorporeal reconstruction may translate to a higher complication rate (as compared to conventional laparoscopy) early in the learning curve.

Similar observations to both the Permpongkosol and Best studies were recently highlighted in a multicenter experience on the complications and conversions of upper urinary tract SPL from members of the NOTES Working Group. In this series, Irwin and colleagues presented data on 125 patients who underwent SPL at six high-volume academic centers [18]. Of these cases, an overall complication rate of 15.2 % was identified. The authors further stratified complications by extirpative/ablative vs. reconstructive SPL cases. In this regard, significant differences were noted. Specifically, of the 77 extirpative/ablative cases, the complication rate was only 7.8 %, with three patients requiring a conversion to conventional laparoscopy. Conversely, among the 48 reconstructive SPL cases, the complication rate was 27.1 %, with four conversions. These authors conclude that SPL is technically feasible for upper tract extirpative, ablative, and reconstructive procedure; however, early experience notes higher complication rates compared to mature conventional laparoscopy series.

Collectively, both single- and multiinstitutional series highlight that SPL is feasible although reconstructive cases present a greater challenge and a greater potential risk of associated complications.

Management and Prevention of Complications

Complications as described above typically occur intraoperatively and postoperatively. Many complications of SPL are similar to those experienced during conventional laparoscopy. In that regard, a comprehensive review is beyond the scope of this chapter. However, several scenarios that present unique challenges with respect to SPL cases are discussed below, with a focus on management and prevention strategies.

Perhaps the most anxiety-provoking complication during SPL (or conventional laparoscopy for that matter) is acute bleeding or hemorrhage. Management of this scenario typically can be approached in a stepwise progression that is predicated in part on the hemodynamic stability of the patient, visualization, and briskness of the bleeding. Preoperative preparation of a vascular "safety stitch," which is loaded and available for use prior to starting a procedure, is essential. In general, such a stitch can utilize any vascular nonabsorbable suture (i.e., 4-0 prolene) with a Lapara-ty® (Ethicon Endo-Surgery, Cincinnati, OH) or Hem-o-lok® Weck clip (Teleflex, Research Triangle Park, NC) loaded at the back such that one pass through the bleeding vessel can potentially cinch and tamponade the injury site without requiring knot tying. At the time of bleeding, an initial first step involves increasing abdominal insufflation pressures from standard levels of 15 to 20 or 25 cm H_2O. An increased abdominal pressure can slow bleeding, thereby improving the operative visibility and identification of the offending site. Hemostatic agents [such as Surgicel® (Ethicon, Somerville, NJ)] can be used for temporary compression while allowing prompt decision making regarding continuation with SPL, conventional laparoscopy, hand-assisted laparoscopy (HAL), or open surgery.

Bowel injury is a particular concern for SPL for a few reasons. First, the angle from the umbilicus to the target organ is typically more horizontal than usual, thereby placing bowel structures in line with instruments entering the abdominal cavity. Second, the inherent increased clashing associated with SPL may obscure obvious intraabdominal resistance that can occur when instruments contact visceral structures. Therefore, careful introduction of instruments angled toward the anterior abdominal wall can potentially prevent iatrogenic injury to small or large intestine. Furthermore, meticulous dissection is necessary during bowel mobilization to limit the potential for thermal injury. The surgeon should thoroughly evaluate the operative field at the conclusion of SPL cases with particular attention to bowel structures adjacent to the portal of entry. Postoperative management should follow standard care although heightened attention to occult signs of bowel injury including focal trocar site pain and leukopenia should alert the clinician [19].

Wound-related complications present a potentially unique complication related to SPL. Ergonomically, one may assume that the local tissue trauma may be analogous to traction during open surgical procedures. This is in part related to attempting to maximize the operative fulcrum at the anterior abdominal wall by stretching the incision as much as possible. Such concerns may particularly occur with use of the GelPOINT® or GelPort® devices (Applied Medical Systems, Rancho Santa Margarita, CA) whereby the Alexis wound retractor can be rotated until the tissues are maximally extended. To date, however, no series have documented permanent tissue damage or trauma during SPL cases. Several groups have noted postoperative incisional hernias, which underscore the need for careful closure at the conclusion of SPL cases. In summary, attention to the incision and wound is crucial to avoid iatrogenic wound complications during SPL procedures.

Conclusions

Careful consideration of pertinent issues associated with SPL is critical to ensure safe and successful completions of cases. Nonetheless, in the setting of complications, surgeons must be prepared to adapt to scenarios with consideration of the unique challenges related to SPL. Learning from the experiences of others often provides a basic framework, which can be tailored to individual practices and surgical experience.

Conflict of Interest   The author has no conflicts of interest or disclosures regarding the subject matter of this chapter.

References

1. Gill IS, Advincula AP, Aron M, et al. Consensus statement of the consortium for laparoendoscopic single-site surgery. Surg Endosc. 2010;24:762–8.
2. Raman JD, Bagrodia A, Cadeddu JA. Single-incision, umbilical laparoscopic versus conventional laparoscopic nephrectomy: a comparison of perioperative outcomes and short-term measures of convalescence. Eur Urol. 2009;55:1198–204.
3. Tugcu V, Ilbey YO, Mutlu B, et al. Laparoendoscopic single-site surgery versus standard laparoscopic simple nephrectomy: a prospective randomized study. J Endourol. 2010;241315–20.
4. Mir SA, Best SL, Donnally III CJ, et al. Minimally invasive nephrectomy: the influence of laparoendoscopic single-site surgery on patient selection, outcomes and morbidity. Urology. 2011;77:631–4.
5. Desai MM, Berger AK, Brandina R, et al. Laparoendoscopic single-site surgery: initial hundred patients. Urology. 2009;74:805–11.
6. White WM, Haber GP, Goel RK, et al. Single-port urologic surgery: single-center experience with the first 100 cases. Urology. 2009;74:801–4.
7. Ylinas E, Ploussard G, Durand X, et al. Evaluation of combined oncological and functional outcomes after radical prostatectomy: trifecta rate of achieving continence, potency and cancer control – a literature review. Urology. 2010;76:1194–8.
8. White WM, Haber GP, Autorino R, et al. Robotic laparoendoscopic single-site radical prostatectomy: technique and early outcomes. Eur Urol. 2010;58:544–50.
9. Skinner EC, Stein JP, Skinner DG. Surgical benchmarks for the treatment of invasive bladder cancer. Urol Oncol. 2007;25:66–71.
10. Huang WC, Levey AS, Serio AM, et al. Chronic kidney disease after nephrectomy in patients with renal cortical tumours: a retrospective cohort study. Lancet Oncol. 2006;7:735–40.
11. Han WK, Kim DS, Jeon HG, et al. Robot-assisted laparoendoscopic single-site surgery: partial nephrectomy for renal malignancy. Urology. 2011;77:612–6.
12. Cindolo L, Berardinelli F, Gidaro S, et al. Laparoendoscopic single-site partial nephrectomy without ischemia. J Endourol. 2010;24:1997–2002.
13. Raman JD, Bensalah K, Bagrodia A, et al. Laboratory and clinical development of single keyhole umbilical nephrectomy. Urology. 2007;70:1039–42.
14. Haber GP, White MA, Autorino R, et al. Novel robotic da Vinci instruments for laparoendoscopic single-site surgery. Urology. 2010;76:1279–82.
15. Choi KH, Ham WS, Rha KH, et al. Laparoendoscopic single-site surgeries: a single-enter experience of 171 consecutive cases. Korean J Urol. 2011;52:31–8.
16. Permpongkosol S, Ungbhakorn P, Leenanupunth C. Laparo-endoscopic single site (LESS) management of benign kidney diseases: evaluation of complications. J Med Assoc Thai. 2011;94:43–9.
17. Best SL, Donnally C, Mir SA, et al. Complications during the initial experience with laparoendoscopic single-site pyeloplasty. BJU Int. 2011;108(8):1326–9.
18. Irwin BH, Cadeddu JA, Tracy CR, et al. Complications and conversions of upper tract urological laparoendoscopic single-site surgery (LESS): multicentre experience: results from the NOTES Working Group. BJU Int. 2011;107(8):1284–9.
19. Bishoff JT, Allaf ME, Kirkels W, et al. Laparoscopic bowel injury: incidence and clinical presentation. J Urol. 1999;161:887–90.

Part IV
Future Perspectives

Chapter 26
Robotic LESS Urological Surgery: Experience and Future Perspectives

Rakesh Vijay Khanna, Mihir M. Desai, and Robert J. Stein

Keywords Laparoendoscopic single site • Single port • Robotic • Natural orifice NOTES • LESS • Laparoscopic • VeSPA

Introduction

Laparoscopy has largely been embraced in urology as it can offer better cosmesis, less bleeding, diminished pain, and faster recovery. Nevertheless, for some time investigators have been exploring techniques to decrease the size and number of incisions even further. In this vain and with the aim to limit pain and decrease complications further, techniques such as NOTES (natural orifice translumenal endoscopic surgery) and LESS (laparoendoscopic single-site) surgery have been developed [1, 2].

R.V. Khanna, M.D.
Department of Urology, SUNY Upstate Medical University,
750 East Adams Street, Syracuse, NY 13210, USA
e-mail: khannara@upstate.edu

M.M. Desai, M.D.
Department of Urology, Keck Medical Center,
University of Southern California Institute of Urology, 1441 Eastlake Avenue,
Suite 7416, Los Angeles, CA 90033, USA
e-mail: adityadesai2003@gmail.com

R.J. Stein, M.D. (⊠)
Center for Robotic and Image-Guided Surgery,
Glickman Urological and Kidney Institute, Cleveland Clinic,
Q10, 9500 Euclid Avenue, Cleveland, OH 44195, USA
e-mail: steinr@ccf.org

A. Rane et al. (eds.), *Scar-Less Surgery*,
DOI 10.1007/978-1-84800-360-6_26, © Springer-Verlag London 2013

"Scarless surgery," with little to no postoperative pain due to the absence of abdominal wall trauma, has been the driving force behind the development of NOTES. Nevertheless, complexity, risk, and the lack of appropriate technology have limited the ability to perform these procedures thus far [3].

LESS appears to provide many benefits of NOTES, including enhanced cosmesis and decreased abdominal wall trauma, without the added risks of traversing a true natural orifice [4]. Postoperative pain may be lessened with the transumbilical approach due to the absence of muscle transection and due to the restriction of painful stimuli to a solitary locus.

Attempts to perform urologic surgery through a single incision began in 2005 with a report by Hirano et al., who used a specialized resectoscope tube and standard laparoscopic instruments to perform a retroperitoneoscopic adrenalectomy [5].

Rane et al. were the first to report laparoscopic urological surgery through a single multi-channel port in the clinical setting [6]. The authors were able to complete a single-port nephrectomy for a nonfunctioning kidney and a transperitoneal ureterolithotomy with a mean operating time of 90 min and no intraoperative complications. In early 2007, Raman et al. reported their initial experience with "keyhole" nephrectomy in pigs and humans using a single incision to introduce three adjacent trocars (one 10-mm and two 5-mm). Using a combination of bent and articulating instruments, they were able to complete the three human nephrectomies with a mean operative time of 133 min through a mean incision of 3 cm with no complications [7].

Since these pioneering reports, groups from different institutions have published several clinical series with LESS so that almost the entire spectrum of urological extirpative and reconstructive laparoscopic procedures has been demonstrated to be feasible [8, 9].

Based on these early experiences, it has been largely recognized that LESS is accompanied by several technical challenges that need to be addressed before this approach might be widely adopted. Difficulties encountered with LESS include (1) a lack of triangulation, (2) counterintuitive instrument movement, (3) clashing of instruments, and (4) challenging visualization secondary to an in-line view.

To reduce some of these limitations, new equipment has been designed, developed, and applied in these early series, including access devices, articulating/flexible instruments, and deflectable scopes [10]. Nevertheless, besides the significant cost considerations of disposable equipment, these devices are usually difficult to master, requiring advanced laparoscopic skills. The surgeon and assistant also need to stand in close proximity, and the technique requires a skilled camera driver and constant coordination.

With the advent and acceptance of surgical robotics has come the natural fusion of this technology with LESS. Benefits of the da Vinci® Surgical System (Intuitive Surgical, Sunnyvale, CA) for LESS include easier articulation using EndoWrist® (Intuitive Surgical, Sunnyvale, CA) instruments, three-dimensional vision, and motion scaling. These features improve ergonomics and range of motion during LESS, especially for fine dissection and suturing.

Robotic LESS: Preclinical Investigation

Box et al. were the first to accomplish a robot-assisted hybrid NOTES nephrectomy in a porcine animal model [11]. They placed the robotic scope through one 12-mm abdominal trocar site, while the right and left arms of the robot were placed transvaginally and transcolonically via 12-mm trocars, respectively. The assistant operated the camera through the midline port. The kidney was dissected and removed intact through the vagina. The total operative time was 150 min, and no complications were reported. Repeated arm collision was noted due to limited port separation. Formerly, the authors were unable to remove the kidney with the standard da Vinci robotic system. However, the da Vinci S system provided an increased range of motion and increased instrument length compared to the previous generation robot. The authors also noted that the EndoWrist technology helped to achieve instrument triangulation while the robotic arms provided strong traction, which were significant advantages over pure NOTES.

Haber et al. reported a large experience with robotic NOTES in the laboratory setting [12]. Using 10 pigs, 30 robotic NOTES procedures were performed, including 10 pyeloplasties, 10 partial nephrectomies, and 10 complete nephrectomies. The first robotic arm and camera were placed through a 2-cm umbilical incision, whereas the second robotic arm was placed though the vagina. The mean operative time was 154 min, with a mean warm ischemia time during partial nephrectomy of 25.4 min. No intraoperative complication occurred. The time to robot preparation was found to be inversely correlated to increasing case number. Due to space limitations around the umbilicus, a considerable restriction in movement was encountered. Furthermore, friction between the robotic arm and camera resulted in unexpected intracorporeal movement of the instruments. While the robotic arm placed through the vagina had a full range of motion, in a third of the radical nephrectomy cases, the instrument was unable to reach the upper pole of the kidney.

Desai et al. reported the technical feasibility of performing transvesical robotic radical prostatectomy in two fresh male cadavers (prostate volume 46 and 30 ml) [13]. In the first procedure, four laparoscopic transvesical trocars and in the second a single-port device were used and placed percutaneously into the bladder. A pneumovesicum was established in both cases and the da Vinci S robotic system was used. All steps of the procedure were performed transvesically and robotically. Both procedures were technically successful, with no need for additional ports or conversion to standard laparoscopy. The operative duration was 3 h for the multiport procedure and 4.2 h for the single-port procedure. Clashing of the da Vinci arms represented the major technical difficulty with the single-port procedure but did not occur in the multiport procedure.

In these preliminary studies, clashing of the robotic instruments remained a significant obstacle. Joseph et al. proposed a novel robotic docking technique to minimize collision of the robotic arms [14]. They described a "chopstick" arrangement in which the instruments are crossed such that the right instrument is on the left side and the left instrument is on the right. The robotic console is then directed to control the left instrument with the right hand, and vice versa. The authors subsequently compared the "chopstick" arrangement to standard single-port placement in a laparoscopic box trainer. They noted that the "chopstick" arrangement improved times and reduced instrument collision, camera manipulations, clutching, and errors across all tasks. It is the author's experience that while this arrangement can be useful in certain situations, it is usually not effective for use during a complete procedure.

Robotic LESS: Clinical Experience

As experience with standard "laparoscopic" single-site surgery has grown, so too has the complexity of the procedures performed. The same holds true for robotic single-site surgery (Table 26.1). Kaouk et al. reported the initial clinical experience with robotic single-port surgery, using the da Vinci S system and a multichannel single port, the R-Port® (Advanced Surgical Concepts, Dublin, Ireland), to perform a radical prostatectomy, pyeloplasty, and radical nephrectomy [15]. The robotic camera and a 5-mm robotic port were placed through the R-Port, while a second 5- or 8-mm robotic trocar was placed alongside the multichannel port though the same incision. Using this robotic setup, surgeons completed all procedures successfully without the need for the placement of additional ports, and no intraoperative complications occurred. Operative times, estimated blood losses, and hospital lengths of stay were within the ranges of those reported with conventional laparoscopy.

From the same group of investigators at the Cleveland Clinic, Stein et al. reported robotic LESS using the GelPort® (Applied Medical, Rancho Santa Margarita, CA) [16]. Two pyeloplasties (mean operative time 235 min), one radical nephrectomy (operative time 200 min), and one partial nephrectomy (operative time 180 min) for an 11-cm angiomyolipoma were performed. No complications were reported. A 12-mm camera port, two 8-mm robotic ports, and a 12-mm assistant port were placed through the GelPort. While use of the robot required a longer incision than for standard LESS procedures, the GelPort allowed for a larger-profile working platform, flexibility for port placement, and easier access for the assistant.

Together with their experience in a cadaveric model, Barret et al. also presented their initial case of a robot-assisted LESS radical prostatectomy [17]. One 12-mm trocar and two 8-mm robotic ports were placed through a 4-cm umbilical incision. Fascial dissection permitted 3–3.5-cm separation between robotic trocars. An additional 5-mm port was placed in the lower abdomen to assist with suctioning and to serve as the drain site. Disadvantages of this configuration included some external clashing of the robotic arms and difficulty with instrument exchange. The operative time was 150 min (5 min to control the dorsal venous complex and 30 min to perform the urethrovesical anastomosis), and final pathologic examination revealed negative surgical margins. The authors pointed out that before embarking on single-site surgery in the clinical setting, it was important to gain experience with the limited working environment using pelvic trainers and cadaver models.

Table 26.1 Robotic LESS: early clinical experience

References	No. of ports	Procedure	Port used	Operative time	Outcome	Complications	Comment
Kaouk et al. [15]	3	1 radical prostatectomy	R-Port® (Advanced Surgical Concepts, Dublin, Ireland)	5 h (45 min for anastomosis)	Margins negative	None	Longer incision required. Allows more flexibility of port placement and easier access for the assistant
		1 pyeloplasty		4. 5 h		None	
		1 radical nephrectomy		2.5 h		None	
Stein et al. [16]	4	2 pyeloplasties	GelPort® (Applied Medical, Rancho Santa Margarita, CA)	235 min		None	
		1 radical nephrectomy		200 min		None	
		1 partial nephrectomy		180 min		1 transfusion	
Barret et al. [17]	1	1 radical prostatectomy	4-cm umbilical incision	150 min (30 min for anastomosis)	Negative margins	None	An additional 5-mm port placed at drain site
Barret et al. [18]	1	1 radical prostatectomy	Umbilical incision with ports placed in a rhomboid fashion	210 min (35 min for anastomosis)	Negative margins	None	
White et al. [19]	20	20 radical prostatectomies	SILS™ port (Covidien, Cupertino, CA)	189.5 min	4 positive margins	1 ileus, 1 transfusion, 1 pulmonary embolus, 1 urosepsis	Retraction difficult and advise liberal use of marionette sutures 30° upward-looking lens, staggering of robotic cannulae helps to reduce instrument clashing Using a combination of 8- and 5-mm instruments maximizes benefits of both

(continued)

Table 26.1 (continued)

References	No. of ports	Procedure	Port used	Operative time	Outcome	Complications	Comment
Kaouk et al. [20]	2	2 partial nephrectomy	TriPort™ (Olympus, Tokyo, Japan)	170 min		None	Pediatric robotic instruments were utilized, resulting in increased range of motion
White et al. [21]	10	10 radical nephrectomy	SILS GelPort/ GelPOINT	167.5 min	Negative magins	1 wound infection	
Choi et al. [22]	73	56 partial nephrectomies	Homemade single-port device	198 min	Mean $T^{1/2}$ 26 min / 2 positive margins	2 conversions / 1 renal vein injury / 1 ureter injury / 1 postoperative bleeding	Single-port device cost-effective, provided adequate range of motion and more cost-effective than other available devices
		12 nephroureterectomies		227 min		1 acute renal failure, 1 retroperitoneal abcess	
		2 radical nephrectomies		248 min		1 conversion	
		1 simple nephrectomy		128 min		1 bowel injury	
		2 adrenalectomies		167 min		Nil	

The same group reported a second case of robotic LESS radical prostatectomy [18]. Again, the operation was performed with the da Vinci interface and standard trocars. Ports were placed in a rhomboid fashion with the endoscope in the upper corner (12-mm), a 5-mm trocar in the lower corner for suction and retraction purposes, and 8-mm working ports on either side. Clashing between instruments was noted externally, and this impaired the assistant's performance. The total operative time was 210 min. Dorsal venous control was accomplished in 3 min, whereas the urethrovesical anastomosis was performed in 35 min. No perioperative complications were observed.

Extensive experience with robotic LESS radical prostatectomy has recently been described by White et al. [19]. They reported 20 cases performed via a 3–4.5-cm periumbilical incision. Optimal port positioning was achieved by placing an 8-mm robotic port on the right side, under finger guidance, at the most caudal portion of the incision directed as far laterally as possible. This same positioning was then repeated on the opposite side with a 5- or 8-mm robotic port. The multichannel SILS™ port (Covidien, Cupertino, CA) was then deployed through the fascial incision into the abdominal cavity. The robotic camera and a 5-mm assistant port were then inserted through the single-port device and a prostatectomy performed with the aid of "marionette" sutures. The mean operative time was 187.6 min, and the EBL was 128.8 ml. Pathology revealed four positive margins, with two occurring during the first three cases. The authors reported that tissue retraction can be difficult secondary to the lack of the fourth robotic arm and advised liberal use of the "marionette" sutures. Furthermore, crowding of instruments and leaking of carbon dioxide through the single-port access device on occasion limited the assistant's ability to suction or retract tissues.

Laparoscopic partial nephrectomy represents a technically demanding procedure under the best of circumstances. Kaouk and Goel reported on their experience with seven LESS partial nephrectomies, two of which were performed with the robot: a 2.8-cm left lower pole tumor and a 1.1-cm right lower pole tumor [20]. Both were excised without hilar clamping using a harmonic scalpel. The multichannel TriPort™ (Olympus, Japan) and 5-mm robotic instruments were utilized for the procedure. The authors noted that the smaller (5-mm) instruments deflect rather than articulate, resulting in an increased range of motion. One 5-mm robotic trocar was placed though the TriPort, whereas the second robotic trocar was placed through the same skin incision alongside the TriPort. This arrangement diminished clashing and improved the second robotic arm's range of motion. The operative time was 170 min. Based on the authors' experience, small, exophytic, anterior, interpolar to lower pole renal masses are best suited to LESS and robotic LESS approaches.

White et al. [21] recently described their technique of robotic LESS radical nephrectomy using either the SILS port or the GelPoint® (Applied Medical, Rancho Santa Margarita, CA). The patient is positioned in a modified flank position and an incision is made extending 1 cm below to 2 cm above the umbilicus. The abdomen is then entered. With the SILS port, the robotic trocars are placed through separate laterally directed fascial stab sites, whereas with the GelPOINT, the trocars are placed through the port itself. The robot is then positioned over the patient's shoulder. A 30° downward directed scope and two 8-mm trocars or an 8-mm trocar and a 5-mm trocar were used to perform the surgeries. The nephrectomy is performed according to standard principles. Ten cases were performed using this technique, and the masses were primarily interpolar or lower pole in location and as such did not require hepatic or splenic retraction. The mean operative time was 167.5 min, and the estimated blood loss was 100 ml. In a retrospective comparison with ten standard laparoscopic nephrectomies, the R-LESS cohort was found to have a decreased mean hospital stay (2.5 vs. 3 days) and reduced narcotic requirements (25.3 vs. 37.5 mg) compared to conventional laparoscopy.

Choi et al. [22] recently reported their results with 171 consecutive LESS cases, 73 of which were performed robotically. This included 56 partial nephrectomies, 12 nephroureterectomies, 2 radical nephrectomies, 1 simple nephrectomy, and 2 adrenalectomies. A homemade single-port device consisting of an Alexis wound retractor and a size 7½ surgical glove was used as the access platform. With the exception of simple and radical nephrectomies, most procedures required the addition of a 12-mm port. The mean WIT during partial nephrectomy was 26 min. Two patients had focally positive margins on final pathology, while in both cases, intraoperative frozen sections were reported as negative. Complications during partial nephrectomy included one renal vein injury, one ureteral injury, and one case of postoperative hemorrhage. Two complications occurred during nephroureterectomy, including acute renal failure and retroperitoneal abscess, and one complication occurred in the patient undergoing simple nephrectomy (bowel injury). The authors noted that their homemade single-port device offered advantages, including flexibility to accommodate a variable number and size of trocars depending on the operation to be performed and an increased range of motion. When comparing conventional LESS to robotic LESS, the authors noted that robotic LESS was more suitable for complex procedures requiring intracorporeal suturing such as partial nephrectomy or bladder cuff resection. The authors felt that the robotic EndoWrist technology made hilar dissection and dissection of the upper and posterior portions of the kidney safer and more expedient. The authors stated that transitioning from conventional to robotic LESS allowed them to treat intraparenchymal, upper pole, and posterior masses.

Robotic laparoendoscopic single-site surgery is also being applied across disciplines. Initial case reports of right colectomy and hysterectomy have been described [23, 24].

Clinical studies have shown that avoiding instrument clashing and external collision of the robotic arms is key to optimizing success with robotic LESS. Aside from the "chopstick" arrangement described previously and/or using 5-mm robotic instruments, additional tips for reducing instrument clashing include use of a 30 degree lens in an upward or downward configuration and setting the da Vinci system to "fine"-tuning to obtain better motion scaling. A major disadvantage of using the present robotic system for LESS is the need to create a larger incision (approximately 4 cm or more) compared to the smaller incisions used for standard LESS.

Robotic LESS: Future Perspectives

The future of both LESS and NOTES depends on technological advances. These improvements can occur in different areas: visual systems, access systems, and instrumentation. The flexible-tip laparoscope has represented a great adjunct in single-site surgery; however, it still occupies some space at the abdominal access site and no deflectable-tip scope exists for use with the da Vinci robotic system. A novel voice- and/or foot-controlled low-profile robot has been developed to control the laparoscope for conventional LESS and tested in the laboratory setting. They noted that the robotic endoscope holder allowed more room for the operating surgeon [25]. In addition, a number of newer access devices designed for LESS have entered or will soon enter the market [26]. The use of magnetic anchoring and guidance systems (MAGS) may also become a valuable tool, permitting the retraction and manipulation of tissues without the addition of extra transabdominal instruments [27] (Fig. 26.1). MAGS instruments are introduced into the peritoneum through an incision in the skin or natural orifice and are controlled with extracorporeal magnets.

While the da Vinci and da Vinci S systems are valuable allies in LESS, this is not what they were specifically designed for. A robot built specifically for single-site surgery, the VeSPA® (Intuitive Surgical, Sunnyvale, CA), with a purpose-built single-port access device and longer bent trocars, has undergone laboratory trials with radical nephrectomy, partial nephrectomy, and pyeloplasty all being successfully completed in the porcine model [28] (Fig. 26.2). The VeSPA instruments are used with the da Vinci Si Surgical System. The multichannel port allows placement of an 8.5-mm scope, a 12-mm assistant trocar, and two crossing curved cannulae for the robotic instruments. In order to be placed through these longer curved cannulae, the VeSPA instruments are semirigid and lack articulation at their distal end. Because the instruments cross, the console is instructed to control the right robotic arm with the left hand, and vice versa. The system was noted to provide a wide range of motion, scope stability, and reasonable ergonomics. Furthermore, instrument clashing was noted to be significantly reduced compared to standard laparoendoscopic single-site surgery. The disadvantages noted with the new system, however, included the loss of articulation, rendering intracorporeal suturing more difficult, leak of pneumoperitoneum, and tearing of the multichannel port.

Flexible Robotics and In Vivo Robots

Despite their advantages, current robotic systems are constrained by a fulcrum effect at the abdominal wall incision. To overcome this restriction, research and development has focused on the development of miniature and flexible robots.

Fig. 26.1 (**a**) Manipulation
of a magnetic anchoring and
guidance systems (*MAGS*)
endoscope using an
extracorporeal magnet; (**b**)
appendectomy as visualized
with a MAGS endoscope
(With kind permission from
Springer Science+Business
Media: Cadeddu et al. [27])

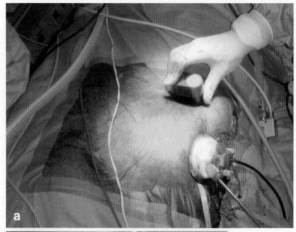

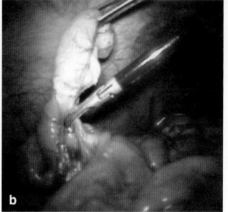

Flexible Robotics

The Sensei® robotic catheter (Hansen Medical System, Mountain View, CA) was
initially developed for cardiovascular applications and has subsequently been
adapted for ureteroscopy. This device is a master–slave system that is composed of
four components: (1) a surgeon console consisting of liquid-crystal display (LCD)
monitors and a master input device (MID); (2) a steerable catheter system; (3) a
remote catheter manipulator; and (4) an electronic rack. The steerable catheter system is composed of a 14/12 Fr outer catheter sheath and a 12/10 Fr inner catheter
guide. The ureteroscope is inserted through the catheter guide. The scope, sheath,
and guide are then mounted onto the remote catheter manipulator. The surgeon uses
the MID to remotely control the tip of the catheter guide. Manipulations can be
performed under endoscopic or fluoroscopic guidance. Desai et al. reported using
this system for robotic ureterorenoscopy in the porcine model [29]. The system was
introduced into ten ureters, two of which required balloon dilation. Eighty-three of

Fig. 26.2 (a) Flexible instruments and curved cannulae of the VeSPA® (Intuitive Surgical, Sunnyvale, CA) single-site robotic prototype; (b) VeSPA robotic prototype docked in the porcine model through a specifically designed single port

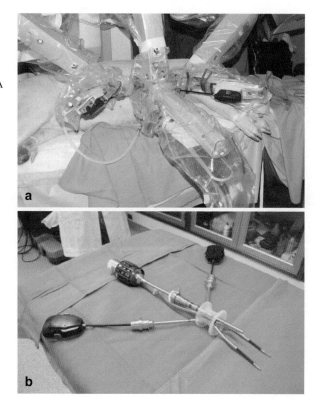

85 calices were inspected, and the mean time to inspect all calices in each kidney was 4.6 min. In addition, calculi placed within the kidney could be successfully managed with holmium laser lithotripsy. A perforation of the ureteropelvic junction comprised the sole complication. Instrument stability and the reproducibility of access into each calyx were rated 10 on a 10-point visual analog scale. The authors report that advantages of this system included an increased range of motion, instrument stability, and improved ergonomics. This group subsequently reported the first clinical application of robotic flexible ureteroscopy in 18 patients [30]. All patients were presented for 2 weeks. All intrarenal maneuvers, including stone localization, repositioning, and lithotripsy, were performed under control of the flexible prototype system. All procedures were successfully completed, with a mean operative time of 91 min. Complications included pyelonephritis in two patients, pyrexia in one patient, and temporary limb paresis in one patient. One patient required repeat ureteroscopy for a residual stone.

The Sensei robotic catheter (Hansen Medical St. Louis, MO) is a flexible catheter manipulator that uses a computer-controlled magnetic field and a custom-designed catheter for steering [30]. Catheter tip manipulations can be made in 1-mm increments with 1° of deflection. This system has been used primarily for cardiovascular applications, and nonvascular applications have yet to be reported.

The NeoGuide® (NeoGuide Systems, San Jose, CA) was developed to overcome the problem of looping encountered during colonoscopy [31]. The system utilizes a computer-controlled insertion tube. This tube allows proximal segments of the colonoscope to follow the path taken by the tip as it is advanced through the colon. A sensor at the tip records the steering commands of the endoscopist while an external position sensor records the depth of insertion. The computer combines this information to articulate each segment of the scope such that it follows the same shape as the tip of the scope and the contour of the colon. The system is currently available for use for colonoscopy.

The Viacath® (EndoVia Medical, Norwood, MA) is a first-generation robot used for endolumenal surgery [31]. It consists of a master console, a slave drive system, and flexible instruments that run in conjunction with a flexible endoscope. The articulated instruments deploy in front of the endoscope, providing triangulation and allowing for surgical manipulation under visual control.

In 2006, the group of Dr. S. C. Low from the Nanyang Technological University, Singapore, reported the MASTER (Master And Slave Transluminal Endoscopic Robot) for gastrointestinal endoscopic procedures. This is a master–slave system that consists of a master controller, a workstation, and a manipulator with two end effectors: a grasper and monopolar hook cautery. The controller is attached to the wrist and fingers of the surgeon and connected to the manipulator by electrical wires. The surgeon's movements are detected and converted to control signals that operate the end effector. Using this system, transgastric wedge hepatic resection was performed in a porcine model [32].

In Vivo Robots

In vivo robots can be inserted into the abdominal cavity. Since they are not constrained by the abdominal incision, miniaturization leads to enhanced intraabdominal mobility.

Current miniature robotic platforms fit into two broad categories: fixed-base and mobile robots. Fixed-base robots cannot self-navigate from their original position, whereas mobile robots possess the capability to navigate the abdominal cavity.

The pan-and-tilt imaging robot is a fixed-base robot that is able to rotate 360° and tilt 45° [33]. The robot rests on spring-loaded platform legs that are abducted after entry into the abdominal cavity. This robot has been used to assist in laparoscopic cholecystectomy in a porcine model and laparoscopic prostatectomy in a canine model. The designers report that it provided additional camera angles that augmented visualization.

Conversely, the mobile imaging robot is capable of forward, reverse, and turning motion. It contains two independently driven helical-profile wheels that provide traction without causing tissue trauma. This device was able to provide enhanced depth perception during a porcine cholecystectomy. Furthermore, the addition of a biopsy forcep to this design has created a mobile biopsy robot that has been used for liver biopsy.

Fig. 26.3 Six-degree-of-freedom multifunctional miniature in vivo surgical robot was designed to be completely inserted into the abdominal cavity through a single incision, yet is capable of performing surgical procedures in multiple quadrants of the abdominal cavity utilizing interchangeable end effectors (Compliments of Dr. Dmitry Oleynikov)

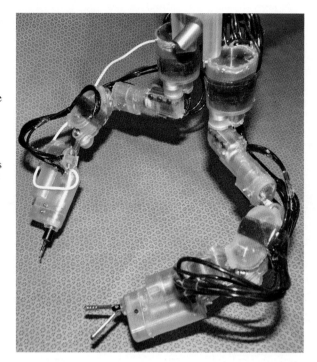

Task-specific robots, including a camera robot, lighting robot, and retracting robot, have been used in combination to perform cholecystectomy in a nonsurvival porcine study [34]. The imaging robot consists of a clear outer tube that houses an inner cylinder containing a lens, camera board, light-emitting diodes (LED) for lighting, and direct-current micromotors capable of rotating the inner housing within the clear outer tube. The robot is held to the anterior abdominal wall by the interaction between magnets fitted on each end of the robot with an external magnetic handle. Similarly, a magnetically anchored lighting robot containing six white LEDs and a retraction robot consisting of a tethered grasping device have also been developed.

The University of Nebraska group has also developed a multiarm, dexterous miniature robot with a remote surgeon interface. The robot consists of two arms, each made up of upper and lower segments, that are connected to a central body. Retraction and extension can be achieved by telescoping the lower arm in and out of the upper arm [33]. End effectors can be interchanged to function as cautery or tissue manipulators. The robot is designed to be inserted through a single incision and contained completely within the peritoneal cavity (Fig. 26.3). The robot is held to the upper abdominal wall using magnets housed in the body of the robot and an external magnetic handle that can be repositioned throughout the procedure.

Wortman et al. used a miniature robotic platform to perform four cholecystectomies in the porcine model [35]. While the authors were able to insert the robot through a 1-in. incision, complete intraperitoneal assembly of the robot was not possible due to limited space. Therefore, a larger incision was made and the robot was suspended to complete the procedure. The authors reported that the primary limitation of the current system remains the size of the device and that this was being addressed in newer designs.

While still in their infancy, these prototypes hold great promise to remedy challenges currently encountered in robotic single-port surgery. As newer instruments are designed that allow for more precise dissection, retraction, and reconstruction, this will ultimately allow more complex procedures to be performed using a LESS or NOTES approach.

Conclusions

LESS is a technically demanding endeavor. Clinical studies have shown it to be safe and feasible; however, a strong laparoscopic skill set is required for both the surgeon and the assistant, and considerable challenges and ergonomic disadvantages exist. Robotics provides substantial promise in terms of improving precision, safety, and surgeon comfort. While the current robotic system is bulky, it nonetheless already offers many of these advantages for LESS. Technological advancements, including the development of novel robotic prototypes and flexible robots, will likely overcome current limitations and usher in the next generation of robotic single-site and NOTES surgery.

References

1. Pemberton RJ, Tolley DA, van Velthoven RF. Prevention and management of complications in urological laparoscopic port site placement. Eur Urol. 2006;50(5):958–68.
2. Box G, Averch T, Cadeddu J, et al. Nomenclature of natural orifice translumenal endoscopic surgery (NOTES) and laparoendoscopic single-site surgery (LESS) procedures in urology. J Endourol. 2008;22(11):2575–81.
3. White WM, Haber GP, Doerr MJ, Gettman M. Natural orifice translumenal endoscopic surgery. Urol Clin North Am. 2009;36(2):147–55, vii.
4. Tracy CR, Raman JD, Cadeddu JA, Rane A. Laparoendoscopic single-site surgery in urology: where have we been and where are we heading? Nat Clin Pract Urol. 2008;5(10):561–8.
5. Hirano D, Minei S, Yamaguchi K, et al. Retroperitoneoscopic adrenalectomy for adrenal tumors via a single large port. J Endourol. 2005;19:788–92.
6. Rane A, Kommu S, Eddy B, et al. Clinical evaluation of a novel laparoscopic port (R-Port) and evolution of the single laparoscopic port procedure (SLIPP). J Endourol. 2007;21 Suppl 1:A1–292.
7. Raman JD, Bensalah K, Bagrodia A, et al. Laboratory and clinical development of single keyhole umbilical nephrectomy. Urology. 2007;70:1039–42.
8. White WM, Haber GP, Goel RK, et al. Single-port urological surgery: single-center experience with the first 100 cases. Urology. 2009;74(4):801–4.
9. Irwin BH, Rao PP, Stein RJ, Desai MM. Laparoendoscopic single site surgery in urology. Urol Clin North Am. 2009;36(2):223–35, ix.
10. Kommu SS, Rane A. Devices for laparoendoscopic single-site surgery in urology. Expert Rev Med Devices. 2009;6(1):95–103.

11. Box GN, Lee HJ, Santos RJ, et al. Rapid communication: robot-assisted NOTES nephrectomy: initial report. J Endourol. 2008;22:503–8.
12. Haber GP, Crouzet S, Kamoi K, et al. Robotic NOTES (natural orifice transluminal endoscopic surgery) in reconstructive urology: initial laboratory experience. Urology. 2008;71: 996–1000.
13. Desai MM, Aron M, Berger A, et al. Transvesical robotic radical prostatectomy. BJU Int. 2008;102(11):1666–9.
14. Joseph RA, Goh AC, Cuevas SP, et al. "Chopstick" surgery: a novel technique improves surgeon performance and eliminates arm collision in robotic single-incision laparoscopic surgery. Surg Endosc. 2010;24:1331–5.
15. Kaouk JH, Goel RK, Haber GP, et al. Robotic single port transumbilical surgery in humans: initial report. BJU Int. 2008;103:366–9.
16. Stein RJ, White WM, Goel RK, et al. Robotic laparoendoscopic single-site surgery using GelPort as the access platform. Eur Urol. 2010;57(1):132–7.
17. Barret E, Sanchez-Salas R, Kasraeian A, et al. A transition to laparoendoscopic single-site surgery (LESS) radical prostatectomy: human cadaver experimental and initial clinical experience. J Endourol. 2009;23(1):135–40.
18. Barret E, Sanchez-Salas R, Cathelineau X, et al. Re: initial complete laparoendoscopic single-site surgery robotic assisted radical prostatectomy (LESS-RARP). Int Braz J Urol. 2009;35(1): 92–3.
19. White MA, Haber GP, Autorino R, et al. Robotic laparoendoscopic single-site radical prostatectomy: technique and early outcomes. Eur Urol. 2010;58:544–50.
20. Kaouk JH, Goel RK. Single-port laparoscopic and robotic partial nephrectomy. Eur Urol. 2009;55(5):1163–9.
21. White MA, Autorino R, Spana G, et al. Robotic laparoendoscopic single-site radical nephrectomy: surgical technique and comparative outcomes. Eur Urol. 2011;59:815–22.
22. Choi KH, Ham WS, Rha KH, et al. Laparoendoscopic single-site surgeries: a single center experience of 171 consecutive cases. Korean J Urol. 2011;52:31–8.
23. Ostrowitz MB, Eschete D, Zemon H, DeNoto G. Robotic-assisted single-incision right colectomy: early experience. Int J Med Robot. 2009;5(4):465–70.
24. Escobar PF, Fader AN, Paraiso MF, et al. Robotic-assisted laparoendoscopic single-site surgery in gynecology: initial report and technique. J Minim Invasive Gynecol. 2009;16(5): 589–91.
25. Crouzet S, Haber GP, White WM, et al. Single-port, single-operator-light endoscopic robot-assisted laparoscopic urology: pilot study in a pig model. BJU Int. 2009;105(5):682–5.
26. Herati AS, Atalla MA, Rais-Bahrami S, et al. A new valve-less trocar for urologic laparoscopy: initial evaluation. J Endourol. 2009;23(9):1535–9.
27. Cadeddu J, Fernandez R, Desai M, et al. Novel magnetically guided intra-abdominal camera to facilitate laparoendoscopic single-site surgery: initial human experience. Surg Endosc. 2009;23(8):1894–9.
28. Haber GP, White MA, Autorino R, et al. Novel robotic da Vinci instruments for laparoendoscopic single-site surgery. Urology. 2010;76:1279–82.
29. Desai MM, Aron M, Gill IS, et al. Flexible robotic retrograde renoscopy: descriptions of novel robotic device and preliminary laboratory experience. Urology. 2008;72:42–6.
30. Aron M, Desai MM. Flexible robotics. Urol Clin North Am. 2009;36:157–62.
31. Karimyan V, Sodergren M, Clark J, et al. Navigation systems and platforms in natural orifice translumenal endoscopic surgery (NOTES). Int J Surg. 2009;7:297–304.
32. Rane A, Autorino R. Robotic natural orifice translumenal endoscopic surgery and laparoendoscopic single-site surgery: current status. Curr Opin Urol. 2011;21:71–7.
33. Tiwari MM, Reynoso JF, Lehman AC, et al. In vivo miniature robots for natural orifice surgery: state of the art and future perspectives. World J Gastrointest Surg. 2010;2(6):217–23.
34. Shah BC, Buettner SL, Lehman AC, et al. Miniature in vivo robotics and novel robotic surgical platforms. Urol Clin North Am. 2009;6:251–63.
35. Wortman TD, Strabala KW, Lehman AC. Laparoendoscopic single-site surgery using a multifunctional miniature in vivo robot. Int J Med Robot. 2011;7:17–21.

Chapter 27
Future Perspectives on Scarless Surgery: Where We Have Been and Where We Are Going

Alexander R. Aurora and Jeffrey L. Ponsky

Keywords Single-incision • Scarless • Transumbilical • NOTES • Needlescopic

Introduction

Surgeons are the directors of the future in surgery. Since the dawn of surgery, surgeons have been pushing the envelope and impatiently awaiting technology to catch up. In the early days of surgery, there was more interest in how large an incision could be made and how much exposure could be achieved. Patients were proud to show off their stem-to-stern incision and brag they survived. In this new era, surgery has taken a 180° turn, and we pride ourselves on doing the most surgery through the smallest incision, or even better, no incision. This has been the birth of scarless surgery. Although laparoscopy has been practiced since the early 1900s, it was not until the advent of the charge-coupled device (CCD) that videoscopic surgery rose to prime time. The CCD catapulted laparoscopic surgery across the country and around the world. The availability of excellent magnified vision of the surgical field gave surgeons the confidence to go beyond where laparoscopy had been before. As so many of the baby boomers and Generation Xers will

A.R. Aurora, M.D., M.Sc. (✉)
Department of General Surgery and Bariatrics,
Harford Memorial Hospital, Upper Chesapeake Medical System,
2027 Pulaski Hwy, Suite 201, Havre de Grace, MD 21078, USA
e-mail: aaurora@uchs.org

J.L. Ponsky, M.D.
Department of Surgery, University Hospitals Case Medical Center,
11100 Euclid Ave LKS-5047, Cleveland, OH 44106, USA
e-mail: jponsky@yahoo.com, jeffrey.ponsky@uhhospitals.org

A. Rane et al. (eds.), *Scar-Less Surgery*,
DOI 10.1007/978-1-84800-360-6_27, © Springer-Verlag London 2013

the rapid evolution of technology and development of new ideas has ‿ outpace our capacity to master the latest and greatest before we are over-run by something new. Most open surgical procedures have now been mastered by the experts in videoscopic surgery. Even as these procedures are still being perfected, new techniques have developed, single-incision laparoscopic surgery (SILS) and natural orifice translumenal endoscopic surgery (NOTES). Now as we affront the twenty-first century, the introductions of SILS and NOTES present themselves for the conquering by surgeons, once again pushing the limits of their skill, restricted only by technology. Surgery has evolved from a colon resection that required a 40-cm incision to a 3-cm single incision, or even to a transvaginal partial colectomy.

Natural Orifice Translumenal Endoscopic Surgery (NOTES)

NOTES was first described in 2004 by Kalloo et al. [1] from Johns Hopkins Hospital in Baltimore. They demonstrated that the peritoneal cavity could be accessed via a transgastric route for potential surgical intervention. In 2005, leaders from the American Society of Gastrointestinal Endoscopy (ASGE) and the Society of American Gastrointestinal and Endoscopic Surgeons (SAGES) met as a group called the Natural Orifice Surgery Consortium for Assessment and Research (NOSCAR). NOSCAR published a white paper of their deliberations and recommended IRB approval before performing any human NOTES procedure. The concept of NOTES rapidly gained interest around the world, and within a few years groups from India and others had already performed NOTES appendectomy, cholecystectomy, and other simple procedures. Surgeons attempted accessing the peritoneal cavity via different routes, including the stomach, vagina, colon, and bladder, all of which have their intrinsic limitations. While these approaches were demonstrated to be safe and effective, they were also laborious, time-consuming, and costly. Additionally, the method suffered from a lack of solution to basic technical problems like suturing, anastomosis, and hemostasis. These are but a few reasons why NOTES has struggled to gain a strong foothold in the general surgeon's toolbox. NOTES is still performed by a select group of surgeons, and much research and development is ongoing, but it is far from prime time. Continued development and refinement of technology as well as application of NOTES to more appropriate procedures may lead to common use of the method in the future. Specifically, the development of a stable surgical platform from which to operate and a dependable closure device will catapult NOTES into the mainstream. Recently, the over-the-scope clip (OTSC) has shown promise in the animal model.

Single-Incision Laparoscopic Surgery (SILS)

On the flip side from NOTES, the drive for scarless surgery has pushed laparoscopic surgeons to go from multiport to single-port surgery and sharpen their laparoscopic skills. Single-incision laparoscopic surgery has become the rage, and industry and patients are there to support it. New devices and instruments appear almost on a weekly basis for surgeons and researchers to make new leaps in the frontier of single-incision laparoscopy.

Laparoscopy began in the early 1900s without video and exploded once video was installed in the 1980s. Since the 1980s, surgeons have become adept at performing virtually any and all procedures that can be done open. On our voyage toward scarless surgery, we have challenged ourselves by decreasing the number of access ports needed to perform a procedure. Single-incision surgeries have blossomed throughout the country and world, from the early simple gallbladder and appendix to sleeve gastrectomies and colon resections. Most of these procedures can now be hidden by using the ideal historical natural orifice, the umbilicus. Transumbilical surgery has made general surgery a scarless domain. The umbilicus can be opened 3–5 cm. Using one of many single-port devices on the market, three to four instruments can be introduced and a dozen procedures performed. Once the procedure is complete, the single port is removed, the umbilicus carefully closed to avoid hernia formation, and a little skin glue applied to cover the umbilical incision. No one can ever tell this person had surgery because the patient remains without a visible scar, scar*less*.

Currently, transumbilical surgery is the most effective platform for performing a multitude of procedures and leaving no visible scar. The domain is already saturated with a multitude of single-access ports, newly developed instruments helping surgeons overcome the coaxial sword fighting by reproducing triangulation. This is made possible by either bending the instruments or making them flexible. The development of new instruments for the field of single-incision laparoscopic surgery is expanding on a daily basis. New video camera devices are also being produced to once again provide more flexibility when working from a single port to be able to view the anatomy from multiple angles, thereby enlarging the working space.

Needlescopic Surgery

Needlescopic surgery is a new form of laparoscopic surgery using instruments that are 2–3 mm in diameter, including the camera. Clearly, this technology is better suited for our pediatric surgery colleagues. However, newer instruments are constructed better and stronger for eventual use in adult patients. This approach allows the surgeon to use standard laparoscopic positioning while making smaller incisions that may be virtually invisible once healed. On the down side, an incision will eventually have to be made to be able to extract the given specimen.

Devices and Instrumentation

Single-Port Devices

There have been a number of single-port access devices developed for entry into the abdominal cavity through a single site, whether it is the umbilicus or through another site of the abdominal wall (Fig. 27.1). The principle is the same: One incision is made in the skin and fascia through which a rigid or spongy 3–5-cm device is inserted. The device may have a fixed number of trocar sites, or they can be placed on an as-needed basis. The most common models currently used employ the use of down-sized, streamlined, low-profile trocars with smaller heads to reduce the clashing of trocars and camera at the fulcrum of entry.

Camera Options

The conventional angled laparoscope is most commonly used for single-incision laparoscopy. Typical adjustments for SILS compared to standard laparoscopy are to use a 5-mm scope with a longer shaft. A 5-mm scope gives you more space at the point of entry and makes the platform less rigid and easier to move other instruments. With the use of a longer scope, the camera head is drawn away from the patient, thereby decreasing external clashing with the operator. Clearly, these benefits are not without the sacrifice of inferior lighting and therefore an overall decrease in image quality. A 5-mm coaxial 30° laparoscope does exist that provides excellent imaging, and this does dismiss the need for a longer laparoscope.

Some authors have described the use of the flexible endoscope to perform single-incision laparoscopic procedures. This technique provides a relatively unstable operating platform and makes triangulation difficult. The advantages of using a flexible endoscope are increased ergonomics, decreasing sword fighting and instrument conflict inside the abdomen, and hassle-free vision with instantaneous camera

Fig. 27.1 Trocars and single-port devices. (**a**) SILS™ port (Copyright © 2012 Covidien. All rights reserved. Used with the permission of Covidien). (**b**) SILS™ port, obturator, cannulas, and obturator/cannula (Copyright © 2012 Covidien. All rights reserved. Used with the permission of Covidien). (**c**) GelPOINT™ (Courtesy of Applied Medical Resources Corporation, Rancho Santa Margarita, CA; all rights reserved)

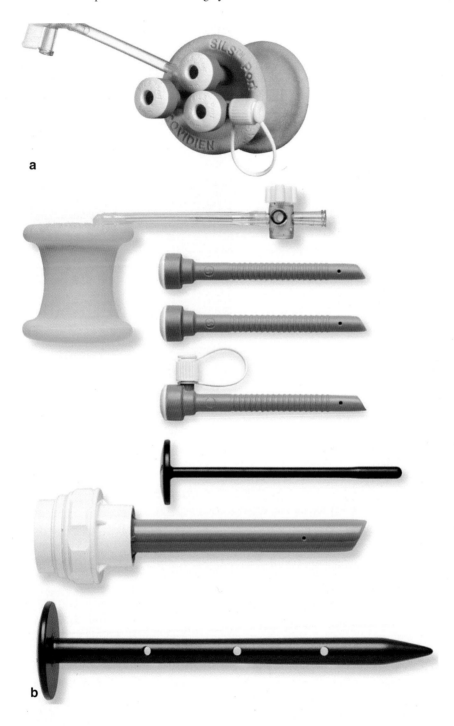

Fig. 27.1 (continued)

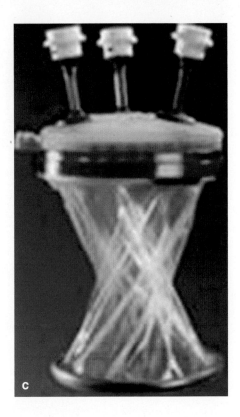

irrigation. However, one must consider the availability of an extra set of trained hands to maneuver the endoscope.

One company has developed an excellent compromise between a rigid laparoscope and a flexible endoscope, known as the EndoEYE™ (Olympus Surgical, Center Valley, PA) (Fig. 27.2). The EndoEYE is a rigid 5-mm high-definition video laparoscope with a flexible tip that provides excellent images. It can be more easily maneuvered than an endoscope and locked in place. This device is more amenable to laparoscopy than an endoscope and its function grasped quickly.

Future endeavors may employ the use of a battery-powered wireless light-emitting diode (LED) camera, which can be placed in the abdomen through a 2-cm incision and then fixed in placed with magnets. This device has been used and provides a view from above, is able to visualize all parts of the abdomen, but often does not provide enough light. Research efforts will certainly overcome this difficulty in the near future. The eventual development of wireless high-definition CCD would be a significant advance in the world of laparoscopy.

Lastly, one can imagine a microcamera fixed in place on the abdominal wall that now has auto tracking technology. The device recognizes the marker on the tip of the instruments and can follow the procedure robotically without external guidance. Currently, this technology is only being used in the security industry but could easily be adapted for use in surgery.

Fig. 27.2 Deflectable-tip
camera EndoEye™ (Courtesy
of Olympus Surgical, Center
Valley, PA)

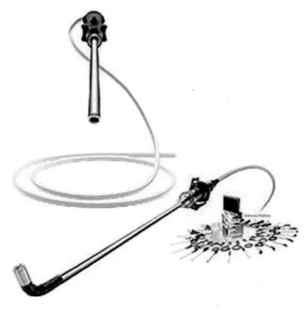

Instruments

The most prevalent difficulties encountered during single-incision laparoscopic surgery are the coaxial movement of instruments, lack of triangulation, and sword fighting. These are worse when using an access device that has predetermined trocar sites and trocar sites that are closer together. The single-port access devices that allow for the operator to decide the trocar position and allow for greater space between trocars are advantageous.

Standard, straight, rigid instruments are commonly used but newer prebent or flexible instruments are available and new ones are in development. Currently, several companies have graspers, electrocautery, scissors, and suturing devices with flexible tips (Fig. 27.3a–d). These instruments provide a degree of freedom with some return to the concept of triangulation that is so important in laparoscopy. However, these instruments are more expensive, nonreusable, and not as robust as standard disposables.

Prebent instruments are more robust and reusable; however, they must be used through a specific access port. These instruments have been found to provide a closer replication of standard laparoscopic movement and technique.

There has been interest in the development of "smart tools" with multifunctional tips. The concept of a robotic device changing the tip of your instrument without having to pull it out and replace it is another possible advance in instrument design on the horizon. Early studies have suggested that this may significantly decrease OR time and may reduce the risk of iatrogenic injury during surgery.

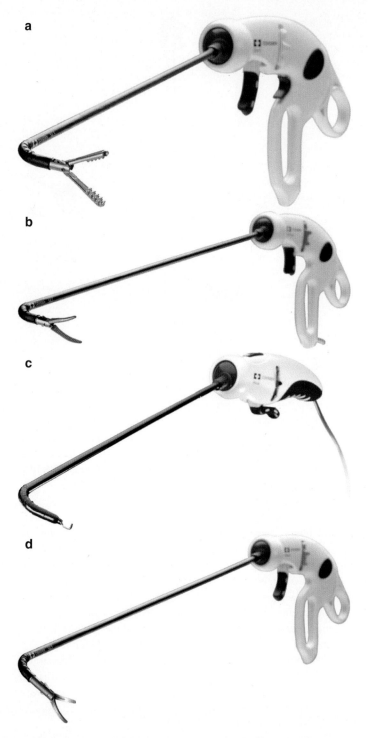

Fig. 27.3 Flexible instruments (SILS™ hand instruments): (**a**) clinch; (**b**) dissector; (**c**) hook; (**d**) shears (All images copyright © 2012 Covidien. All rights reserved. Used with the permission of Covidien)

Fig. 27.4 Single-Port
Instrument Delivery
Extended Research
(SPIDER®) device used for
single-incision surgery
(Courtesy of TransEnterix,
Durham, NC)

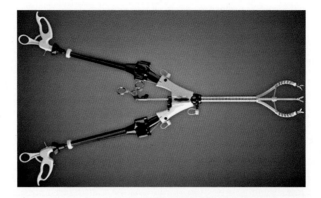

Advanced instruments for hemostasis and energy delivery are currently only available in straight and rigid forms, i.e., harmonic and ligasure devices. These devices will need to be developed in a flexible form. There is currently only a flexible hook-cautery device available.

A newcomer to the single-incision laparoscopy scene is the Single Port Instrument Delivery Extended Research (SPIDER®; TransEnterix, Durham, NC), which is essentially a delivery system from a rigid platform of three 5-mm instruments that are curved on the inside of the abdomen (Fig. 27.4). The SPIDER provides a good rigid platform and does have easy maneuverability, triangulation, and a 360° range of motion. It is currently undergoing clinical testing in humans.

Robotics

The current surgical robotic system in use provides an excellent platform for a limited number of minimally invasive laparoscopic procedures. Some are starting to employ the robot for single-incision laparoscopic surgery although the bulkiness of the current robot makes this challenging. There is development of motion-sensitive gloves that can be worn by the surgeon, who can then control the movement of robotic end effectors by simply moving his or her hands. One could also imagine a robotic device that can hold and control an endoscope after its introduction by the surgeon to the appropriate location. This would leave the surgeon's hands free for use of the instrumentation that could be passed via the endoscope.

The Face of Surgery 2025

True scarless surgery will not happen until technology catches up with our imagination. The development of wireless electricity by Marin Soljacic and Eric Giler (WiTricity™; WiTricity Corp., Watertown, MA) that is now available for simple household items is the launch pad for the future of surgical devices (Google WiTricity). If one can deliver wireless energy precisely, to a focal point across a distance, it will be the dawn of a new surgical era once again. One can imagine a patient laying on the OR table with an active real-time 3D MRI virtual image device providing instantaneous imaging of the inside of the patient (without a camera). A robotic device would be placed beside the patient with access to a simple pencil-like instrument that delivers wireless energy across the body wall to a desired focal point inside the patient without touching the body. The surgeon would sit at a console with 3D imaging provided by the MRI device in real time and be able to see and direct the focal point of the energy device (i.e., red spot) inside the patient. Initially, simple cases such as cholecystectomies and appendectomies could be done where the organ in question could just be vaporized and the lumen sealed. Eventually, other devices would need to be developed for more complex interventions. The key is that the imaging technology and the wireless electricity already exist, and it is therefore a relatively short leap to what is described here.

Conclusions

Regardless of the current financial climate in medicine and surgery, one can be sure that surgeons will not stop pushing the boundaries of what is possible and going beyond it. It is almost innate in the human spirit to search for the undiscovered and forge ahead into the unknown. We hope this chapter has provided some information as to what is available out there and stimulated some interest in pushing the limits of surgery further than currently known.

Reference

1. Kalloo AN, Singh VK, Jagannath SB, et al. Flexible transgastric peritoneoscopy: a novel approach to diagnostic and therapeutic interventions in the peritoneal cavity. Gastrointest Endosc. 2004;60(1):114–7.

Index